CLEFT LIP AND PALATE

CLEFT LIP AND PALATE

Plastic Surgery, Genetics and the Team Approach

Edited by

FRANK W. PIRRUCCELLO, M.D.

Surgeon-in-Chief
Northwestern University Cleft Palate Institute
Clinical Associate Professor, Plastic Surgery
Northwestern University Medical School
Clinical Associate Professor,
Northwestern University Dental School
Clinical Professor, Plastic Surgery
University of Wisconsin, Madison
Chief, Division of Plastic Surgery
Evanston Hospital
Senior Staff
St. Francis Hospital, Evanston, Illinois
Former Plastic Surgeon in Charge
Shriners' Hospital for Crippled Children
Diplomate, American Board of Plastic Surgery
The American Society of Plastic and Reconstructive Surgery, Inc.
Fellow, American College of Surgeons
The American Society of Aesthetic Plastic Surgery, Inc.
The American Society of Maxillofacial Surgeons

With Illustrations by Ruth Mark

CHARLES C THOMAS • PUBLISHER
Springfield • Illinois • U. S. A.

Published and Distributed Throughout the World by

CHARLES C THOMAS • PUBLISHER
2600 South First Street
Springfield, Illinois 62794-9265

ISBN 0-398-05348-0

Library of Congress Catalog Card Number: 87-6529

With THOMAS BOOKS *careful attention is given to all details of manufacturing and design. It is the Publisher's desire to present books that are satisfactory as to their physical qualities and artistic possibilities and appropriate for their particular use.* THOMAS BOOKS *will be true to those laws of quality that assure a good name and good will.*

Printed in the United States of America
Q-R-3

Library of Congress Cataloging in Publication Data

Cleft lip and palate.

Includes bibliographies and index.
1. Harelip. 2. Cleft palate. I. Pirruccello, Frank W.
[DNLM: 1. Cleft lip. 2. Cleft Palate. WV 440 C62155]
RD524.C53 1987 617'.522 87-6529
ISBN 0-398-05348-0

CONTRIBUTORS

M. Hugh Bailey, M.B.

Fellow of the Royal College of Surgeons
Resident in Plastic Surgery, Northwestern University Medical School, Chicago, Illinois

Lora B. Baum, M.D.

Genetic Counselor for Northwestern Memorial Hospital, Chicago, Illinois
Section on Human Genetics

Stanley G. Biel, D.D.S., M.S.

Assistant Professor of Orthodontics
Northwestern University Dental School, Chicago, Illinois

Kenneth Bzoch, Ph.D.

Professor and Chairman, Department of Communicative Disorders,
College of Health Related Professions, University of Florida, Gainesville, Florida

John Cook, M.D.

Resident in Plastic Surgery, Northwestern University Medical School
Formerly Chief Resident in General Surgery, St. Luke's Presbyterian Hospital, Chicago, Illinois

R. William Cornell, D.D.S.

Professor of Pedodontia and Head of Department of Pedodontia,
Northwestern University Dental School, Chicago, Illinois

Jordan Gottlieb, M.D.

Former Resident at Northwestern University Medical School
Assistant Professor, University of Washington
Chief, Plastic Surgery, VA Hospital, Seattle, Washington

Jeannette Israel, M.D.

Assistant Professor, Rush Medical College, Chicago, Illinois
Diplomate of the American Board of Medical Genetics

Peter E. Johnson, M.D.

Clinical Instructor of Surgery, Division of Plastic, Reconstructive and Maxillofacial Surgery, Northwestern University Medical School, Chicago, Illinois

Roger H. Kallal, D.D.S.

Associate Professor of Clinical Orthodontia, Northwestern University Dental School, Northwestern University Cleft Palate Institute, Chicago, Illinois

Norman Olsen, D.D.S., M.S.D.

Professor of Pedodontia and Dean, Northwestern University Dental School, Chicago, Illinois

Harold T. Perry, M.D., Ph.D.

Professor of Orthodontia and Head of Department of Orthodontia, Northwestern University Dental School, Chicago, Illinois

John Tanner, D.D.S.

Former Resident in Oral and Maxillofacial Surgery, Northwestern University Medical School, Chicago, Illinois

Mort Rosen, D.D.S.

Professor of Prosthodontics and Head of Department of Prosthodontics, Northwestern University Dental School, Chicago, Illinois

Harry Staffileno, Jr., D.D.S.

Professor of Dentistry, Northwestern University Dental School, Chicago, Illinois
Chief, Dental Division and Director of Dental Residency, Evanston Hospital, Evanston, Illinois

To

John S. Latta, Ph.D.
Emeritus Professor of Anatomy
University of Nebraska

and to

Marilyn Hanson Pirruccello

". . . at fifteen, I had set my heart upon learning.
At thirty, I had formed my character.
At forty, I no longer suffered from perplexities.
At fifty, I knew what was the mandate of heaven.
At sixty, I heard it with docile ear.
At seventy, I could follow the dictates of my own heart
for what I desired no longer overstepped the boundaries of right."

Confucius

FOREWORD

IT SEEMS TO ME that both medicine and dentistry have gone through growth periods during which they moved away from general practice into a bewildering variety of specialization. The resulting professional compartmentalization often caused both disciplines to lose communication with one another. Indeed, they often became the object of ridicule. Now, I am pleased to observe that, having achieved a maturity of their own, the specialties within medicine and dentistry have joined hands under the rubric of health sciences. Perhaps no better example of this is in the area of cleft lip and palate treatment.

At Northwestern University Dental School, where author and editor Frank W. Pirruccello, MD has been associated with the faculty for 31 years, the great and complex problems of cleft palate are addressed by a cleft palate team. Dr. Pirruccello, who is also a member of the medical faculty, is a plastic and reconstructive surgeon. He works with a team that includes a pedodontist, a speech pathologist and representatives from other involved disciplines. For the purposes of this book, Dr. Pirruccello has also consulted a geneticist. The result is a volume drawn from a vast amount of clinical and experimental research by people with substantial experience in their chosen fields and a commitment to a team approach to treatment.

Dr. Pirruccello's objective is to present a book that represents the state-of-the-art in learning and experience. He hopes he has produced an uncluttered text and reference book, that, in his words, "would separate the chaff from the wheat." Clearly, he has accomplished his purpose.

Dr. Pirruccello, who has been Chief of the Division of Plastic and Reconstructive Surgery at Evanston Hospital for over 30 years, has succeeded admirably in finding competent professionals — including genetic and speech experts — to present a variety of essays on the general topic of management of cleft lip and palate treatment. The result is an excellent study of an interdisciplinary approach to the total rehabilitation of the cleft palate child.

I congratulate Dr. Pirruccello and his colleagues. They have joined their talents in an exercise that represents health services at their best.

Norman H. Olsen
Dean, Dental School
Northwestern University
Member, Cleft Palate Institute

FOREWORD

A TEXTBOOK on cleft lip and palate is a natural for a surgeon of the stature of Dr. Frank W. Pirruccello to write. As a journalist, I've known Dr. Pirruccello for fifteen years. He is an important media source because of his excellent medical reputation, his ability to communicate his thoughts and ideas; and one more thing—his humanity and his concern for other human beings. Because of these factors and his outstanding artistic abilities, Dr. Pirruccello, a noted teacher, can weave together with words and illustrations the facts and techniques that will lead to the diminishing of pain and suffering.

His humanizing of cleft lip and palate surgery will change lives for the better, which is Frank W. Pirruccello's raison d'etre.

Carol Kleiman
Associate Financial Editor
The Chicago Tribune

PREFACE

NO BOOK covers everything about anything, and this collection of treatises on cleft palate is no exception. These authors are experts in their fields and, therefore, they deserve your attention.

Hugh Bailey, MD, Peter Johnson, MD and John Cook, MD, my residents from Northwestern University Medical School, are my associates in practice, and they deserve thanks for their help and support.

Ruth Mark is one of the brightest, most capable artists I have worked with.

Patricia Wold, Karen Wold, Nancy Scharfe and Chris Gritschke handled the tough jobs of typing, correcting and assembling this material. Invaluable assistance by Mary Jane Herlocker, Lynn Pirruccello Kanter and Ann Pirruccello must be acknowledged. C C Cheng, the owner of the Peking Book House in Evanston, Illinois, gave me valuable assistance with the Confucius sayings and the Chinese symbols for cleft lip and palate.

The editors at Charles C Thomas have been understanding and helpful. They have been great.

Thank you all.

F.W.P.

CONTENTS

CLEFT LIP AND PALATE

CHAPTER 1

THE TEAM CONCEPT AND CLEFT MANAGEMENT

JOHN COOK and FRANK W. PIRRUCCELLO

> *. . . The man who loves truth is better than the man who knows it, and the man who finds happiness in it is better than the man who loves it.*
>
> *. . . Confucius*

THE PATIENT with a cleft of the lip or palate requires the skill of a variety of specialists in order to obtain optimum appearance and function. For this reason the team approach to cleft management has evolved, as exemplified by this book, most of whose authors are either members or alumnae of one such team, the Northwestern University Cleft Palate Institute. There are several advantages to the team approach. The parents of a cleft infant, often confused by vague feelings of guilt, are comforted by a format where precise answers can be provided regarding all aspects of their child's future treatment. Once they realize that an apparently monstrous cosmetic and functional deformity can be conquered by a logical sequence of treatments, they can concentrate their energies on providing a healthy and supportive environment for their child. As with so much in medicine, once the fear of the problem is overcome, the problem itself becomes more manageable.

An additional advantage of the team concept is that it allows for efficient coordination of the specialists' services. For example, an otolaryngologist should be present when the patient undergoes general anesthesia for a lip repair, so that the tympanic membrane can be examined and treated if necessary with polyethylene (PE) tubes. Also, situations can be avoided where specialists are actually working at cross purposes. The orthodontist and maxillofacial surgeon must work together if a patient develops midface retrusion; otherwise, the work of one may compromise the work of the other.

It is a rare person who enjoys a visit to a doctor's office, and this problem is compounded when the services of many specialists are required—especially with the prospect of sitting in so many waiting rooms for so many hours. This time burden for the parent can be reduced by bringing the specialists together in conference format. The more convenient we make our services, the better will be the rapport and followup with our patients. Hopefully, we can avoid the situation where a patient "slips between the cracks" and misses a beneficial intervention, such as speech therapy during the critical early years of language development.

Logistically, it is easier to gather and analyze data about a large group of patients when they are treated at a cleft palate center. This increases the likelihood that this information will be communicated to other professionals in the form of books and articles, so that all patients will benefit. It is also easier to keep track of complications and unfavorable results; these can be compared with the results of other groups to make certain that optimum care is provided.

A final benefit of the team approach to cleft palate management is a selfish one from the standpoint of the specialist affiliated with a cleft palate center. Working in concert with other skilled professionals, that specialist will find that a free flow of ideas will contribute to his or her own professional development. The goal of any health care specialist, no matter what his or her training, should be continued professional growth and refinement of skills. The healthy interchange that takes place in a cleft palate team ensures that this growth takes place.

A glance at the chapter headings of this book shows the variety of skilled specialists who make up a cleft palate team. The plastic surgeon, geneticist, pedodontist, orthodontist, prosthodontist, oral surgeon, speech therapist and otolaryngologist are essential team members. In addition, a variety of administrative support staff are vital to the smooth function of a cleft palate center. In each chapter of this book there is a concise, in-depth summary of one aspect of treating the patient with a cleft. In this chapter the key points raised by each author are stressed and placed within a chronological framework. This gives the reader an idea of how the various treatment modalities are interrelated, and, in a general sense, how one cleft palate center manages its patients.

The initial evaluation by the cleft palate team can do much to allay the concern of parents who are confronted by a child with a cleft. The geneticist is perhaps the key member of the team at this point, from the parents' standpoint, since they have so many questions regarding the cause of the cleft and its likelihood of occurrence in future pregnancies. It is important that the parents as well as the patient be examined and questioned, since clefts that occur as part of a genetic syndrome are much more likely to appear in future siblings. In addition, associated anomalies may affect the aggressiveness or course of treatment. Chromosome disorders such as Trisomy 13 and Trisomy 18 may include clefts. Clefts are also present in specific monogenic syndromes that are autosomally dominant (Van der Woude, EEC, Hay-Wells) or autosomally recessive (Mechel-Gruber, Roberts). A careful history regarding exposure to medications or industrial agents is also important. One of the geneticist's most crucial roles is to record and analyze data obtained from patient interviews in order to increase scientific understanding of the etiology of cleft lip and palate.

The otolaryngologist and audiologist are similarly important in the early care of the cleft patient. Audiologic screening can detect aural pathology even in the early months of life with such measures as the speech awareness threshold and the pure tone sound field measure. Each visit to the cleft palate team will afford the otolaryngologist an opportunity to visualize the tympanic membranes, and early visits to the operating room should include a microscopic ear examination and insertion of PE tubes if necessary. There is evidence, as Dr. Bzoch discusses in his chapter, that an aggressive approach of this sort will lead to a decrease in permanent aural abnormalities so that the best possible ground is established to develop normal speech and language abilities.

Many surgeons still follow the rule of tens (weight of 10 pounds, hemoglobin at least 10 grams, white cell count under 10,000 and age greater than 10 weeks) to establish when cleft lip repair should be done, but there is a trend towards earlier repair in some centers. A majority of surgeons use one of three established methods for repair of the unilateral cleft lip: the Tennison triangular flap, the Millard rotation advancement method or a modified straight line closure. It is generally accepted that the lip repair must include reapproximation of the orbicularis to avoid an unsightly lateral bulge when the patient purses his lips. Repair of a bilateral cleft lip is more complicated because of the protruding premaxilla, deficient columnella and absence of functional muscle in the prolabium with complete defects. Some authors advocate presurgical orthopedics in order to narrow wide unilateral or bilateral cleft lips, but these methods increase the likelihood of crossbite and growth deficiency of the premaxilla. Occasionally a preliminary lip adhesion procedure is helpful for wide unilateral clefts, especially if the surgeon plans to use the rotation advancement method of closure. The timing of repair of cleft lip nasal deformities is controversial. Some authors advocate early repositioning of the alar cartilage on the cleft side in the hope that the nose ultimately will assume a more symmetric shape. Others advise waiting until the time of school admission for nasal modification; this is also a good time to repair the secondary lip deformities which occur in even the most competent hands.

The pedodontist's role in the care of the cleft palate patient begins before the primary dentition erupts. The patient is provided with an intraoral appliance prior to lip repair, and the appliance is maintained until closure of the palate. This appliance makes feeding much easier and helps prevent collapse of the maxillary segments. Once the primary dentition erupts, the pedodontist's skill is required almost continuously. Frequently the lateral incision on the cleft side is congenitally absent; in this case space must be maintained for the permanent dentition. Supernumerary teeth should be maintained as long as they are not in the path of proposed surgery. Other tasks for the pedodontist include the restoration of malformed anterior teeth, the prevention of premature loss of the primary second molar, the application of adhesive sealants to prevent caries and the treatment of caries with restoration dentistry. The pedodontist should initiate a program of comprehensive preventive dentistry with reduction of cariogenic food intake and instruction in oral hygiene.

When the patient is between nine months and one year of age, surgery is necessary to close the palate. Some authors advocate closure of only the soft palate at this time, and delay closure of the hard palate until later in order to avoid diminished midface growth. Most feel that poorer speech results from this approach, however, and it is generally policy to close the hard and soft palates at the same time.The two most common methods of closure are the von Langenbech palatoplasty, which is especially useful in narrow clefts, and the Wardell-Kilner pushback, which employs the V-Y advancement principle. The functional part of the repair is the soft palate closure, and it is important to free the palatal muscles to redirect them medially and to make certain that they are accurately approximated. Considerable controversy exists regarding primary bone grafting of the alveolar aspect of the cleft; most surgeons delay this procedure until later due to concern regarding a deleterious impact on midface growth. Some patients require secondary palatal surgery either to correct a palatal fistula or to eliminate velopharyngeal incompetence.

Velopharyngeal incompetence is but one of the disorders of speech, language and hearing which affect patients with cleft lip and palate. The otolaryngologist can aid the patient with early diagnosis and treatment of middle ear disease and the plastic surgeon can improve speech with functional closure of the lip and palate supplemented by a pharyngeal flap when indicated. However, the main orchestrator of optimal speech and language is the speech therapist. Working in conjunction with an audiologist, the speech therapist assesses communicative disorders with speech evaluation tests, language assessment tests and audiologic tests. Correction may be necessary in any or all of the following categories: nasal emission distortions, hypernasal distortions, grimacing, hyponasal resonance distortion, gross sound substitutions, aspirate voice production, hoarse voice, articulation disorders, delayed language development and misarticulation disorders. Since disorders of speech and language set children apart from their playmates, as surely as the visible deformity of a cleft lip, correction must be approached with the same degree of care and finesse necessary for artistic closure of a lip.

Secondary deformities of the lip occur frequently, no matter what method of primary lip repair is used and no matter how skilled the surgeon. These are best corrected before the patient enters school because they can be the source of much teasing and unhappiness. Several problems with the reconstructed lip are discussed in the chapter on lip repair: The scar may be unsatisfactory; there may be inadequate functional muscle across the cleft; the vermillion may be irregular; the lip may be tight due to deficient soft tissue; and, there may be a discrepancy between the amount of tissue medially and laterally, especially following triangular repair. Residual deformities of the alar region and columnella may be corrected at this time, but a more extensive rhinoplasty should be deferred until the usual age for that procedure.

Alveolar bone grafting is accomplished between the ages of nine and twelve, prior to the eruption of the maxillary canine when its root is one-quarter to one-half formed. This insures that the tooth will erupt into the grafted areas and the alveolar height will be increased by physiologic osteogenesis. By this age the grafting procedure will have minimal effect on maxillary growth.

To insure maximal patient compliance, it is best to delay orthodontia until the eruption of the permanent dentition. A treatment plan is formulated with the aid of plaster study casts and radiographs. Frequently the orthodontist must expand the maxillary dental arch and then maintain position with a retainer. The orthodontist also works in conjunction with the maxillofacial surgeon if corrective mandibular of maxillary surgery is necessary. Unless compelling psychological problems exist, correction of midface hypoplasia should be delayed until growth is complete. This corresponds to age 18 in men and age 17 in women. At this time a maxillary advancement with accompanying orthodontia optimizes the appearance and function of the midface.

The remaining chapters of this book provide in-depth discussion of the skills necessary to render optimum care to the patient with cleft lip and palate. Ideally, the skills should be integrated into a cleft palate team so that the course of therapy is uninterrupted and free of conflict among specialists. The goal is to provide every patient with the best of current techniques and to analyze constantly the results of therapy so that the standard of care may be even higher in the future.

CHAPTER 2

HISTORY OF CLEFT LIP SURGERY

JORDAN GOTTLIEB and FRANK W. PIRRUCCELLO

> . . . *Rotten wood cannot be carved, nor a wall of dried dung troweled.*
>
> . . . *Confucius*

OUR KNOWLEDGE of the earliest operations for correction of the cleft lip is fragmentary. Most surgeons made no record of their work. What records do survive are a sporadic but tantalizing collection of reports from here and there with a number of historic "firsts"—"firsts" of which we are aware. Evidence of the occurrence of cleft lip and palate among ancient people exists in their art. However, little attention was given to the cleft lip deformity or its treatment by the earliest medical writers, as Rogers has noted.[1] There is no mention in the papyri of Ebers nor in Edwin Smith nor in the writings of Hippocrates, Celcus, Galen nor Antyllus.

A Chinese surgeon performed the first recorded closure of cleft lip.[2] The history of the Chin Dynasty (317-420 AD) was written some three centuries later from official archives. Included is this story of a young farmer named Wei Yang-Chi, who was born with a cleft lip (t'u ch'ueh = harelip). A fortune teller predicted:

> "From your physiognomy I can foretell that later in life you will have wealth and honor."

At age 18 Wei Yang-Chi heard of a doctor who could cure the cleft lip deformity. He met with his family and told them:

> "With this ugly deformity of mine, there is no future for me. What is the use of existing?"

He next went to meet the governor of the state of Chu, because the doctor he had heard of worked for the governor. The doctor was called, examined the patient and said:

> "I can cure your condition by cutting and stitching the edges together. However, after the operation it will be necessary for you to rest the affected part for 100 days. During this time you can ingest only thin gruel and you cannot smile or talk."

Wei answered:

> "What is 100 days when for relief of my condition I would remain silent for half of my lifetime?"

Wei's lip was repaired, and, as was prophesied in his youth, he went on to a successful military and civil career.

During the Tang Dynasty (618-907 AD), the period in which the Chin Annals were compiled, there is mention of a surgeon, Fang Kan, who had earned a reputation as a "doctor of lips." Fang Kan seems to be the first named surgeon to have closed clefts of the lip.

The Leech Book of Bald is thought to have been written in about 950 AD. This manual was a handbook for the Saxon leeches, the surgeons of pre-Norman Britain. The operation for cleft lip is described:

> "For harelip, pound mastic very small; add the white of an egg and mingle as thou dost vermillion; cut with a knife the false edges of the lip, sew fast with silk; then smear without and within with the salve, ere the silk rot. If it draws together, arrange it with the hand; anoint again soon."[1]

Who was the surgeon who inaugurated the "modern" era in cleft lip closure? That surgeon would have written a description of the deformity and discussed its repair. His work would have started a steady trend of progress in the case of patients with cleft lip. There are several candidates for this recognition. One is the Flemish surgeon Jehan Yperman (1295-1351).[3] He described the defects of the unilateral and bilateral clefts of the lip and a method of repair. The borders of the cleft were freshened with a bistouri (knife), and then repaired with a wax suture on a triangular needle. This was reinforced by the placement of a harelip needle which passed through the lip at a distance from the cleft margin. Other surgeons of the day would not suture the margins, but relied upon the needle alone. The harelip needle was then secured with a wraparound figure-of-eight suture. Some surgeons made relaxing incisions in the cheek in order to close wide clefts. Yperman himself discouraged this maneuver because the resulting facial scarring might "compromise the reputation of the surgeon."

Another candidate is a Bavarian surgeon, Heinrich von Pfolsprundt, who wrote a surgical text (1460) which described an operation for cleft lip using interrupted sutures through the full thickness of the lip. Hieronymus Brunshwig, an Alsatian army surgeon, wrote (1497) of the necessity of strapping the patient to the table with towels, then operating with scissors, using interrupted sutures. He described a pinch clasp and a self-retaining clamp to aid in dressing wider clefts.

The Renaissance had an impact on all fields of human endeavor, including medicine. The Renaissance principle of drawing conclusions based upon observation and experience rather than upon preconceived dogma encouraged progress. Surgery began to rise to the level of a profession in this era. The great practitioners were two Huguenots, both trained outside the universities which were reserved for "medicine." Ambrose Pare (1510-1591) trained first as an apprentice barber-surgeon and later as a house surgeon in Paris at Hotel Dieu. Pierre Franco (1500-

1561) trained as a provincial *inciseur,* a still lower rank of itinerant surgeon. That these two men became famous reflects the basis of their knowledge—observation and experience. This was different from the basis of their "professional" colleagues' knowledge—dogma from their masters. Franco said, commenting on his work:

> "Neither books nor men taught me this method. . .but experience, mistress in all things, showed me."[4,5]

Both wrote in French, rather than in Latin, the language of the university medical schools. Their teachings, therefore, were available to all the surgeons of their day. Franco wrote a clear description of cleft lip and palate in his *Petit Trait* (1556):

> "Cleft lips are sometimes congenital, through a defect of nature. At times they are caused by an accident which befalls them. Furthermore, they are sometimes cleft without a cleft of the jaw or palate, sometimes the cleft is only slight, and at times the cleft is as long and wide as the lip. Or so wide as to expose the incisors. . .and occasionally even the canine teeth as well. It sometimes happens that small cartilaginous and thin sutures in the nostrils called alae, are lacking. When the palate is also cleft, the patient must talk through his nose, so that he can be understood only with difficulty, all the more because the mouth, which shapes the words, is defective. When this opening is closed he speaks fairly well."

Although he did not operate for cleft palate, he was aware of the benefit of obturation. He described a method of lip closure:

> "The entire skin of the margins which are to be joined must be cut with a razor or scissors, or with the cautery. Then put on dressing to ease the pain, and leave them for one or two days. And if the cautery is used, after the dressings are put on, the eschar will have to be loosened with fresh butter or something similar before proceeding further. For otherwise it would generally be a waste of effort and hurt the patient needlessly, especially when the margins are far apart. After this is accomplished, the margins must be brought together so that there is no portion of one which does not touch the other. This can be done in two ways, one with needles, as I show later, and the other with pieces of cloth triangular in shape and suitable in size for the patient. The latter (method) is preferable as causing the least pain and the least scarring. This is very desirable in these areas, especially when (the patient) is a girl."

He also described bilateral clefts and recommended excision of the prolabium to make closure easier. Pare wrote about lip repair in his *Works* (1575), and included what seems to be the first published illustration of a repaired lip.

Pare became the more successful, the more influential of the two. He became a surgeon to kings, while Franco practiced in the provinces. The writings of each include works borrowed from the other. It seems, according to Barsky, that Pare's writings on the cleft lip are borrowed from Franco. It is the work of Pare that ultimately received the wider circulation and had the greater lasting effect on surgeons who followed. Pierre Franco has been called the "Father" of cleft lip surgery. It is not clear that he had done anything that had not already been done by Yperman and perhaps by other surgeons whose names have been lost. But he clearly described the anomaly, its repair and postoperative care. He and Pare practiced surgery during the time it became a profession, and they wrote their text in the era of the printing press. Thus, their works were distributed widely as never before and their influence on later surgeons has been lasting.

Gaspare Tagliacozzi of Bologne suggested the use of interrupted sutures (1597):

> "First we will begin with the Hare-lip, because this is the most simple evil, and easiest to cure. If both lips be such, the same method of cure must be used for both. . .Let the Artist therefore take up that part of the Lip, which must be excoriated, in his Left Hand, and then take off the Skin equally with a very sharp knife, till the blood comes to the very Angle of the *Hiatus,* and then he must smoothe the Wound. This Operation may also be done very quickly and safely with a pair of Scissors. The same must be done on the other side. Then we must draw the parts together with his Hand, and stitch them. We must observe this, not to take our stitches superficially, but through all."[1]

Tragliacozzi's body was taken from its consecrated grave and moved when a controversy developed in the Church regarding his operations for altering what was described as "the creation of God." Hieronymus Fabricius of Aquapendente advised using buccal mucosa or alveolar tissue to close the cleft lip. He observed the feeding difficulties of babies with cleft palate. Hendryk von Roohuyse (1674) recommended cleft lip closure at the early age of three to four months.[6] John Philip Hoffman (1686) described a headcap that could be adjusted to reduce the tension on the repaired lip.[6]

Speech difficulties of children with cleft palate were more widely recognized during the 18th century. Leviett (1772) reported on the importance of the oral muscle sphincter in the infant with cleft lip and palate. He noted that adults with unrepaired lips had more widely separated palatal shelves. He appreciated the need for maxillary orthopedics in using a linen band to realign the maxillary arch as well as to remove tension from the repaired lip. Girard (1787) used a linen band preoperatively to set back a protruding premaxilla, which enabled a repair which included the prolabium. He later wrote about the effect of lip closure on spontaneous closure of the palate. This work predated palatal repairs, which were not performed until the early 19th century by Carl Frederich von Graefe and Philibert Roux.

Many early surgeons alluded to methods of minimizing the pain of lip operations. They discussed methods of immobilizing the patient during operations and attempts at sedation. John Cook of Warwick (1693) wrote:

> . . ."To operate in, choose a very clear place, and put the Child in the Lap of a discreet person, and let one stand behind to hold the Head, the Child's Hands being ty'd down, and if possible to keep it from Sleep for ten or twelve hours before the Operation, that it may be disposed to sleep presently after. For it have ready a glass of Wine or Cordial, in case of fainting upon the loss of Blood."[6]

One patient described the agonies of his operations in a psalm:

> "In the month of April sweet, On the Sixteenth day of it,
> Did the Doctor me attend, My deformity to mend.
> Put before me then a Chair, And I sat me gladly there;
> Held my Face and with knife-tip, Cut into my deformed Lip.
> Soon I held my Eyes closed tight, And my Hands with all their might,
> On my Heart together pressed, Fingers twisted in Distress.
> Felt a sharp and dreadful Pain, Felt the agony again,
> So my Flesh shivers and shakes, All my Body the pain takes. . ."[7]

It seems that most cleft lips went unrepaired: Further progress in the cleft lip surgery had to wait for the development of good anesthesia.

From the beginnings of cleft lip surgery, through the early 19th century, the operation remained relatively crude despite some of the progress that has been outlined. Efforts were directed toward the closure of a hole, with a minimum of attention to the preservation or creation of those landmarks by which we recognize a normal lip. Attention to the inadequacy of the simple paring of the cleft edges with straight line closure, and a systematic attempt to improve results came later.

The lack of vertical length of the lip on the cleft side was perhaps the first problem noted. Von Graefe (1816) designed a curved incision around the cleft margins to lengthen the straight line closure,[8] but this was at the expense of more radical excision of tissue from both sides of the cleft. This operation is, however, the forerunner of the present day straight line repairs, which are still used most commonly for the closure of the bilateral cleft.

Further progress had to wait for recognition of areas of relative tissue deficit and excess and the development of techniques of shifting that tissue. Joseph Francis Malgaigne of Paris (1843) complained that persistent notching occurred because of scar contracture of the straight line closure.[9] His creative thinking, which led to the development of his operation, was based on his recognition of the absence of substance at the labial border. The previous operations discarded tissue. He preserved as much as possible and borrowed from neighboring tissue. He created two flaps, turning vermillion down from each side of the cleft. This, unfortunately, created a new deformity which caused lip asymmetry.

Germanicus Mirault (1844) of Anger wrote to Malgaigne applauding his technique and, at the same time, added a modification that discarded one of the two flaps. This produced a triangular flap from one side to set into the other.[10] It is unclear from which side the flap actually came. Claude Bernard (1850) revised the procedure and published it in his text. Here it is clear that the flap from the cleft side slides to insert into the medial portion. This triangular flap is the predecessor of many modifications, including those of Blair and Brown (1930) and Brown and McDowell (1950).

Werner Hagedorn (1884) of Magdeberg, Germany, described his operation in which a quadrilateral flap was developed.[11] He designed this to correct the asymmetry of the vermillion resulting from other operations. His procedure resulted in a small protuberance corresponding to the middle of the upper lip and more fullness at the vermillion border. This created the first Cupid's Bow in lip repairs, albeit an artificial one. Though Hagedorn's method had some popularity, it was soon lost until modified a half-century later by LeMesurier.

This era in the 19th century was marked by the development and promotion of a number of flaps of varied geometric design. Although the patterns were complex and intricate, the incisions were crude and indelicate in most hands and surgeons had to struggle against sitting, awake and unanesthetized patients. Sir William Ferguson of London began to operate on cleft lip patients under general anesthesia.[12] His student, William Rose, continued the work and reverted to a simple V-excision and straight line closure. His results were the best to date, undoubtedly because of his excellent execution with the use of anesthesia. However, the lesson learned by other surgeons was that it was also the straight line closure that was superior. This became dominant through the first one-third of the 20th century.

But dissatisfaction with cleft lip surgery and cycle of lip repairs, which developed in the 19th century, arose again 80 years later with some new modifications. Blair and Brown were unhappy with some of the postoperative results of straight line repair that had troubled Malgaigne and Mirault—the lip was either pulled up or too long, was retruded and the nose was poor. They discovered that a similar flap had been designed by Mirault, adapted later by Bernard and again by Henry Hollingsworth Smith. This repair gave some of the best results to date with the nostril. Brown and McDowell (1950) later modified the triangular flap with a small flap because of dissatisfaction with earlier results as the young patient grew up.[13] The markings for this revised operation were more reproducible than those of the Blair-Brown procedure. The Brown-McDowell triangular flap became the predominant technique, producing improved lip closure. The primary criticism of this repair is the unnatural appearance of the lip due to failure to create a Cupid's bow. In 1948, LeMesurier presented his series of lip repairs,[14] accomplished with a quadrilateral flap technique that could be traced back to Hagedorn's design. The square flap lowers the prolabium to create a simulated Cupid's bow. The results, based on 13 years' experience and followup, were a further improvement upon the previous triangular flap procedures.

The primary criticism concerned the vagueness of marking technique, which was inexact and difficult to duplicate. In 1952, Tennyson presented a similar flap design, marking out the flap with a bent wire to serve as template.

Millard remained displeased with the postoperative results and noted that the lip repair and low z-plasty were unappealing because the cleft side of the philtrum was not straight. Furthermore, he felt that the true tissue deficit was high in the lip, rather than low, and that the tissue was being brought into the wrong area in both the triangular and quadrilateral flap repairs. He felt that the more natural line for the philtrum could be created by carrying the noncleft side incision down from under the columnella. This permitted the natural landmarks of the upper lip that created the Cupid's bow to rotate downward and toward the cleft and into the natural position. This left a tissue deficit high in the lip. This deficit was filled by a flap of tissue from the cleft side, a flap that was designed to carry the abnormal alae to a corrected position. This design was appealing because it did not require fixed geometric patterns which could not be revised during the operation.

The pathological anatomy of the muscle in the cleft lip was reported by Fara in 1965, and later by others. Randall (1974) drew attention to the importance of orbicularis reconstruction in repair of the cleft lip. This has become generally recognized and is done as part of most techniques.

REFERENCES

1. Rogers BO: Harelip repair in colonial America. *Plast Reconstr Surg,* 34:142, 1964.
2. Boo-Chai K: An ancient Chinese test on a cleft lip. *Plast Reconstr Surg,* 38:89, 1966.
3. Vrebos J: Jehan Yperman, medieval cleft lip surgeon. *Plast Reconstr Surg,* 70:762, 1982.
4. Barsky AJ: Pierro Franco, father of cleft lip surgery: His life and times. *Br J Plast Surg,* 17:335, 1964.
5. Franco P: The cure of cleft lip in 1561, in McDowell F (ed): *The Sourcebook of Plastic Surgery.* Baltimore, Williams & Wilkins, 1977.
6. Rogers BO: History of cleft lip and palate treatment, in Grabb W, Rosenstein SW, Bzoch K (eds): *Cleft Lip and Palate.* Boston, Little Brown & Co, 1972.
7. Rintala AE: How a patient experienced a cleft lip operation in 1763, in McDowell F (ed): *The Sourcebook of Plastic Surgery.* Baltimore, Williams & Wilkins, 1977.
8. Millard DR Jr (ed): *Cleft Craft: The Evolution of its Surgery.* Boston, Little Brown & Co, 1976, vol 1: *The Unilateral Deformity.*
9. Malgaigne JF: New method for the harelip operation (1884), in McDowell F (ed): *The Sourcebook of Plastic Surgery.* Baltimore, Williams & Wilkins, 1977.
10. Mirault G: Letter on operation for harelip (1884), in McDowell F (ed): *The Sourcebook of Plastic Surgery.* Baltimore, Williams & Wilkins, 1977.
11. Hagedorn WH: A modification of the harelip operation (1884), in McDowell F (ed): *The Sourcebook of Plastic Surgery.* Baltimore, Williams & Wilkins, 1977.
12. McDowell F: The aftermath, in McDowell F (ed): *The Sourcebook of Plastic Surgery.* Baltimore, Williams & Wilkins, 1977.
13. Brown JB, McDowell F: Small triangular flap operation for the primary repair of single cleft lips. *Plast Reconstr Surg,* 5:392, 1950.
14. LeMesurier AB: A method of cutting and suturing the lip in the treatment of complete unilateral clefts. *Plast Reconstr Surg,* 4:1, 1949.
15. Tennyson CW: The repair of the unilateral cleft lip by the stencil method. *Plast Reconstr Surg,* 9:115, 1952.
16. Fara M, Chlumska A, Hrivnakova J: Musculus orbicularis oris in incomplete hare lip. *Acta Chir Plast,* 7:125, 1965.
17. Randall P, Whitaker LA, LaRossa D: The importance of muscle reconstruction in primary and secondary cleft lip repair. *Plast Reconstr Surg,* 54:316, 1974.

CHAPTER 3

GENETIC ASPECTS OF CLEFT PALATE AND CLEFT LIP AND PALATE

JEANNETTE ISRAEL and LORA D. BAUM

> *. . . Learn as if you were following someone whom you could not catch up with, as though it were someone you were frightened of losing.*
>
> *. . . Confucius*

THE COMPLEX care of the patient with cleft lip (CL) with or without cleft palate [CL(P)] or cleft palate alone (CP) can be managed well by a team approach, and the geneticist is a unique and important member of that team. The geneticist's role may include answering the family's questions regarding etiology, recurrence risk, associated anomalies and prognosis, as well as many others that may arise. The nature of the counseling setting lends itself to providing emotional support to the family members in a time of crisis when they are dealing with numerous uncomfortable feelings such as anxiety, guilt and despair. The geneticist also can identify the family that will need additional psychological counseling in order to deal with the emotional aspects of this traumatic situation.

The geneticist can make an initial contact at the time of birth of the child and explain the role of the geneticist in regard to the patient, the evaluation and the future discussion of recurrence risks. Other meetings with the patient and the family, at a time during which the situation is less stressful, can be more conducive to a discussion or rediscussion of the diagnosis, prognosis and recurrence risks. Naturally, each situation is individual and depends on the immediate needs of the family and the patient. Some families are eager to know the recurrence risks at the first visit; for others, the projections are best discussed at another meeting.

The geneticist can be a part of a cranofacial or CP clinic. In this setting the geneticist, in this situation, can provide services after a considerable amount of care of the patient is underway. The approach to the patient and the family may be somewhat different under these circumstances. Whatever the setting, the geneticist continues to have a unique position in the care of the patient with CL(P) or CP.

The formation of the oral facial structures is very complex, as are the factors that cause the disruption of the areas that result in CL(P) or CP. No single discussion can prepare the individual reader totally to perform comprehensive genetic counseling for these etiologically hetereogeneous defects. In addition, controversies and new discoveries continue to arise about certain genetic aspects of these conditions. The purpose of this discussion is to provide some insights into the concepts and complexities of the topic.

Cleft Lip (P) and CP are structurally and embryologically related, but various studies[1] have indicated that they are genetically distinct entities, i.e., there are different empiric recurrence risks for each defect. In addition, certain syndromes may present with only one or the other of these defects or sometimes with both.

Incidence and Epidemiology of CL(P) and CP

The epidemiology of CL(P) and CP is very complicated. There have been numerous studies of the incidence of these conditions, involving many population groups.[1,2] The analysis of data may be difficult because ascertainment may be different in the various studies and reporting methods can vary. Some studies include stillborn as well as liveborn infants, and some fail to specify single anomalies versus multiple anomalies. In addition, CP is not always discovered in the newborn period. The very small cleft of the soft palate may be missed on initial newborn examination. These facts may influence data.

Oka[3] reviewed the extensive body of epidemiologic studies with reference to the distinct racial gradient in the incidence of CL(P) and minor differences in the incidence of CP. He concluded that Orientals (Japanese) have the highest incidence of CL(P) with 1.61 per 1,000, Caucasians have an intermediate incidence with 0.9 per 1,000 and American blacks have the lowest with 0.31 per 1,000.

Oka[3] also reports several differences in sex ratios among patients with clefts: (1) More males are born with CL(P)—60-80 percent in various studies;[4] (2) Of all CL(P) patients, males have more severe clefts than females; (3) More females are affected with CP alone. There are various theories to explain these phenomena, including differences in embryologic timing and sex influences in multifactorically inherited conditions.

Another interesting finding is the physical presentation of the cleft. Two-thirds of unilateral clefts of the lip with or without CP occur on the left side. Cleft palate occurs with bilateral CL 86 percent of the time, with unilateral CL 68 percent of the time.

Studies of twins are indicative of the genetic factors in clefting. In twins with CL(P) concordance is greater in monozygotic twins (35%) than in dizygotic twins (7%). In twins with CP the concordance is not so different—28 percent for monozygotes and 10 percent for dizygotes.[5]

Genetic Heterogeneity and Genetic Evaluation

Etiologic heterogeneity, the concept of multiple causes for an entity, is important in genetics. The formation of the craniofacial area is very complex because of the interaction of many genes and environmental factors. It is understandable that a variety of factors may interfere with the normal development of this complicated area and result in the defects of CP and CL(P). These disruptive factors (summarized in Table 3-1) may be in the form of chromosome abnormalities, single gene mutations (dominant, X-linked, recessive), multifactorial factorial inheritance (multiple genes and environmental factors), teratologic agents and other known, unknown or undefined etiologies.

Table 3-1

Cause of Birth Defects

I. Chromosomal Disorders

II. Single Gene Mutations
   A. Autosomal Dominant
   B. Autosomal Recessive
   C. X-Linked Dominant
   D. X-Linked Recessive

III. Multifactorial Inheritance

IV. Teratologic

V. Sporadic

VI. Syndromes of Unknown Causes

One of the most important steps in the genetic evaluation of a patient with CP or CL(P) is to ascertain whether the patient has only the anomaly of CP or CL(P) or also has other anomalies. The presence of other anomalies, major or minor, makes a significant difference in how the remaining evaluation, counseling and, frequently, the treatment will proceed.

Cleft palate or CL(P) without other anomalies is the most common situation and many authorities feel that these solitary defects of CP or CL(P) are inherited in a multifactorial manner to which empiric recurrence risks can be applied. The presence of other anomalies must make one suspect that a pattern other than multifactorial inheritance may be operating, including the possibility of an underlying chromosomal disorder or a known or unknown genetic syndrome.

Searching for other anomalies, both major and minor, is critical in the genetic evaluation of patients with clefts. A thorough physical examination is mandatory and other testing such as radiographs may be helpful. In addition, the evaluation should include a complete pedigree, pregnancy history, drug and environmental history and examination of the parents. Abnormalities found through these evaluations may affect the direction of further investigations and counseling.

It is estimated that 9 percent of the infants with CL(P) are stillborn and 12 percent die within the first 10 days of life.[6] These infants are likely to be affected with other severe anomalies or syndromes since the defect of CL(P) alone does not, for the most part, result in early death. Clearly a comprehensive evaluation, as well as additional studies such as a complete autopsy, radiographs and chromosome studies, should be pursuant in stillborn infants and infants who die in the neonatal period. These studies reveal valuable information to be used in genetic counseling.

As stated before, families of patients who have CP or CL(P) without other anomalies, a negative environmental and drug history and a pedigree that does not indicate a single gene disorder may have a multifactorial mode of inheritance at work. Empiric recurrence risks are available and can be given to these families.

Multifactorial Inheritance

Many authorities feel that multifactorial inheritance is the most important and most common type of inheritance pattern operating in most disorders and traits that have a genetic predisposition.[7] Numerically, multifactorial inheritance accounts for the largest number of genetically influenced disorders or traits. Unfortunately, multifactorial inheritance is the least understood pattern of inheritance. Perhaps this is because of the complexity of the hypothesis on which it is based and the complexity of the organism in which these disorders or traits are manifested.

The concept of multifactorial inheritance involves multiple genes and environmental factors operating together to bring about the formation and function of the organism and the presence of traits and defects. The exact number of genes, their interaction and the environmental factors are unknown. The concept is based on a model in which the multiple genes and environmental factors are distributed continuously (or quasi-continuously),[8] and a threshold is important in determining the presence or absence of a quantitative trait or anomaly. Just as height is distributed among a continuum and arbitrary thresholds are determined for tallness or shortness, a developmental threshold or endpoint near the tail of the curve determines the presence or absence of a defect such as a cleft.

Cleft Lip(P), CP and Multifactorial Inheritance

Evidence from many sources has shown that CL(P) and CP may fit the multifactorial model of inheritance.[9] These studies observe CP or CL(P) that appear to match a prescribed multifactorial mode or inheritance criteria.

Predictions of Multifactorial Threshold Model in CP or CL(P)[10]

1. **Population Frequency and Frequency in Relatives.**

   A feature of multifactorial inheritance is the relationship between population frequency of the trait and the frequency in relatives of the affected individuals. For CL(P), using a population frequency of 1/2,500, expected sib recurrence is 2 percent, which fits the observed data.[10]

2. **Decrease in Frequency with Decreasing Degree of Relationship.**

   This concept reveals the fact that the incidence of a trait falls off rapidly with the degree of relationship. It is related to the number of shared genes among first, second, third, etc. degree relatives.

3. **Increased Risk with Increased Number of Affected Relatives.**

   The risk for a child being affected increases with the number of relatives who also have the trait: there are more genes in the family to allow for the threshold to be exceeded.

4. **Recurrence Risk Related to Sex.**

   The recurrence risk for an individual of the less commonly affected sex will be higher than for the more commonly affected sex. This is because the less affected sex has to have more genes to have been affected, i.e., to have reached the threshold.

5. **Recurrence Risk Varies with the Severity of the Defect in the Proband.**

   If the proband has bilateral CL(P), the risk for recurrence is higher than if the proband is affected with unilateral CL(P).

6. **Consanguinity.**

   Because blood relatives share a portion of their genes, one would expect the same increased consanguinity in multifactorial inheritance as is found in autosomal recessive inheritance.

7. **Microforms.**

   There have been suggestions that the presence of microforms in relatives of the proband or "minor degrees of CL(P) or CP" increases the risk of recurrence in CL(P) and CP. Examples of microforms in CL(P) and CP are nonsurgical scar in appropriate place, notched alveolus, submucous CP, bifid uvula and congenital palatal pharyngeal incompetence.

Table 3-2 is an example of empiric risk data used in counseling families and patients with clefts. It is Gorlin's[5] interpretation of Tolarova's[11] data. Other risk data, such as Gorlin's[5] modification of Woolf's[12] data, include other factors such as the sex and degree of severity in the proband. In this data 8.59 percent of sibs with bilateral CL(P) were affected; 4.1 percent of sibs of females with unilateral CL(P); 5.5 percent of sibs of males with bilateral CL(P) and 3.7 percent of sibs of males with unilateral CL(P). Other tables are available[5] which have data that include more distant relatives. This empiric risk data appears to support many of the concepts of multifactorial inheritance such as (1) higher risk related to less commonly affected sex [females with CL(P) have a higher recurrence risk because they are the less commonly affected sex]; and (2) decreasing degree of relationship and decreased recurrence risk (more distant relatives share fewer genes and are at a lower risk).

Table 3-2

Recurrence Risk for Clefts

		CL(P)%	**CP%**
Normal Parents:			
affected sibs	normal sibs		
1	0	4.0	3.5
1	1	4.0	3.0
2	0	14.0	13.0
One Parent Affected:			
affected sibs	normal sibs		
0	0	4.0	3.5
1	0	12.0	10.0
1	1	10.0	9.0
2	0	25.0	24.0
Both Parents Affected:			
affected sibs	normal sibs		
0	0	35.0	25.0
1	0	45.0	40.0
1	1	40.0	35.0
2	0	50.0	45.0

In using this sort of data to counsel families the admonition[5] must be heeded to examine carefully other family members for microforms of clefting such as bifid uvula, submucous cleft and velopharyngeal insufficiency. In a family with a positive history for clefting, an individual with a microform should be treated as affected.

Although CP and CL(P) have been recognized since early times, conflicts continue as to the precise genetics of these conditions when they occur without other anomalies. Multifactorial inheritance is one attractive model, and empiric data in CL(P) and CP appear to support that theory. But there are criticisms of application of that mode of inheritance to CL(P) and CP. Geneticists continue to use population data and other theoretic models to explore the possibility of other modes of inheritance and other factors in the inheritance of these conditions.[13,14]

Bixler[13] summarized the specific criticisms of the various aspects of multifactorial inheritance as it relates to the occurrence of CL(P) and CP without other anomalies. His paper reviewed significant data and his analysis contradicts all of the predictions of the multifactorial inheritance model in the entities of CL(P) and CP. Bixler feels that the data do not reject the multifactorial inheritance model, but that the CL(P) and CP data do not conform to the offered predictors. He suggests that an explanation of these results is that CL(P) and CP, without other anomalies, are both etiologically heterogeneous.

He goes on to propose that the data presented in his paper suggest that there are at least three groups of CL(P) and CP: (1) *Syndromic,* including 1 percent of CL(P) and 8 percent of CP. These cases encompass monogenic, chromosomal and environmental etiologies. (2) *Familial,* including kindreds with two or more affected first, second or third degree relatives. This accounts for 25 percent of CL(P) and 12 percent of CP cases. (3) *Isolated* (nonfamilial), kindreds with only the proband affected. This group encompasses 75 percent of CL(P) and 80 percent of CP cases.

He suggests that this information and classification can be used in counseling. Known syndromic cases should be identified and counseled as such. Familial cases should be identified and pooled data should not be used because these families indeed have a higher risk than previously indicated in empiric risk data. The third group—isolated cases—can be given the recurrence risk of much less than 1 percent with the stipulation that familial cases with only one affected member cannot be identified in this group.

Obviously, genetic counseling is not always simple nor easy, and choices have to be made in order to serve best and counsel accurately the patient and the family. Certainly the possibly higher risk than indicated in empiric data is worthy of note and of clinical significance in counseling. But, many clinical geneticists may find it difficult to abandon the use of the somewhat higher recurrence risk for a family with only one individual affected in favor of less than 1 percent risk. This reluctance may come from the personal experience of counseling "low risk families" with only one affected child who subsequently go on to become high risk families with the birth of a second and third affected child. It is always wise to warn the family with one affected individual of this possibility. Some cases may indeed be sporadic, but it would be unfair to advise any family that the risk is nearly zero.

Clefts Associated with Other Anomalies and Syndromes

The presence of other anomalies with clefts can change the picture for prognosis, treatment and genetic counseling. Other anomalies are reported to be associated with 13-50 percent of cases of CP, 7-13 percent of CL and 2-13 percent of CL(P).[5] More malformations are reported in individuals with bilateral CL than in those with unilateral CL. Associated anomalies are more common in patients with a negative family history.[5] Reports indicate that in those patients surviving the neonatal period, the incidence of other anomalies drops to 2 percent.[15] The population of a craniofacial center may show other anomalies in 54 percent of patients with CP and 35 percent of patients with CL(P).[16]

Genetics and the Patient with Other Anomalies

Because other anomalies happen with relative frequency in individuals with CL(P) and CP, one must approach the diagnosis, management and genetic counseling of such a patient differently from a patient with CL(P) or CP alone. Obviously, when other major anomalies are present, the team that cares for the patient is expanded to include specialists in those particular areas. The other defects that are present may influence the timing of procedures and general care of the patient. For instance, the presence of a severe cardiac problem may cause the child to fail to thrive. The general care of the infant may move in a completely different direction, such as achievement of adequate weight gain or treatment of congestive heart failure.

The role of the geneticist can be to help identify those conditions which may imply a poor or relatively lethal condition such as Trisomy 13 or Trisomy 18. Once a syndrome is identified, the treatment plan must be individualized. Communication among team members at all times is critical in the management of patients with multiple anomalies.

The recognition of other anomalies is extremely important in the care of the patient and in the genetic counseling. Many geneticists have faced the uncomfortable experience in informing a falsely reassured family that their child instead has a severe and for the most part lethal condition such as Trisomy 13. Individuals who care for patients with CL(P) and CP must recognize the broad picture of the patient and look beyond the cleft in a physical as well as psychological sense.

Clefts and Syndromes

Fraser[10] reported that less than 3 percent of clefting cases were associated with syndromes. Bixler[13] suggested that 1 percent of CL(P) and 8 percent of CP cases are associated with syndromes. If indeed as high as 50 percent of clefts[5] have associated anomalies, there may be many syndromes yet to be identified. A *syndrome* can be defined as multiple anomalies thought to be pathologically related and not representing a sequence.[17,18] A syndrome usually, but not always, implies a single etiology.[18] A *malformation sequence* (complex) may be defined as multiple defects derived from a single known or presumed structural defect.[19] The *Robin complex* is an example of a malformation sequence. Sorting out those cases of CL(P) and CP associated with syndromes is critically important for genetic counseling purposes. Cohen[20] provides an excellent review of the subject of syndromes with clefts. His paper delineates 154 syndromes associated with clefts, gives a review of the subject and provides tables that can be used in diagnosis. Presented are 28 syndromes with CL(P), 77 syndromes with CP, 18 syndromes associated with Robin complex, 29 chromosome disorders with clefts, 7 associated with median CL, 17 with associations, 39 autosomal recessive, 5 X-linked, 6 environmentally induced and 40 of unknown genesis.

Chromosome Disorders and Clefts

Cleft Lip(P) and CP can be associated with numerous chromosome abnormalities. A patient presenting with CL(P) or CP along with other anomalies is certainly a candidate for this type of study. Chromosome disorders tend to cause complexes of major and minor anomalies, abnormalities in size (usually smallness) and neurologic findings such as mental retardation and hypotonia or hypertonia.

Trisomy 13 is one of the classic trisomy syndromes that can present with CL, CP or CL(P). Cleft lip is present in 60-75 percent of cases.[6,21,22] In addition, holoencephaly (incomplete development of the forebrain), which can be associated with CL(P), also is found frequently in Trisomy 13.[23,24,25] As with all autosomal anomalies, multiple system involvement and mental deficiency occur in Trisomy 13. Other frequent anomalies in this condition are: (1) a characteristic facial appearance with broad, thick nose and nasal bridge, eye anomalies and abnormal ears; (2) polydactyly; and (3) congenital heart disease (80%).[21] Although fairly characteristic in appearance, this syndrome can on occasion be subtle and not recognized as the severe defect that it is. The prognosis for this condition is extremely poor—50 percent die in the first month and 66 percent by the sixth month.[26] Those that survive are usually severely retarded.

Trisomy 18 is another classic chromosome syndrome with (1) growth deficiency, (2) classic facies, (3) mental deficiency and (4) clenching of the hands and fingers. Cleft lip(P) or CP also occurs in numerous other chromosomal anomalies including *Turner Syndrome,*[6,28] *Down syndrome,*[5] *Cri du Chat syndrome,* (5p-),[29] *Wolf-Hirschhorn syndrome* (4p-),[30] *XXXXY syndrome*[31,32] and *Triploidy.*[33] In the genetic evaluation of a patient with multiple congenital anomalies, a normal chromosome study is important in the pursuit of other possible syndromes.

Monogenic Syndromes Associated with Clefts

Van der Woude syndrome of lip pits-cleft lip[34] is a notable syndrome because it illustrates the need for a very thorough and meticulous examination of both the patient and the parents. In this syndrome the only manifestation that an individual carries the gene for this condition may be a very subtle lip pit or fistula. Discovery of this defect is significant because the condition is autosomal dominantly inherited, which makes a considerable difference in the recurrence for the family. In autosomal dominant conditions the risk for a carrier of the gene to have an affected child is 50 percent per pregnancy. Eight percent of carriers of Van der Woude syndrome will express it physically (the penetrance is 80 percent),[35] and up to 80 percent have CL(P).[34]

There are two other syndromes with clefts that are autosomal dominantly inherited and are seen with some frequency. One is the *EEC syndrome.*[36] This syndrome includes a hand/foot anomaly (ectodactyly, a decreased number of digits in a certain pattern), ectodermal dysplasia and CL(P). There is variable expression and even lack of penetrance.[36,37] The other is *Hays-Wells syndrome.* This syndrome, also known as *AEC syndrome,* includes ankyloblepharon (adhesions between the eyelids), ectodermal dysplasia and clefting.[38]

The counseling of an autosomal dominant condition is complicated by the fact that there is variability of expression of the trait and lack of penetrance involved in this type of inheritance pattern. Lack of penetrance means that a person carries a gene but shows no manifestation of it. A geneticist may never feel completely comfortable in counseling a couple with a child affected with what appears to be a new dominant mutation because the possibility exists that the gene is nonpenetrant in one of the parents.

In autosomal recessively inherited conditions both parents carry one gene for the condition, but it is only manifest in their children who have two doses of the gene. The recurrence risk in each pregnancy for another affected child is 25 percent. These conditions can be severe in nature.

One of the more frequently occurring autosomal recessive conditions that has CL(P) is the *Meckel-Gruber syndrome.*[39] This syndrome includes encephalocele (neural tube defect), polydactyly and polycystic kidneys. The patient may have either CL(P) or CP and occasionally holoprosencephaly.[40] The prognosis in this condition is poor and it may simulate Trisomy 13.

The *Roberts syndrome* is another autosomal recessive condition that has multisystem involvement. It includes shortened extremities, craniofacial anomalies [including CL(P)] and growth deficiency. Many of these infants are stillborn or die shortly after birth. They also may simulate conditions caused by teratogens.[41]

Cleft lip(P) or CP may occur in association with anomalies of any other organ system. *Camptomelic dysplasia syndrome* features skeletal anomalies (bowed extremities, rib and scapular defects) and craniofacial anomalies such as CP.[42] This syndrome also is inherited in an autosomal recessive manner.

Syndromes of Undefined/Unknown Etiology and Complex Heterogeneous Etiologies

There are numerous syndromes of unknown or undefined etiology. One that is rather common (1/2,000 births) is the curious *amnionic band syndrome.*[29] In this condition there is extreme variability of anomalies. One of the primary findings involves amputations or disruptions affecting the extremities. Numerous other areas of the body may be involved in various ways, including usual or unusual types of CL(P). This syndrome has been the source of many theories of etiology. One involves the notion than the amnion ruptures and forms bands that wrap around parts of the body or may be swallowed, thus forming the CL(P).[43] For the most part, this condition is sporadic in nature and must be identified for counseling purposes.

The *Robin sequence* (complex) which includes micrognathia, glossoptosis and cleft of the soft palate, is a common and heterogeneous condition.[5] It may occur in otherwise normal individuals but also can be part of another broader diagnosis such as Stickler syndrome or Trisomy 18. Cohen[20,44] reports 18 conditions that may be associated with the Robin complex. The identification of the underlying condition is critical for genetic counseling and prevention of other associated problems. *Stickler syndrome,* for instance, is an autosomal dominant condition with a high frequency of retinal detachment.[45]

Holoprosencephaly is an extremely interesting defect. The frontal lobes of the brain fail to divide and form normally because of a defect in the precordial mesoderm. This in turn prevents the normal formation of the midface.[46] The premaxillary area deficiency may be associated with a severe CL(P) deformity and hypotelorism.[47] The most severe manifestation of this defect is cyclopia. Holoprosencephaly occurs in about 1/5,000 births.[23,29,40] If a syndrome cannot be identified in the patient with holoprosencephaly, the empiric recurrence risk is about 6 percent.[5] Some cases are inherited in an autosomal recessive manner or even autosomal dominantly.[48]

Cleft and Other Anomalies

One of the most important aspects of finding the first anomaly is that it should alert the specialist to search for other anomalies. Cohen[18] reports that 3 percent of all newborns have significant malformations and approximately 1 percent have multiple malformations. Myrianthopoulus[2] reports that 34 percent of infants with any malformations will have multiple malformations. This concept is important in CL(P) and CP.

Clefts frequently are found in association with other anomalies. Fraser[10] suggests the concept of generalized developmental instability of the organism to account for the increase of other major malformations found in children with CL(P) and CP. This situation, he says, may result from a specific teratogen with a familial tendency affecting the face and other organ systems that may be susceptible. This concept may extend to other family members as well. Fraser[49] reports anomalies including CL(P) and CP in sibs of patients with neural tube defects (NTD). In four independent sets of data the frequency of NTD in sibs of children with CL(P) was higher than expected.

Opitz[50] reviewed the concept of midline developmental field defects to explain such anomalies as neural tube defects, oral clefts, omphalocele and diaphragmatic hernia. There may be factors that tie together anomalies that are midline developmental field defects.

Anencephaly is associated with CL(P) in 10 percent of cases.[15] Czeizel[51] reported 26 cases of anencephaly with CL(P) in his series. These two anomalies may be related in the previously mentioned midline developmental field defects.

Congenital heart disease (CHD) and clefts may be associated with a specific syndrome, a single gene mutation such as *facio-cranio-renal syndrome*[52] or a chromosomal disorder such as Trisomy 13. Cleft lip(P) or CP are reported in 2 percent of congenital heart disease cases.[15] A weak recurrence pattern has been reported between atrial septal defect and CP. These two entities have occurred more than once in unrelated individuals but usually do not occur together. Individually they are common.[18] Cleft lip(P) amd CP have uncommonly been reported with many cardiac anomalies.[53] Geis et al.[54] report a tenfold increase in prevalence of CHD in the Tufts New England Medical Center Cleft Palate Clinic. Of patients with bilateral CL(P), 12.5 percent had CHD and of CP patients only 4.3 percent had CHD. In another study of 150 living patients with clefts, 1.3 percent had CHD.[55] Six cases out of 39 (15.4%) with Robin complex had CHD.[56] Other anomalies reported with CL(P) or CP include clubbed foot, anomalies of the vertebrae and forearm bone hypoplasia.[15]

Teratogens in CL(P) or CP

A teratogen is a substance or condition that causes a birth defect. Drugs and infections are two major causes of environmentally caused birth defects. Because teratogens can be important in the etiology of CL(P) or CP, a thorough pregnancy history should be taken. For most teratogens involved in CL(P) or CP the exposure to a teratogen causes a specific birth defect in only a small fraction of cases. The effect of a teratogen is mediated by both the maternal and fetal genotype, as well as by the timing and dose of the drug. Drugs taken after the closure of the lip and palate cannot be implicated as factors in CL(P) or CP. Teratogens in CL(P) or CP can cause a cleft without any other anomaly, a cleft with possible other associations or a recognizable malformation syndrome, including a cleft. These three categories will be discussed separately.

Teratogens Producing CL(P)/CP Without Other Anomalies

Several studies have shown an increased risk of CL(P) following maternal ingestion of diazepam (Valium). Saxen[57] showed a threefold increase in CL(P) in mothers taking antineurotic drugs, mostly diazepam. The association remained when the subgroup benzodiazepines was analyzed.[58] Safra and Oakley[59] showed a fourfold increase in CL(P) with ingestion of diazepam during the first trimester of pregnancy. However, Czeizel[60] found no significant difference in the frequency of diazepam intake between mothers who had babies with CL(P) and the control group of mothers having babies with anencephaly or spina bifida babies. More recently, Shiono and Mills[61] found no increased frequency of oral clefts in a prospective study of[33,249] pregnant women. Other groups also have supported this conclusion.[62,63] Although it appears unlikely that Valium is a strong teratogen, if an increased risk of as much as fourfold exists, the risk for a mother who took diazepam during the first trimester of pregnancy of having a baby with CL(P) is less than 1 percent.

There are several reports in the literature that steroids taken during pregnancy may cause a slightly increased risk of CP in a baby without other anomalies. Bongioranni and McPadden[63] found two infants with CP out of 260 women who had taken corticosteroids during pregnancy, an incidence of 0.7 percent. Serment and Ruf[65] also found an incidence of 0.7 percent of CL(P) in their study of 428 corticosteroid exposed women. In addition, Fraser[66] reviewed the literature and arrived at a figure of 1.9 percent of pregnancies treated with corticoids resulted in a child with CP when a background rate of 0.4 percent is expected. Although the studies show conflicting numbers, corticosteroids may have a low level effect on the production of CP when taken during early pregnancy.

Teratogens Producing CL(P) with Other Possible Anomalies

Milkovich and Van den Berg[67] performed a prospective study examining anorectic drug use during pregnancy. They found that of 175 infants exposed to amphetamine within the first 50 days of pregnancy, one had CL(P) and two had CP, but no other anomalies. This rate of 1/58 is an 8.5-fold increase over their control group incidence of 1/500. Erikson et al.[68] found four infants of 71 amphetamine addicted mothers to have significant malformations; none of these had CL(P) or CP. Amphetamines also have been implicated as possible teratogens in congenital heart disease (CHD).[69]

Interestingly, CHD and CL(P) or CP are associated in a nonrandom manner. Geis et al.[54] found an approximate tenfold increase in CHD in children with CL(P) or CP when patients with severe mental retardation, holoprosencephaly and trisomies were excluded. In addition, Noonan[70] notes that in children with CL(P) or CP there is a sixfold increase in CHD. Perhaps there are other environmental teratogens working to produce CHD and CL(P) or CP in a single infant.

Infants of diabetic mothers (IDM) have a two- to threefold increased rate of all malformations when compared to controls.[71,72] Pederson[73] found a twofold increase in CL(P), as well as the more well known 600-fold increase in the caudal regression syndrome. Also of interest is the fact that of 14 IDMs with multiple malformations two had CL(P) and two had CP.[74] The significance of these findings is unclear, but maternal diabetes is a condition that may produce CL(P) or CP with other anomalies present.

Medications Producing a Recognizable Syndrome, Including CL(P)

Perhaps the most well known medications that cause clefts in association with a recognizable malformation pattern are the seizure medications—hydantoin and trimethadione. Originally an association was found between seizure disorders in mothers and clefts in their infants.[75] The estimated risk for a mother with a seizure disorder to give birth to a baby with an oral cleft was 1 percent. Some authors believe that it is the underlying maternal epilepsy which is the cause or partial cause for this association.[76,77] However, in 1975 Hanson and Smith described the *fetal hydantoin syndrome.*[78] Cleft lip(P) is considered a frequent anomaly, although it must be present with the history of hydantoin during pregnancy to make the diagnosis.[29] Hanson et al.[79] estimate that of mothers who take hydantoin during pregnancy, about 10 percent of their offspring will have the full syndrome, with the risk of some feature of the syndrome being an additional 33 percent.

Trimethadione is an anticonvulsant that is used much less frequently during pregnancy, but it also produces a recognizable phenotype. The major features include high arched or cleft palate, dental abnormalities, low set and posteriorly rotated ears, V-shaped eyebrows, congenital heart disease, spleen problems and mild mental retardation.[80] Feldman et al.[81] note that 83 percent of women taking trimethadione during pregnancy will give birth to infants with at least one congenital abnormality and that mental deficiency is present in about 50 percent.

Alcohol is a frequently used and abused social drug and is also the cause of birth defects and mental retardation if taken in large quantities during pregnancy. Clarren and Smith[82] summarize the findings in 245 cases of *fetal alcohol syndrome* (FAS). The major abnormalities fall into the four classes of central nervous system dysfunction, growth deficiency, dysmorphic facial features and variable major and minor malformations. Cleft lip or CP were observed in between 1-25 percent of patients with FAS.[82] The risk for FAS in children born to chronically alcoholic women is estimated to be 20 percent and the risk for mental deficiency is close to 50 percent.[83]

As with most other drug-induced malformations FAS is totally preventable through adequate patient and physician education and compliance. It is important to remember that women who have been exposed to a potential teratogen for CL(P) or CP generally have a low risk of actually giving birth to a child with CL(P) or CP. They should be reassured of their low risk if ascertained early in pregnancy. Women who have taken seizure medications or large amounts of alcohol run a higher risk of more severe problems. They should be given complete information and support to facilitate a comfortable decision regarding the pregnancy.

Genetic Counseling of Clefts and Other Anomalies

Because patients who have clefts and other anomalies occur with considerable frequency,[5] the geneticist's dilemma is how to counsel a family with a cleft and other anomalies in terms of prognosis and recurrence risk. Naturally a thorough search of the syndrome literature[5,15,20,29] and possible cytogenetic evaluations are indicated. Studies reveal that a definitive diagnosis can be made in only 40 percent of cases and 60 percent are of unknown etiology.[16,24,84]

The geneticist cautiously approaches the counseling of a couple with a child with multiple anomalies of unknown etiology. He is faced with the always present possibility that birth defects can recur. Studies show that a couple with a child affected with multiple congenital anomalies of unknown etiology has a recurrence risk of 5 percent (BD Hall, unpublished Pediatric Syllabus, University of California, San Francisco, 1980). Because of this data it is prudent to advise families that there is always the possibility the complex of anomalies may occur again.

Alternatively, there are several other possibilities. The first is that the complex of anomalies represents a new "private" syndrome. That is, it is the first identified in that family. In this situation, there is the possibility that the condition has been inherited as a new autosomal recessive syndrome with a recurrence risk of 25 percent. In these families with a child with multiple congenital anomalies of undefined etiology, the empiric recurrence risk is 5 percent, with the possibility that it could be as high as 25 percent if caused by a new autosomal recessive condition. It is advisable to discuss this with the parents; every geneticist has seen a family in which a "new" syndrome has recurred and appears to be inherited as an autosomal recessive condition. A couple who have been noted to have consanguinity, of course, would sway the genetic counselor to consider that the anomaly complex has that higher recurrence risk due to shared genes. One of the factors that suggests a trait or complex is inherited in an autosomal recessive manner is the presence of consanguinity.[85,86]

Another possibility in the causation of multiple congenital anomalies is that of a new dominant mutation. In this case the recurrence risk is very low or, theoretically, the mutation rate for the condition is low. Although this situation must occur, one must be cautious in explaining that a new autosomal dominant mutation is what occurred in that family. It is also possible that this condition may indeed be a new dominant disorder, but as discussed earlier, one of the parents may be a carrier of the gene (even a nonpenetrant gene) and thus have a 50 percent recurrence risk.

Still another situation involves the possibility of a teratogen operating that could interfere with multiple organ system development. A careful and thorough investigation of this possibility is indicated in all families of children with anomalies. New teratogens still are being discovered, and the alert practitioner may be the first one to note an association. Some investigators suggest that temporal anomalies are more likely to be environmentally induced. Temporal anomalies are defects that occur in different organ systems developing at the same time. An agent acting during this time could cause the birth defect complex. These environmental factors, known or unknown, may or may not be present in future pregnancies.

Geneticists are, needless to say, reluctant to counsel families that a given condition will not happen again. It is only fair to share their own experiences and those of other geneticists that birth defects can and frequently do recur.

The Importance of Genetic Counseling from the Parent's Perspective

As stated previously, examination of a child with CL(P) or CP is important to identify syndromes with different genetic factors in order to give accurate recurrence risks for future children. This is a concern for every geneticist. However, the parents of a newborn with CL(P) or CP may have other immediate concerns. This section will outline parental motivation for seeking genetic counseling, proceed to the structure of a genetic counseling session and culminate in a discussion of prenatal diagnostic procedures that may help in future pregnancies.

The immediate concern of many parents is, "What does this mean for my child?" Usually this is addressed in the newborn period, in the bustling hospital environment and during the shock after the birth of a child with a congenital defect. Later, with some distance from the newborn period, parents find themselves asking questions previously raised but not fully answered. The genetic counseling session can be a time to review and expand this information.

Immediately following the delivery of a baby with a birth defect, parents begin to experience a series of emotions and adjustments which may go on for years. In the genetic counseling session parents can receive validation that these feelings are normal and can begin to verbalize their anxieties. The first reaction parents usually have is shock. In the case of the baby with CL(P) this feeling can be intensified because the face is the locus of the majority of visual contact. The birth of a child with CL(P) or CP is a twofold disappointment for the parents—the image of the hoped for perfect child is gone, and in its place is a "feared, threatening and anger-evoking child."[87]

Following an initial period of shock, denial of the event is a common reaction. Anxiety is generated when facts outweigh the capacity to deny, and this may be turned outward in the form of anger or inward in the form of guilt, shame or embarrassment. Depression may occur before resolution is reached. Some people oscillate in a cycle between denial, anxiety and depression before reaching an emotional adaptation to their situation.[88]

Because the birth of a child is often a culmination of parental hopes and desires, a child with a birth defect represents a blow to parental self esteem. Parents may be struck with the inherent fairness of the situation, and come to genetic counseling asking, "Why me?" Additionally, the child with CL(P) or CP can cause a deleterious effect on marriage in the form of blame and can cause a disruption of the entire family unit with the shift in focus to a newborn with problems. Individuals in a dysfunctional relationship may seek genetic counseling as a way of talking with their spouses.

Only after the concerns for the present child are alleviated do the parents turn their thoughts to the possible consequences for future children. Occasionally patients who have had a previous child with CL(P) or CP will return for counseling after again becoming pregnant, only to hear the recurrence risk is significantly different from what they remembered. Perhaps these couples were not prepared to deal with the possibility of problems with another child when they were counseled initially.

The Structure of a Session

Ideally, the genetic counseling session should provide an environment in which parents feel comfortable asking questions about their child's condition and the future. It should be a place to air feelings that may otherwise go unacknowledged. The geneticist may have a separate agenda, such as obtaining information about family history and giving recurrence risks. It is important that these agendas be merged and that both are fully covered. Rather than launching into a one-sided informational speech, it is often helpful to outline at the beginning of the session what may lie ahead for the family and the patient and to encourage an interactional format. In this way the patient can know better how to fit his questions and concerns into the session without leaving important issues unaddressed.

Generally, a session should begin with a pregnancy and birth history. Particular attention should be paid to medications taken during pregnancy, especially seizure medications. A three-generation family history also should be taken, with specific questioning concerning the presence of other family members with CL(P) or CP, family members with lip pits and other minor anomalies.

At this point a shift in focus to the child occurs. A helpful approach to this topic is to ask the parents what they know about their child's condition. This allows the parents a chance to verbalize their feelings and serves as a takeoff point for information about the condition. A decision must be made by the counselor when to explore parents' feelings. If this is done at the wrong time, it may preclude parents from hearing information being given; or it may muddle the session sufficiently to make information giving useless.

Cleft lip(P) or CP should be approached as a developmental event. It should be explained that the lip and palate are formed by the fusion of different parts of the face early in development (9-10 weeks). In some fetuses this fusion does not take place fully, and the result is a cleft. It is very important to emphasize that in CL(P) or CP, without other anomalies, it is only this one step in the developmental process that is abnormal. The baby is normal; it is only the lip or palate that is defective. This attitude can help parents accept their child as a complete person, rather than perceiving him as a defective baby.

Of great importance to many parents is, "Why did this happen?" In any genetic condition this is a difficult question to answer because often the answer is not known or is poorly understood. Multifactorial inheritance is a difficult concept to grasp because of its many ambiguities. The fact that genes and environment combine to produce a birth defect allows for misunderstanding, undeserved blame and irrational guilt. Important points to emphasize are that genes from *both* parents influence development and that the nongenetic factors involved are unknown. When a pregnancy history revealing no teratogens is obtained, this can be used as "evidence" for the parents to help reassure them that it was nothing they did that caused the CL(P) or CP.

Often parents have their own ideas about why the birth defect has occurred. Well-meaning friends and relatives also may have influenced the parents of the affected child. This may be the time for further exploration and clarification of these notions because they can lead to ventilation of parental concerns and an alleviation of inaccurate theories.

In explaining the recurrence risk for CL(P) without other anomalies, emphasis on the fact that the number is derived from empiric data helps to make the idea easier to understand. Patients who have trouble with the concept of percentages or fractions may grasp the meaning better if it is stated as, "Of 100 couples exactly like yourselves, four of them will go on to have another child with CL(P)." After the number has been given, it is important to ask the parents their feelings about the magnitude of the risk. Even a short discussion can create the basis for more extended discussion between parents later. At the present time little more can be done to predict future affected children other than risk figures. A type of prenatal diagnosis for CL(P) and CP will be discussed in a later section.

In closing the session, mention should be made of the future care for the child. Reinforcement of the importance of an integrated CL(P) or CP clinic, if available, is warranted. A chance for questions and then a capsule of the session should be presented. The recurrence risk can be stated as a 96 percent chance that the next baby will not have CL(P) or CP. This turning around of the number often encourages parents to view the situation in a more hopeful manner. A summary letter should be sent to the family after the session, and an open door attitude maintained, if future questions should arise.

The Outcome of Genetic Counseling

The outcome of genetic counseling can be beneficial for both parents and child. An increase in knowledge about the condition allays fears and leads to a decrease in anxiety. Several articles have examined parental self-esteem prior to and after genetic counseling.[89,90] The concensus is that self-esteem is higher, as measured by standard tests, after genetic counseling. Higher parental self-esteem will be translated into better acceptance of their child's condition. A positive parental attitude toward the cleft will help the child to accept the defect in a healthier way. Starr and Heiserman[91] found that higher acceptance of the cleft was associated with higher self-esteem in children with clefts.

Self-esteem in children (average age = 12.38 years) with clefts was examined by Kapp,[92] who found that particularly girls reported significantly less global happiness and satisfaction than children without clefts. Starr[93] tested older children (average age = 15.36 years) and found no significant differences between teenagers with and without clefts in measures of self-esteem, activity level, inhibition, sleep disturbances or somatization. The only difference was that teenagers with clefts were less aggressive than their peers without clefts. In a later study Starr[94] compared two groups of teenagers with CL and CP, one aged 13 and 14, the other aged 15 to 18. He found that the younger teenagers were significantly more aggressive, more active and had more somantic complaints than the older teens with clefts. Perhaps both parent and child continue to adapt positively as time progresses.

Prenatal Diagnosis in CL(P) or CP

Although a recurrence risk is helpful in predicting the probability of having another affected child, the uncertainty involved in taking a risk can be unsettling and anxiety provoking. For these parents prenatal diagnosis can be helpful as a means for either relieving anxiety or preparing for the birth of a child with CL(P) or CP. The largest group with a potential for using a prenatal test for CL(P) or CP would be the parents of a child with CL(P) or CP without other anomalies. Prenatal diagnosis of syndromes involving CL(P) or CP also will be discussed.

Ultrasound provides the safest, if not the most accurate, method of prenatal diagnosis. The noninvasive technique uses high-frequency sound waves to construct an image of the fetus and project it on a cathode ray tube-like screen. The image is examined by an experienced sonographer for possible abnormalities of structure. Christ and Meininger[95] described the first method for prenatal diagnosis of CL(P) using ultrasound. The authors contend that diagnosis of CP also is possible by evaluating tongue movement. Since that time, Frigoletto et al.[96] described the identification of a large facial cleft using ultrasound, and Seeds and Cefalo[97] describe a protocol for diagnosis in the second trimester. Because the accuracy of this method depends on the experience of the sonographer, caution should be used in referring families for this test, generally referred to as Level II ultrasound.

Certain syndromes that carry a higher recurrence risk than does CL(P) or CP without other anomalies are amenable to prenatal diagnosis by ultrasound. Van der Woude syndrome[98] carries a risk as high as 50 percent for some features of the syndrome. Another dominant syndrome with a slightly higher burden, EEC syndrome (ectrodactyly, ectodermal dysplasia and clefting), also has a very high incidence of CL, and could be diagnosed with ultrasound. Roberts syndrome is an autosomal recessive syndrome which includes CL and shortening of the extremities in addition to other abnormalities.[99] Most infants with Roberts syndrome who are not stillborn have a very poor prognosis. By using standards for limb length measurements in conjunction with looking for the CL, diagnosis of a fetus with Roberts syndrome has been made early enough in pregnancy to offer parents the option of termination of pregnancy.[100]

Cleft lip(P) or CP is a feature of several chromosome abnormality syndromes, including 4p- and Trisomy 13. Amniocentesis is a standard test capable of diagnosing chromosome abnormalities, neural tube defects and biochemical abnormalities prenatally, with an estimated fetal loss of approximately 0.5 percent.[101] The risk of recurrence for 4p- is low because most parents of these children are not carriers of a balanced translocation.[102] Tests of blood chromosomes on both parents should be done to rule out this possibility. Trisomy 13 has an empiric recurrence risk of 1 percent for any trisomy if the mother is less than 30 years of age at the time of birth of the affected child. Otherwise, it is what would be expected on the basis of her age alone.[102]

Meckel syndrome is an autosomal recessive syndrome with variable features including CL(P) or CP (32%), cystic dysplasia of the kidneys (100%), occipital encephocele (63%), polydactyly (55%) and anencephaly (13%).[104] Amniocentesis for alpha-fetoprotein (AFP) determination has been used to diagnose Meckel syndrome in the second trimester.[105] Interestingly, cystic kidneys as well as an encephalocele or anencephaly can cause an elevated amnionic AFP.[106] However, to increase accuracy, Wapner et al.[107] have developed a protocol for Level II ultrasound as an adjunct to AFP determination in the prenatal diagnosis of Meckel syndrome.

Apert syndrome is a dominantly inherited condition involving craniosynostosis, CP and syndactyly of hands and feet, commonly resulting in what is called a "mitten hand."[108] Most cases are due to new mutations and therefore do not pose significant recurrence risks for unaffected parents. Prenatal diagnosis for the parent with Apert syndrome is available through the use of fetoscopy. This technique uses a fiberoptic endoscope that is inserted through a cannula into the uterus.[109] Direct visualization of fetal parts such as the head, torso and limbs is possible. The major risk of the procedure is an estimated 5 percent fetal loss rate and an increased chance of premature delivery. Leonard et al.[110] reported the successful second trimester fetoscopic diagnosis of Apert syndrome in a patient with known Apert syndrome.

As previously stated, holoprosencephaly is a developmental defect in which the prosencephalon fails to divide into two hemispheres. The empiric recurrence risk has been calculated as 6 percent,[111] although families with dominant inheritance also have been reported.[112] Median CL is found in many cases of holoprosencephaly. Theoretically the most useful tool in the prenatal diagnosis of holoprosencephaly is level II ultrasound. Potentially diagnostic features of holoprosencephaly include cyclopia, cebocephaly, microcephaly, hypotelorism and median cleft lip. Two cases of the suspicion of holoprosencephaly detected by ultrasound in the third trimester have been reported.[113,114] As both the resolution and the experiences of persons in the field of ultrasonography increase, many conditions previously thought to require fetoscopy can be diagnosed using ultrasound.

Summary

Each patient with CL(P) or CP and immediate family members deserve genetic counseling. The genetic etiologies of CL(P) and CP are many, so the counseling must be on an individual basis. Thorough physical examination of the patient and the parents, history, pedigree and drug and environmental exposure help clarify the course that the counseling takes. The counseling session itself provides information and support.

Patients with known syndromes, environmental or drug etiologies must be sorted out and counseled accordingly. The remaining group comprises most of the patients with clefts. Empiric recurrence risk data is available for these patients. Some authors recommend use of multifactorial inheritance numbers. Others sort out those cases with positive or negative family histories and use other empiric recurrence risk data. Whatever the genetic etiology, good genetic counseling can be a rewarding and informative experience for the patient and/or the family.

REFERENCES

1. Fogh-Anderson P: *The Inheritance of Hare Lip and Cleft Palate.* Copenhagen, Nyt Nordisk Forlag, 1942.
2. Myrianthopoulos NC, Chung CS: Congenital malformations in singletons: Epidemiologic survey. *Birth Defects Original Article Series,* 10(11): 1974.
3. Oka SW: Epidemiology and genetics of clefting, with implications for etiology, in Cooper JR, Spencer SM (eds): *Cleft Lip and Palate: A Team Approach to Clinical Management of the Patient.* Philadelphia, W B Saunders Co, 1979.
4. Drillien CM, Ingram TTS, Wilkinson EM: *The Causes and Natural History of Cleft Lip and Palate.* Edinburgh, Livingston, 1966.

5. Gorlin RJ, Pindborg JJ, Cohen MM Jr: *Syndromes of the Head and Neck.* New York, McGraw-Hill Book Co, 1976.
6. Warkany J: *Congenital Malformations: Note and Comments.* Chicago, Year Book Med Pub, 1971.
7. Carter CO: Genetics of common single malformations. *Br Med Bull,* 32:21, 1976.
8. Gruneberg H: Genetics studies on the skeleton of the mouse. IV. Quaiscontinuous variation. *J Genetics,* 51:95, 1952.
9. Carter CO: The inheritance of common congenital malformations. *Prog Med Genet,* 4, 1965.
10. Fraser FC: The genetics of cleft lip and cleft palate. *Am J Genet,* 22:336, 1970.
11. Tolarova M: Empirical recurrence risk figures for genetic counseling of clefts. *Acta Chir Plast,* 14:234, 1972.
12. Woolf CM: Congenital cleft lip: A genetic study of 496 prospositi. *J Med Genet,* 8:65, 1971.
13. Bixler D: Genetics and clefting. *Cleft Palate J,* 18:10, 1981.
14. Melnick M, Shields E, Bisler D, Conneally PM: Facial clefting: An alternative biologic explanation for its complex etiology. *Birth Defects Original Article Series,* 13(3A):93, 1977.
15. Bergsma D: *Birth Defects Compendium,* ed 2. New York, Alan R Liss, 1979.
16. Rollnick BR, Pruzansky S: Genetic services at a center for craniofacial anomalies. *Cleft Palate J,* 18:304, 1981.
17. Benirschke K, Cohen MM Jr, Hall JG, et al: Terms pertaining to morphogenesis and malformations. Read before the Birth Defects Meeting, June 8-11, 1980.
18. Cohen MM Jr: *The Child With Multiple Birth Defects.* New York, Raven Press, 1982.
19. Spranger JW, Benirschke K, Hall JG, Lenz W: Errors of morphogenesis: Concepts and terms. *J Pediat,* 100:160, 1982.
20. Cohen MM Jr: Syndromes with cleft lip and cleft palate. *Cleft Palate J,* 15:306, 1978.
21. Smith DW: The 18 Trisomy and 13 Trisomy. *Birth Defects Original Article Series,* 5:67, 1969.
22. Taylor AI: Autosomal trisomy syndrome: A detailed study of 27 cases of Edward's syndrome and 27 cases of Patau's syndrome. *J Med Genet,* 5:227, 1968.
23. Conen PE, Erkman B, Metaxotou C: The "D" syndrome. *Am J Dis Child,* 111:236, 1966.
24. Halbrecht I, Kletzky O, Komlos L, et al: Trisomy D in cyclopia. *Obstet Gynecol,* 37:391, 1971.
25. Fujimoto A, Ebbin AJ, Towner J, Wilson MG: Trisomy in two infants with cyclops. *J Med Genet,* 10:294, 1973.
26. Magenis RE, Hecht F, Mulham S Jr: Trisomy 13(D-1) syndrome: Studies on parental age, sex ratio, and survival. *J Pediatr,* 73:222, 1986.
27. deGrouchy J, Turleau C: *Clinical Atlas of Human Chromosomes.* New York, John Wiley & Sons, 1977.
28. Haddad HM, Wilkins L: Congenital anomalies associated with gonadal aplasia: Review of 55 cases. *Pediatrics,* 23:885, 1959.
29. Smith DW: *Recognizable Patterns of Human Malformation: Genetic Embrylogic and Clinical Aspects.* Philadelphia, W B Saunders Co, 1982.
30. Taylor AI: Short arm deletion, chromosome 4 (4p-), a syndrome? *Ann Hum Genet,* 34:137, 1970.
31. Miller OJ, Berg WR, Smickel RD, Tretter W: A family with an XXXXY male, a leukemic male and two 21-trisomic mongoloid females. *Lancet,* 2:78, 1961.
32. Sacrez R, Clavert J, Klein L, et al: Dysgenesic gonadosematic XXXXY. *Arch Fr Pediatr* 22:41, 1965.
33. Niebular E: Triploidy in man: Cytogenetical and clinical aspects. *Humangenetik,* 21:103, 1974.
34. Van der Woude A: Fistula labii inferioris congenital and its association with cleft lip and palate. *Am J Hum Genet,* 6:244, 1954.

35. Cervenka J, Gorlin R, Anderson V: The syndrome of pits of the lower lip and cleft lip and/ or palate: Genetic considerations. *Am J Hum Genet,* 19:416, 1967.
36. Walker JC, Clodius L: The syndromes of cleft lip, cleft palate and lobster-claw deformities of hands and feet. *Plast Reconstr Surg,* 32:627, 1963.
37. Cockaynes AE: Cleft palate, hare lip, dacrocystitis and cleft hand and feet. *Biometrika,* 28:60, 1936.
38. Hay RL, Wells RS: The syndrome of amkyloblepharon, ectodermal defects, and cleft lip and palate: An autosomal dominant condition. *Brit J Dermatol,* 94:277, 1976.
39. Meckel S, Passagre E: Encephalocele, polycystic kidneys, and polydactyly as an autosomal recessive trait simulating certain other disorders: The Meckel syndrome. *Ann Genet,* 14:97, 1971.
40. Fried K, Liban E, Lurie M, et al: Polycystic kidneys, associated with malformations of brain, polydactyly, and other birth defects in newborn sibs. *J Med Genet,* 8:285, 1971.
41. Roberts JB: A child with double cleft of lip and palate, protrusion of the intermaxiallary portion of the upper jaw and imperfect development of the bones of the four extremities. *Ann Surg,* 70:252, 1979.
42. Hall BD, Spranger JW: Camptomelic dysplasia. *Am J Dis Child,* 134:285, 1980.
43. Torpin R: *Fetal Malformations Caused by Amnion Rupture During Gestation.* Springfield, Ill, Charles C Thomas, 1968.
44. Cohen MM Jr: Dysmorphic syndromes with craniofacial manifestations, in Stewart RE, Prescott GH (eds): *Oral Facial Genetics.* St. Louis, C V Mosby Co, 1976.
45. Herrmann J, France T, Spranger J, et al: The Stickler Syndrome (Hereditary Arthroophthalmopathy). *Birth Defects Original Article Series,* 11(2):76, 1975.
46. deMeyer W, Zeman W, Palmer CG: The face predicts the brain: Diagnostic significance of median facial anomalies for holoprosencephaly (arrhinencephaly). *Plast Reconstr Surg,* 32:256, 1964.
47. Brucker P, Hoyt C, Thrusler H: Severe cleft lip and arrhinencephaly. *Plast Reconstr Surg,* 32:527, 1963.
48. Cohen MM Jr: Holoporscencephaly revisited. *Am J Dis Child,* 127:597, 1974.
49. Fraser FC, Czeizel A, Hanson C: Increased frequency of neural tube defects in sibs of children with other malformations. *Lancet,* 2:145, 1982.
50. Opitz JM, Gilbert EF: Editorial comments: CNS anomalies and the midline as a "developmental field." *Am J Med Genet,* 12:443, 1982.
51. Czeizel A: Schisis-association. *Am J Med Genet,* 10:25, 1981.
52. Eastman JR, Bixler D: Facio-cardio-renal syndrome: A newly delineated recessive disorder. *Clin Genet,* 11:424, 1977.
53. Stewart RE, Prescott GH: *Oral Facial Genetics.* St. Louis, C V Mosby Co, 1976.
54. Geis N, Seto B, Bartoshesky L, et al: The prevalence of congenital heart disease among the population of a metropolitan cleft lip and palate clinic. *Cleft Palate J,* 18:19, 1981.
55. Shah CV, Pruzansky S, Harris VS: Cardiac malformations with facial clefts. *Am J Dis Child,* 119:238, 1970.
56. Smith JL, Stowe FR: The Pierre Robin syndrome (glossoptosis, micrognathia, cleft palate): A review of 39 cases with emphasis on associated ocular anomalies. *Pediatr,* 27:128, 1961.
57. Saxen I: Association between oral clefts and drugs taken during pregnancy. *Int J Epidemiol,* 4:37, 1975.
58. Saxen I, Saxen L: Association between maternal intake of diazepam and oral clefts. *Lancet,* 2:498, 1975.
59. Safra M, Oakley G: Association between cleft lip with or without cleft palate and prenatal exposure to diazepam. *Lancet,* 2:478, 1975.
60. Czeizel A: Diazepam, phenytoin, and aetiology of cleft lip and/or palate. *Lancet,* 1:810, 1976.

61. Shiono PH, Mills JL: Oral clefts and diazepam use during pregnancy. *N Eng J Med,* 311:919, 1984.
62. Rosenberg L, Mitchell AA, Parsells JL, et al: Lack of relation of oral clefts to diazepam use during pregnancy. *N Engl J Med,* 309:1282, 1983.
63. Entman SS, Vaughn WK: Lack of relation of oral clefts to diazepam use in pregnancy. *N Engl J Med,* 310:1121, 1984.
64. Bongiovanni AM, McPadden AJ: Steroids during pregnancy and possible fetal consequences. *Fertil Steril,* 11:181, 1960.
65. Serment, Ruf H: Corticotherapie et grossesse. *Bull Fed Soc Gynecol Lang Fr,* 20:77, 1968.
66. Fraser FC: Pregnancy and adrenocortical hormones. *Br Med J,* 2:479, 1962.
67. Milkovich L, Van den Berg B: Effects of antenatal exposure to anorectic drugs. *Am J Obstet Gynecol,* 129:637, 1977.
68. Erikson M, Larsson G, Zetterstrom R: Amphetamine addiction and pregnancy. *Acta Obstet Gynecol Scand,* 60:253, 1981.
69. Nora J, Vargo T, Nora A, et al: Dexamphetamine: A possible environmental trigger in cardiovascular malformations. *Lancet,* 1:1290, 1970.
70. Noonan J: Association of congenital heart disease with syndromes or other defects. *Ped Clin North Am,* 25:797, 1978.
71. Dignan P: Teratogenic risk and counseling in diabetes. *Clin Obstet Gynecol,* 24:149, 1981.
72. Mills J: Malformations in infants of diabetic mothers. *Teratology,* 25:385, 1982.
73. Pederson J: *The Pregnant Diabetic and Her Newborn.* Baltimore, Williams & Wilkins, 1977.
74. Grix A: Malformation in infants of diabetic mothers. *Am J Med Genet,* 13:131, 1982.
75. Erikson JD, Oakley G: Seizure disorder in mothers of children with orofacial clefts: A case-control study. *J Pediatr,* 84:244, 1974.
76. Kelly TE, Rein M, Edwards F: Teratogenicity of anticonvulsant drugs. IV. The association of clefting and epilepsy. *Am J Med Genet,* 19:451, 1984.
77. Dalessio D: Seizure disorders and pregnancy. *N Engl J Med,* 312:559, 1985.
78. Hanson J, Smith D: The fetal hydantoin syndrome. *J Pediatr,* 87:285, 1975.
79. Hanson J, Myrianthopoulos NC, Harvey MAS, Smith DW: Risks to the offspring of women treated with hydantoin anticonvulsant, with emphasis on the fetal hydantoin syndrome. *J Pediatr,* 89:662, 1976.
80. Zackai E, Mellman W, Neiderer B, Hanson J: The fetal trimethadione syndrome. *J Pediatr,* 87:280, 1975.
81. Feldman G, Weaver D, Lovrien E: The fetal trimethadione syndrome. *Am J Dis Child,* 131:1389, 1977.
82. Clarren S, Smith D: The fetal alcohol syndrome. *N Engl J Med,* 298:1063, 1978.
83. Smith D, Jones K, Hanson J: Perspectives on the cause and frequency of the fetal alcohol syndrome. *Ann NY Acad Sci,* 273:138, 1976.
84. Marden PM, Smith DW, McDonald MJ: Congenital anomalies in the newborn infant including minor variations. *J Pediatr,* 64:357, 1964.
85. Nora JJ, Fraser FC: *Medical Genetics: Principles and Practice.* Philadelphia, Lea & Febiger, 1981.
86. Murphy EA, Chase GA: *Principles of Genetic Counseling.* Chicago, Year Book Med Publ, 1975.
87. Solnit A, Stark M: Mourning and the birth of a defective child. *Psychoanal Study Child,* 16:523, 1961.
88. Targum S, Weiss J: A genetic disease in the family. *Psychiatr Opin,* 17:23, 1980.
89. Antley M, Antley R, Harlage L: Effects of genetic counseling on parental self-concepts. *J Psychol,* 83:335, 1973.
90. Corgan R: Genetic counseling and parental self-concept change. *Birth Defects Original Article Series,* 15(5C):281, 1979.

91. Starr P, Heiseman K: Acceptance of disability by teenagers with oral clefts. *Rehabil Coun Bull,* March 1977, p. 198.
92. Kapp K: Self-concept of the cleft lip and/or palate child. *Cleft Palate J,* 16:171, 1979.
93. Starr P: Self-esteem behavioral functioning of teenagers with oral facial clefts. *Rehabil Lit,* 39:233, 1978.
94. Starr P: Cleft type, age, and sex differences in teenagers' rating of their own behavior, self-esteem, and attitude toward clefting. *Rehabil Lit,* 41:177, 1980.
95. Christ J, Meininger M: Ultrasound diagnosis of cleft lip and cleft palate before birth. *Plast Reconstr Surg,* 68:854, 1981.
96. Frigoletto F, Birnholz J, Greene M: Antenatal treatment of hydrocephalus by ventriculoamnionic shunting. *JAMA,* 248:2496, 1982.
97. Seeds JW, Cefalo RC: Technique of early sonographic diagnosis of bilateral cleft lip and palate. *Obsete Gynecol,* 62:25, 1983.
98. Janku P, Robinow M, Kelly T, et al: The Van der Woude syndrome in a large kindred: Variability, penetrance, genetic risks. *Am J Med Genet,* 5:117, 1980.
99. Freeman M, Williams D, Schimke RN, et al: The Roberts syndrome. *Clin Genet,* 5:1, 1974.
100. Hobbins JC, Grannum PAT, Berkowitz RL, et al: Ultrasound in the diagnosis of congenital anomalies. *Am J Obstet Gynecol,* 134:331, 1979.
101. Verp M, Gerbie A: Amniocentesis for prenatal diagnosis. *Clin Obstet Gynecol,* 24:1007, 1981.
102. Guthrie R, Aase J, Asper A, Smith D: The 4p- syndrome. *Am J Dis Child,* 122:421, 1977.
103. Simpson JL, Golbus MS, Martin AO, Sarto GE: *Genetics in Obstetrics and Gynecology.* New York, Grune & Stratton, 1982.
104. Fraser FC, Lytwyn A: Spectrum of anomalies in the Meckel syndrome. *Am J Med Genet,* 9:67, 1981.
105. Friedrich U, Hansen KB, Hauge M, et al: Prenatal diagnosis of polycystic kidneys and encephalocele (Meckel syndrome). *Clin Genet,* 15:278, 1979.
106. Chemke J, Miskin Z, Rav-Acha A, et al: Prenatal diagnosis of Meckel syndrome: Alpha-fetoprotein and beta-trace protein in amnionic fluid. *Clin Genet,* 11:285, 1977
107. Wapner R, Kurtz A, Ross RD, Jackson L: Ultrasonographic parameters in the prenatal diagnosis of Meckel syndrome. *Obstet Gynecol,* 57:388, 1981.
108. Blank CE: Apert's syndrome (a type of acrocephalosyndactyly): Observations on British series of thirty-nine cases. *Ann Hum Genet,* 24:151, 1960.
109. Mahoney MJ, Hobbins JC: Fetoscopy and fetal biopsy, in Lubs HA, DelaCruz F (eds): *Genetic Counseling.* New York, Raven Press, 1977.
110. Leonard C, Diakoku N, Winn K: Prenatal fetoscopic diagnosis of the Apert syndrome. *Am J Med,* 11:5, 1982.
111. Roach E, deMyer W, Conneally PM, et al: Holoprosencephaly: Birth data, genetic and demographic analysis of 30 families. *Birth Defects Original Article Sereis,* 11:294, 1975.
112. Cantu J, Fragoso R, Garcia-Cruz D, Sanchez-Coronar J: Dominant Inheritance of holoprosencephaly. *Birth Defects Original Article Series,* 14(6B):215, 1978.
113. Hill L, Breckle R, Bonebrake C: Ultrasound findings with holoprosencephaly. *J Reprod Med,* 27:172, 1982.
114. Elejalde B, deElejalde M, Hamilton P, et al: Prenatal diagnosis of cyclopia. *Am J Med Genet,* 14:15, 1983.

CHAPTER 4

THE CLEFT LIP

M. HUGH BAILEY & FRANK PIRRUCCELLO

. . .Do not worry about people not knowing your ability, but worry that you have not got it.

. . .Confucius

Introduction

THE CLEFT LIP is the most common type of facial clefting. It is a syndrome distinct from isolated cleft of the secondary palate (see chapter on genetics). Cleft lip may be accompanied by cleft palate and varies greatly in degree of expression. The incidence of cleft lip is approximately 1 per 1000 births,[1] though it is somewhat less common in American Negroes[2] and more common in the Mongolian races.[3,4] The left side, the right side and both sides are involved in a 6:3:1 ratio,[5] and there is a male preponderance of about 2:1.[6] The incidence appears to be increasing.[7]

The usual form of cleft lip, i.e., occurring at the philtral border, represents about 99 percent of facial clefts involving the lip.[8] Repair of the rarer facial clefts is outside the scope of this chapter; however, the clinician must seek evidence of occult Tessier type 1, 2 and 3 clefts in the patient with a cleft lip.[9]

Cleft lip is associated with about 150 syndromes, discussion of which is also outside the scope of this chapter. The clinical assessment should include a careful search for significant family history or other physical abnormalities. However, in the absence of any clinical findings, further investigative procedures are not indicated.

Embryology

Understanding of the events leading to the defect of cleft lip is useful in a critical approach of methods of repair.[10] Unfortunately our understanding of the embryology is imperfect.

Whether the cleft represents a failure of fusion[11] or a deficiency of mesenchyme leading to a breakdown of an existing membrane[12] is still in dispute. As Veau stated, the presence of Simonart's bands seems to support the latter theory.[13] Standard texts[14,15,16] agree on most other points.

From 15 to 20 days postconception, the milaminar embryo develops a mesodermal layer from the ectodermal primitive streak. A notochordal process develops from Hensen's node, and cells from both of these processes migrate cranially to an area of columnar endoderm called the prochordal plate. During mesodermal migration this plate remains firmly fused to ectoderm, forming the oropharyngeal membrane. At this time the neural crests form and fuse, the intraembryonic and extraembryonic coelomic spaces arise in the mesoderm and the embryo develops mesodermal somites.

At about 21 to 23 days, as the neural crests enlarge and fuse, the embryo starts to flex. Then the mesodermal masses of the first (mandibular) and second (Hyoid) branchial arches develop, probably from neural crest cells, and fuse in the midline. The maxillary prominences, which form the lateral borders of the oropharyngeal membrane, develop from the first arch.

By 28 days nasal placodes, separated by a single frontonasal eminence of mesoderm, form the superior borders of the pit lined by the oropharyngeal membrane. This pit is called the stomodeum. Further mesodermal migration and proliferation form medial and lateral nasal prominences and the oropharyngeal membrane disintegrates, joining the stomodeum to the foregut.

The frontonasal eminence becomes superior to the nasal prominences and develops the nasoseptal and paired nasozygomatic portions. The philtrum is thus formed by the merging of the medial nasal prominences, with a small contribution in the midline from the nasoseptal portion of the frontonasal eminence. The remainder of the lip forms from the merging of the maxillary prominences with the developing philtrum. The muscles, and their innervation, result from migration of mesenchyme from the second branchial arch.

Thus, the primary problem is a failure of mesodermal migration or ingrowth. The tissues adjacent to the actual cleft also show derangement of normal anatomy, and there is an overall shortage of tissue.

Myology of the Cleft Lip

The normal anatomy of the upper lip and nose is well known. A single muscle, the orbicularis oris, encircles the mouth, while the remaining muscles are arranged in radial fashion about the oral opening. These muscles of expression insert into the orbicularis and the overlying skin. The orbicularis oris consists of two portions.[17] The deep portion, whose fibers run horizontally, provides oral continence. It is curled upon itself to form the vermillion. The superficial portion, consisting of two bundles, originates from and is functionally a part of the muscles of facial expression. The philtrum and Cupid's bow are formed by the decussation and by contralateral insertion of orbicularis fibers and the insertion of the levator labii at the vermillion border.[18]

In the cleft lip patient the picture is less clear. The orbicularis oris is the most important muscle, and investigation has been directed almost exclusively toward the derangement of its anatomy. The classic theory, based on dissections by Fara,[19,20] describes a relatively orderly arrangement of muscle fibers, in most cases, sweeping up both sides of the cleft. These fibers are then stated to insert into the alar base and columnella.

A minority of cases are said to show a different pattern. The fibers cross, intertwine or spread horizontally like a fan, enter the margin of the cleft and disappear in the connective tissue. Fara correlates these findings with the arrangement of the vasculature, as shown by angiograhy.

Electrical stimulation of the unrepaired lip *in vivo* failed to confirm these findings.[21] More recently, reconstructing a three-dimensional model from histological sections, Kernahan also reported a chaotic arrangement of muscle fibers running transversely, obliquely and anteroposteriorly, with a medial paucity of transverse fibers.[22]

Nicolau[23,24] has reached conclusions through electrostimulation that appear partially to confirm both Fara and Kernahan. He describes the deep portion of the muscle sweeping horizontally until interrupted by the cleft. The superficial portion follows parallel to the border of the cleft, to insert laterally on the piriform aperture and alar base and medially on the septal area. Unfortunately Nicolau's study was not accompanied by anatomic dissections, but it seems to explain the conflicting nature of other reports.

Most recently, a study of nine cleft human embryos[5] has lent further support to Kernahan's view. No evidence of muscle fibers paralleling the cleft was found. Asymmetry and abnormal insertion of the fibers were noted.

Restoration of normal orbicularis function, with adequate muscle bulk across the line of repair, is probably the most important facet of successful cleft lip repair. Failure to achieve this primarily is a frequent indication for a secondary revision.

Preoperative Care

The preoperative care of the cleft patient consists of assessment for other anomalies, as discussed above, and maintenance of satisfactory hydration and nutrition. The latter is most important in order to reduce complications. For many cleft infants a low resistance nipple (i.e., with a large hole) is all that is needed to use to obtain nourishment. Various types of low resistance nipples are available, labeled premature nipple, cleft palate nipple and lamb's nipple. A crosscut on the end of a normal nipple will achieve the same goal.

Where breast feeding is planned, the mother should pump her milk and feed it to the infant via a bottle if the infant is unable to suckle. A soft bottle can be used to squeeze and dribble the milk into the infant's mouth. In the sick or premature infant, gavage feeding and parenteral nutrition may be necessary.

As with any operation involving the oral cavity, there are good theoretical reasons to use antibiotic prophylaxis, though the infection rate is generally low. If used, a cephalosporin, given for one dose preoperative and for 24 hours postoperative, is a good choice.

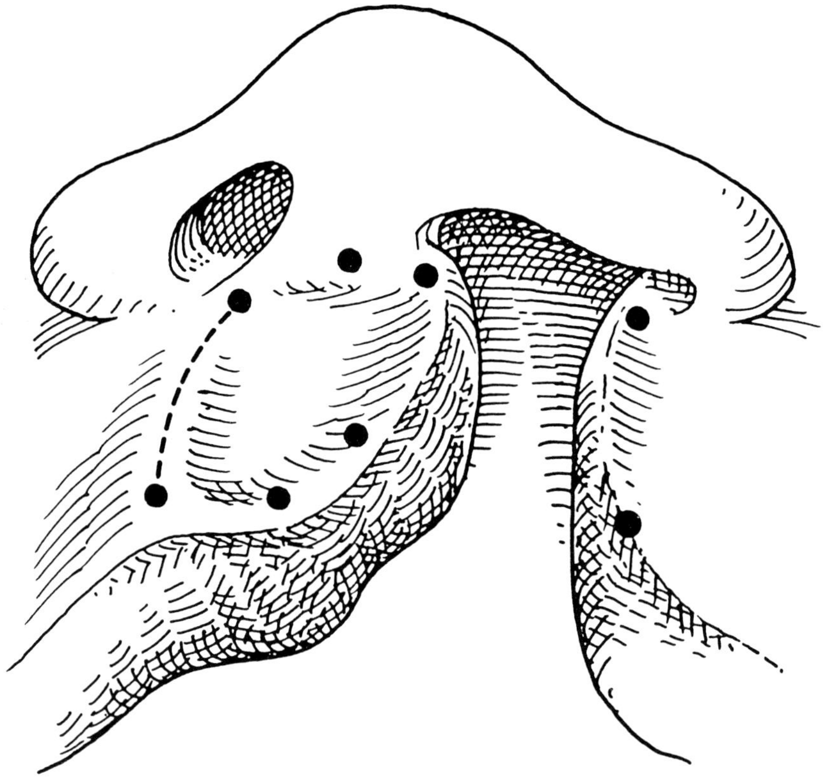

Figure 4-1. Key landmarks tattooed: High point of Cupid's bow on normal and cleft side; midpoint of Cupid's bow; point where white roll gives out on cleft side; nasal threshold on normal and cleft sides; midpoint of columnella (from Barclay T, Kernahan DA (eds): *Plastic Surgery,* ed 4. (Rob & Smith's Operative Surgery Series) London, Mosby, 1986).

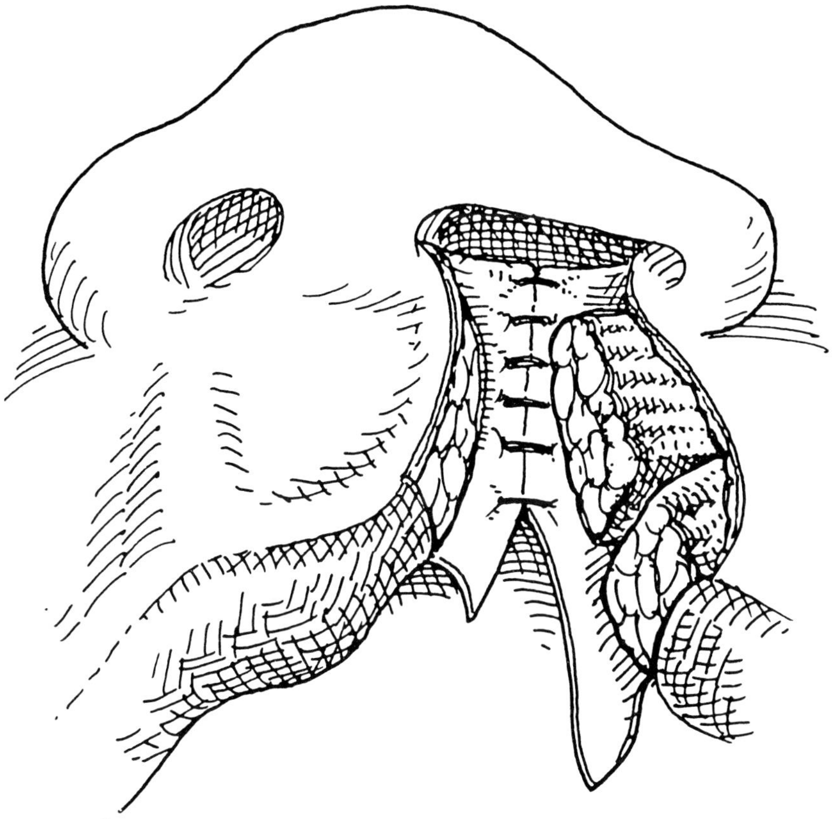

Figure 4-2. Mucosal flaps trimmed and approximated (from Barclay T, Kernahan DA (eds): *Plastic Surgery,* ed 4. (Rob & Smith's Operative Surgery Series) London, Mosby, 1986).

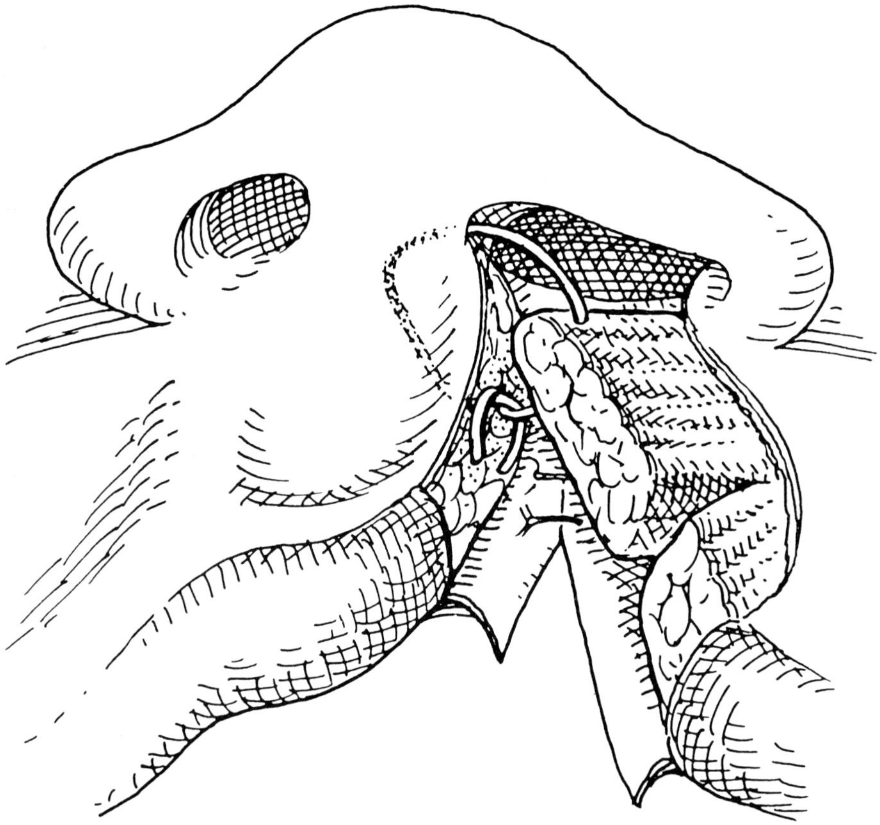

Figure 4-3. Upper part of muscle flap advanced and sutured with clear nylon into pocket at nasal spine (from Barclay T, Kernahan DA (eds): *Plastic Surgery,* ed 4. (Rob & Smith's Operative Surgery Series) London, Mosby, 1986).

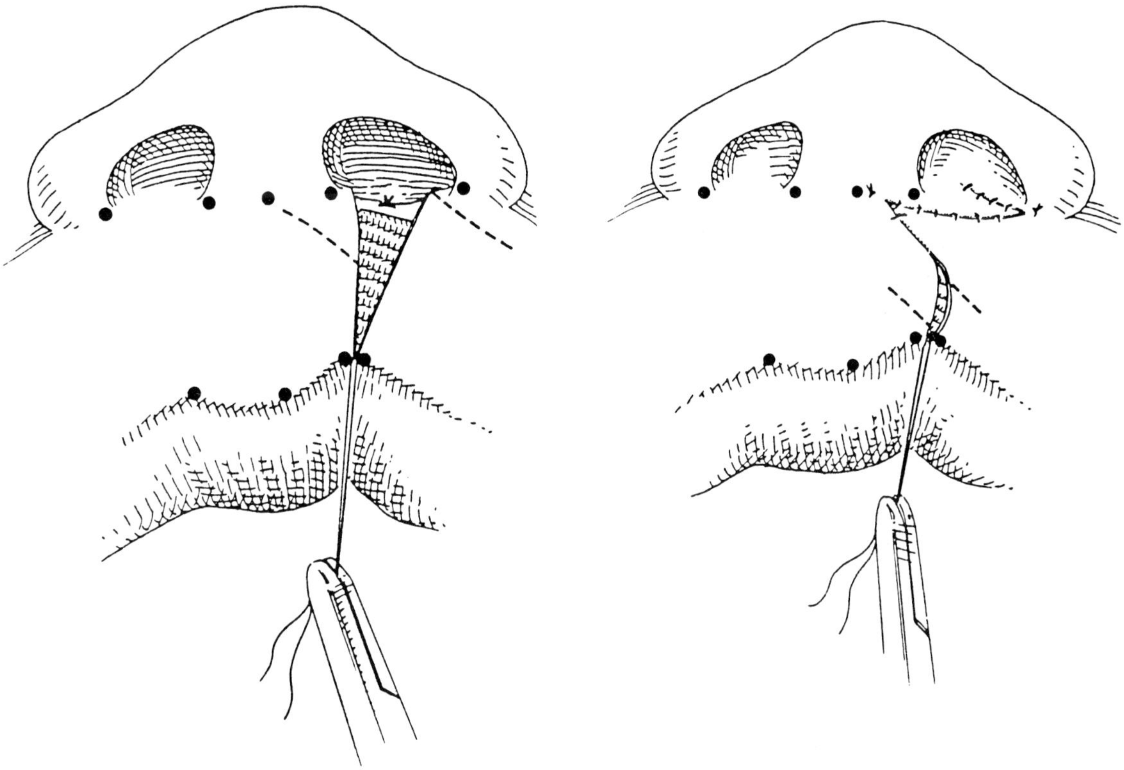

Figure 4-4. Z-plasty designed at nostril sill to lengthen skin repair line. Second Z-plasty designed just about mucutaneous junction if additional length needed (from Barclay T, Kernahan DA (eds): *Plastic Surgery,* ed 4. (Rob & Smith's Operative Surgery Series) London, Mosby, 1986).

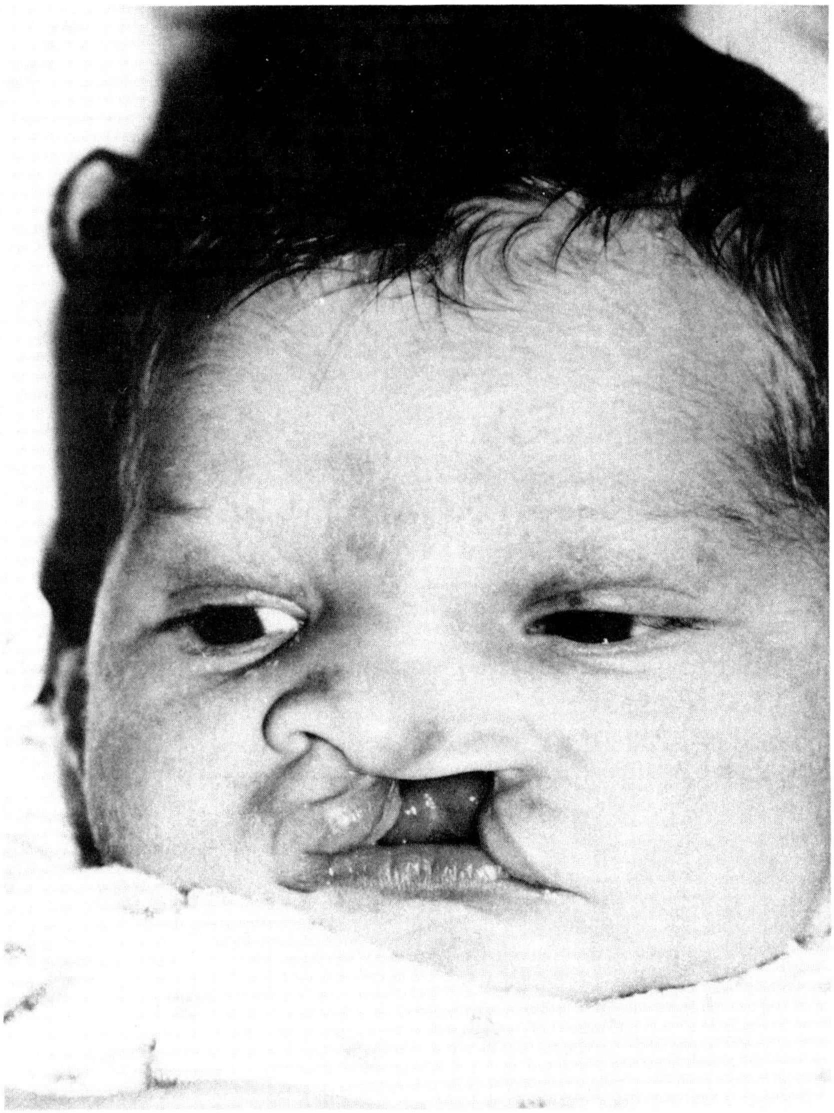

Figure 4-5. Unilateral complete cleft lip (from Kernahan DA and Bauer BS: Functional cleft lip repair: A sequential, layered closure with orbicularis muscle realignment. *Plast Reconstr Surg,* 72:459, 1982).

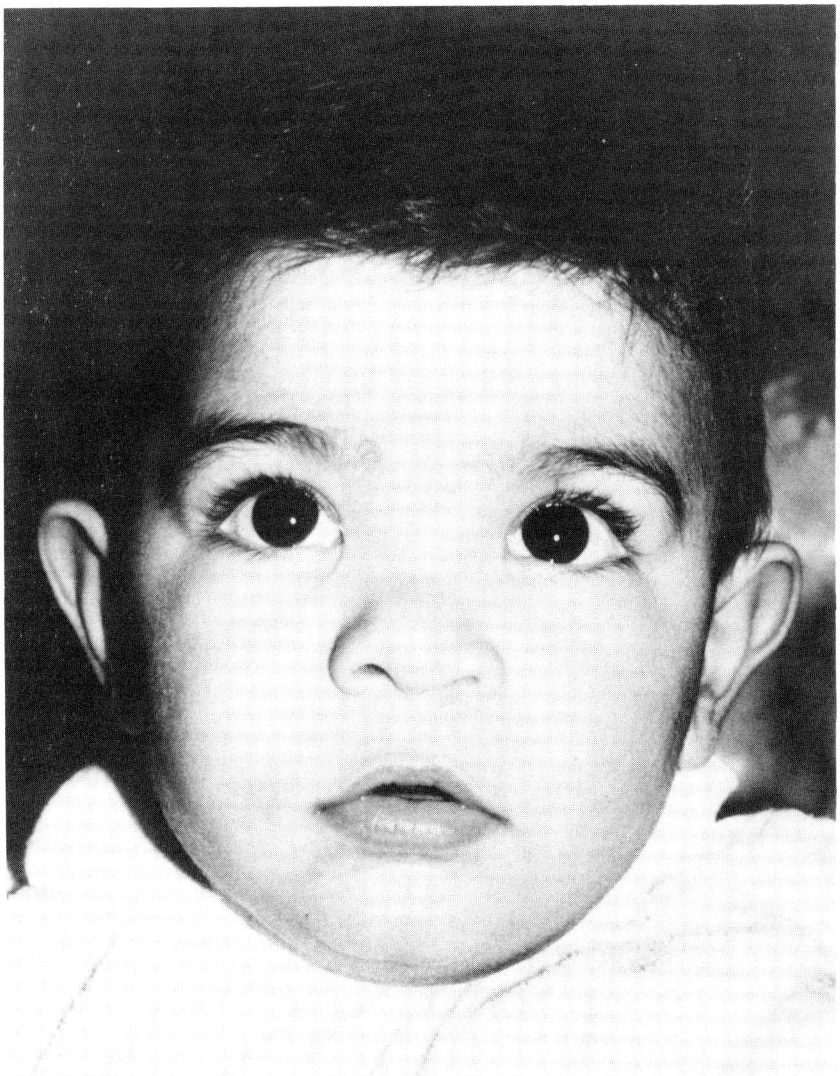

Figure 4-6. Repaired unilateral lip (from Kernahan DA and Bauer BS: Functional cleft lip repair: A sequential, layered closure with orbicularis muscle realignment. *Plast Reconstr Surg,* 72:459, 1982).

Timing of Surgical Repair

In deciding the timing of primary repair, several opposing factors have to be balanced against each other. The parents wish the earliest repair possible, both for appearance and ease of feeding.

Unrepaired unilateral clefts show normal maxillary growth unless they extend into the palate.[26] Lip pressure upon the premaxillary segment following repair is higher than in the unclefted child.[27] Where the cleft extends into the palate, lip repair may worsen any preexisting growth retardation.[28,29] This also has been suggested experimentally.[30]

In wide unilateral or bilateral clefts extending into the palate, presurgical orthopedic maneuvers have been advocated prior to repair of the lip. However, caution is needed. In the unilateral cleft there may be some benefit to controlling a flaring premaxilla, but the lateral maxillary segment may collapse and produce a crossbite.[31] In the bilateral cleft restraint on the premaxilla may worsen a preexisting growth deficiency in this area.

The technical ease of surgical repair increases with the size of the infant, though surgical magnification with the use of lenses allows earlier repair. Similarly, improvements in pediatric anesthesia have lessened the risks of surgery in small infants. Some surgeons favor performance of the surgery under sedation and local anesthesia in the first two weeks of life.[32] The prospect of intrauterine diagnosis[33] and correction[34] of facial clefts has been approached experimentally.

Classically, timing was decided by the rule of tens, i.e., weight of ten pounds, hemoglobin over ten grams, white cell count under 10,000 and age greater than ten weeks. In a healthy, full-term infant early repair at 1 to 14 days of age is now justified. Obviously the surgical setting, level of available anesthetic care, presence of other abnormalities, severity of the cleft and the general health, social circumstances and progress of the patient all will modify the decision.

In timing secondary procedures most surgeons are guided by the social landmark of school admission and the biological landmark of cessation of growth. Depending upon the degree of residual deformity, soft tissue work may be performed at either time. Bony work is best left until a later time.

Lip Adhesion Procedures

Where the cleft is wide, a preliminary closure may be helpful. Where a definitive rotation-advancement repair is planned, a period of molding of the maxilla and premaxilla and stretching of the deficient tissues of lip and cheek is particularly useful.[35] Millard advocates a lip adhesion in most complete clefts.

Lip adhesion was originally proposed as a minimal procedure with minimal dissection or lateral release and closure with mucosal flaps and side to side muscle approximation.[36,37] More recently Furnas has proposed substituting straight line closure for lip adhesion[38] as a preliminary to a rotation-advancement repair. He advocates a more extensive undermining of the cheek and nose on the affected side with rotation of a flap of buccal mucosa and side-to-side muscle apposition.

Furnas uses this approach on all complete unilateral clefts and bilateral clefts with a forme fruste on one side. The disadvantages include the need for a second procedure, performance of the definitive procedure in the presence of scar and the possibility of excessive scarring from multiple surgical procedures in the same area. It may be better to reserve this technique for cases where the definitive repair of the surgeon's choice cannot be performed without distortion of excessive tension.

Surgical Repair of the Unilateral Cleft—Muscle

In the lip, form follows function and restoring orbicularis function is an important part of an aesthetically satisfying repair. Anatomically aligned, functional orbicularis muscle must be advanced into the medial area of deficiency. Clearly, adequate dissection of the muscle laterally is the first step. The plane immediately above maxillary periosteum can be developed laterally beyond the displaced alar base and superiorly to the orbital rim, if needed. Naturally, the infraorbital nerve is preserved.

Whether this wide dissection affects maxillary growth is unclear; to date this has not been reported. However, until a large prospective study is performed the possibility remains. The medial muscle mass should be dissected more conservatively. Some authors feel that the nasal muscles, depressor septi nasi and nasalis, also should be dissected and repaired,[39] though the importance of this is not widely accepted.

Judging the alignment of the dissected muscle frequently is difficult, and electrical stimulation before dissection may be helpful. The repair should involve advancement medially of the lateral muscle mass and overlapping of the medial and lateral masses.

At least five methods of managing the muscle repair are widely used.[40] The methodology reflects the disagreement about the anatomy of the cleft orbicularis. Randall's repair[36] derives from Fara's description of the anatomy. The medial and lateral muscle forms triangular flaps after dissection which are overlapped—medial anterior and lateral posterior—after downward rotation to realign the fibers.

Kernahan[41] uses a direct advancement of the lateral muscle mass in keeping with his description of the anatomy. The lateral mass is split: the upper two-thirds are attached from the nasal spine down and the lower third to the muscle of the normal side at the vermillion border (Figure 4-2).

Adequate dissection of the lateral muscle mass is the key to a good result, whatever repair is used.[42] (The importance of adequate lateral mobilization will be mentioned again in relation to correction of the nasal deformity.) Equally important: if the muscle is advanced too much, an overly tight upper lip will result.

Surgical Repair of Unilateral Cleft—Skin

A multiplicity of repairs for the unilateral cleft has been described. Many have fallen into disuse because of the secondary deformities they frequently produce. Currently three major methods, with adaptations, are widely used: the Tennison triangular flap, the Millard rotation-advancement and the straight line closure. The latter may be adapted with z-plasties (Kernahan) or a wavy line closure (Pfeifer). All three are readily adapted to include formal muscle repair, as outlined. The Tennison requires formal preoperative marking. The Millard, as originally described[43] and in his revision,[44] allows for intraoperative flexibility, though he has described precise mathematical marking of the lip.[45] The straight line closure and its adaptations allow the surgeon great freedom following muscle repair.

The surgeon also should understand the quadrilateral flap repair, first described by Hagedorn,[46] and popularized by LeMesurier[47] with modifications. The method raises a quadrilateral flap on the lateral side of the cleft, and brings it down to join the medial Cupid's bow in the midline. As can be seen, the method results in substantial tissue discard and poor esthetic scar placement.[48] Some surgeons have reported that this method results in an overly-long lip as the patient grows, though this may represent a failure to use proper technique, since it is not universally observed.[49] The method is still used by some practitioners, and the long lip is one of the more challenging problems for secondary correction.

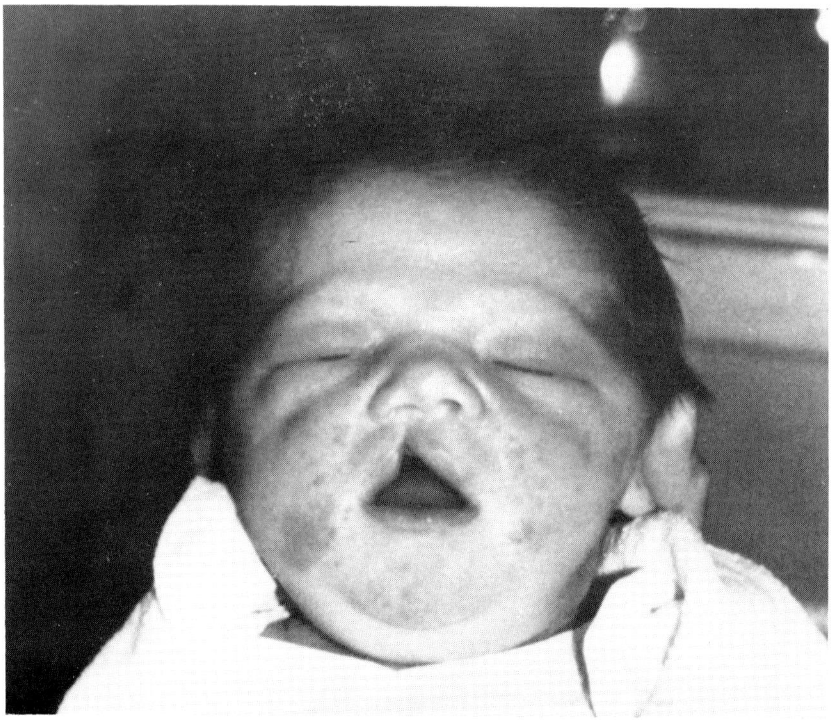

Figure 4-7. Newborn with right unilateral cleft of lip (from Pansky B: *Review of Medical Embryology,* p. 45. New York, MacMillan Pub, 1982).

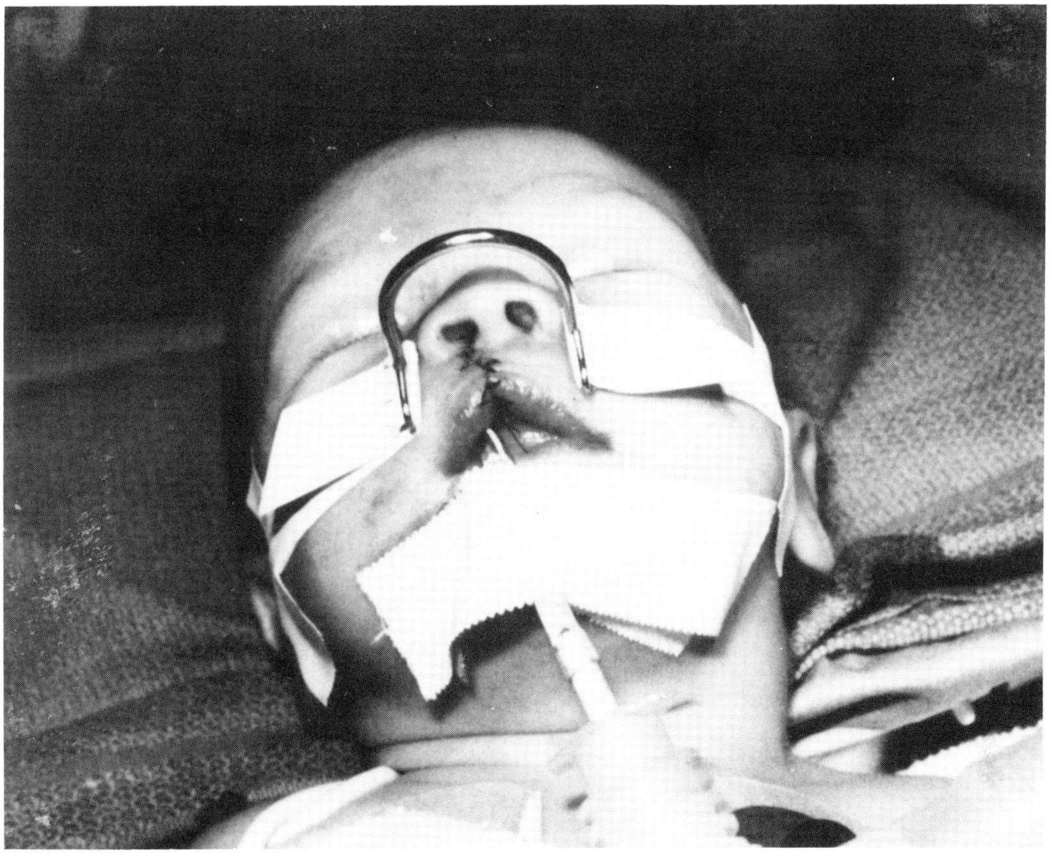

Figure 4-8. Repair completed after modified Hagedorn technique. Right nostril slightly flattened. Endotracheal tube remains in place (from Pansky B: *Review of Medical Embryology,* p. 141. New York, MacMillan Pub, 1982).

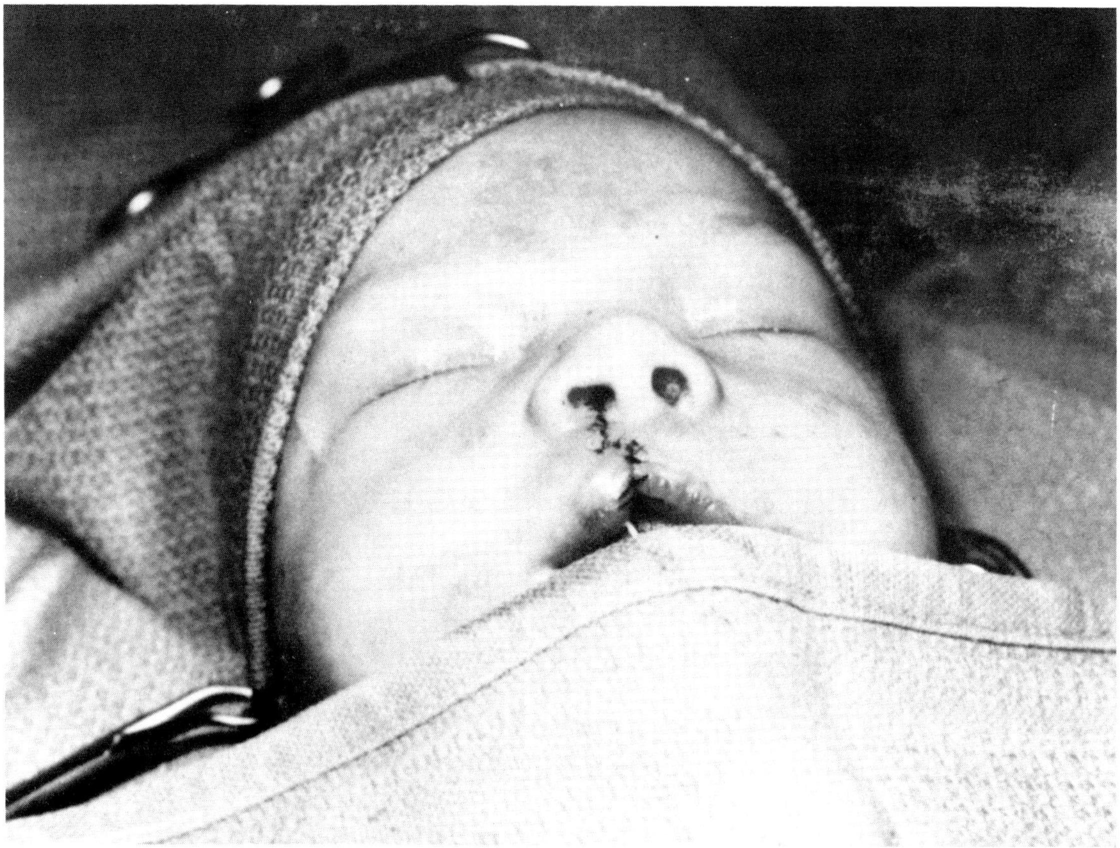

Figure 4-9. View taken immediately after repair has been completed. Endotraceal tube in position. Logan bow placed over lip so that wound remains open and available to the nurse for cleansing and application of antibiotic ointment (from Nicolau PJ: The orbicularis oris muscle: A functional approach to its repair in the cleft lip. *Brit J Plast Surg,* 36:143, 1983).

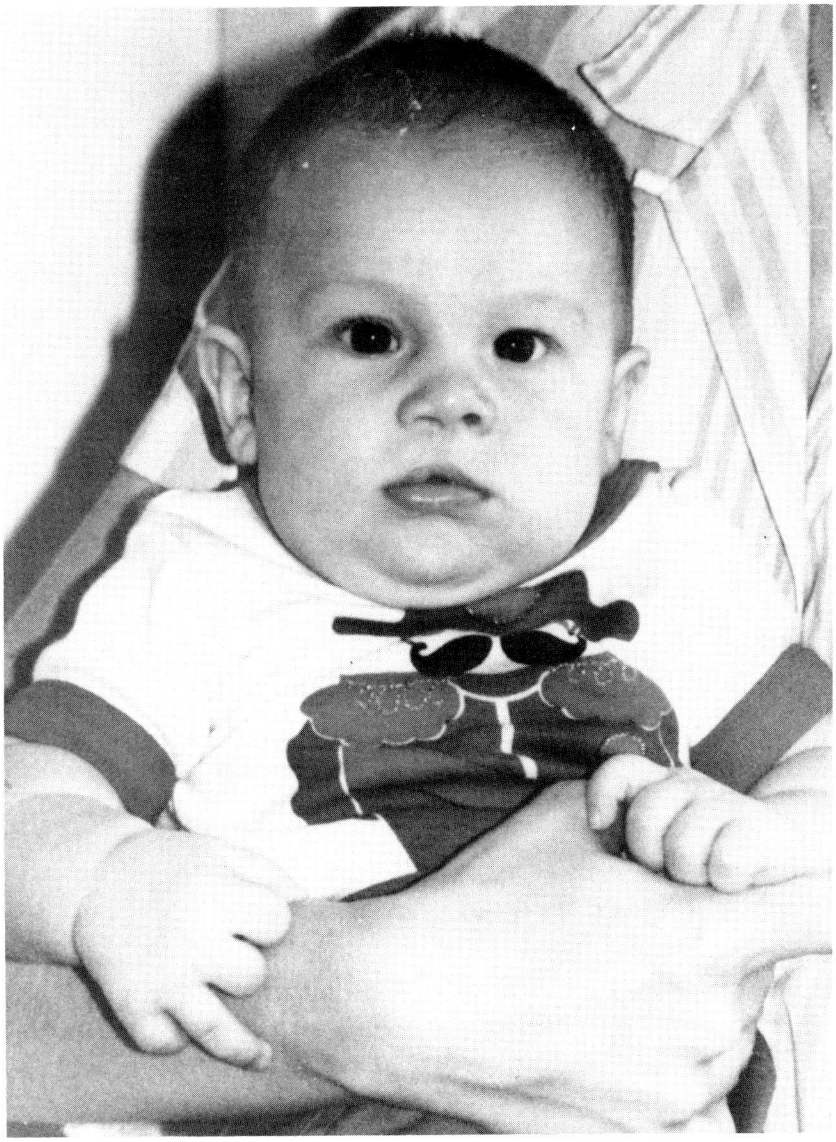

Figure 4-10. Postoperative view of infant (from Randall P: Cleft lip. *Clin Plast Surg,* 2:220, 1975).

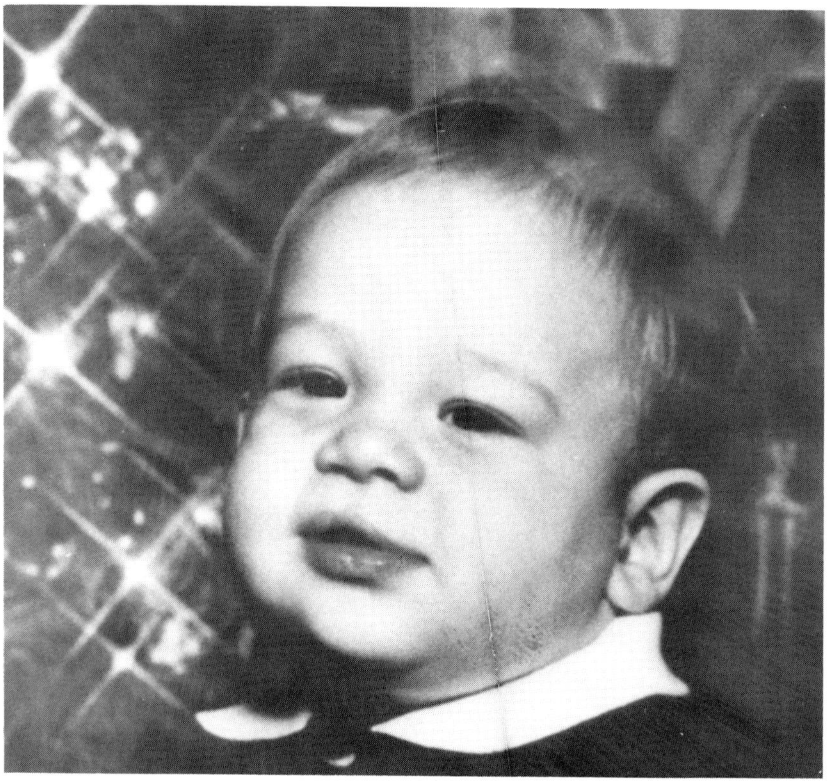

Figure 4-11. Postoperative view of child received on Christmas card, 1985 (from Musgrave RH, Garrett WS Jr: The unilateral cleft lip, in Converse JM (ed): *Reconstructive Plastic Surgery,* p. 2033. Philadelphia, W B Saunders Co, 1977).

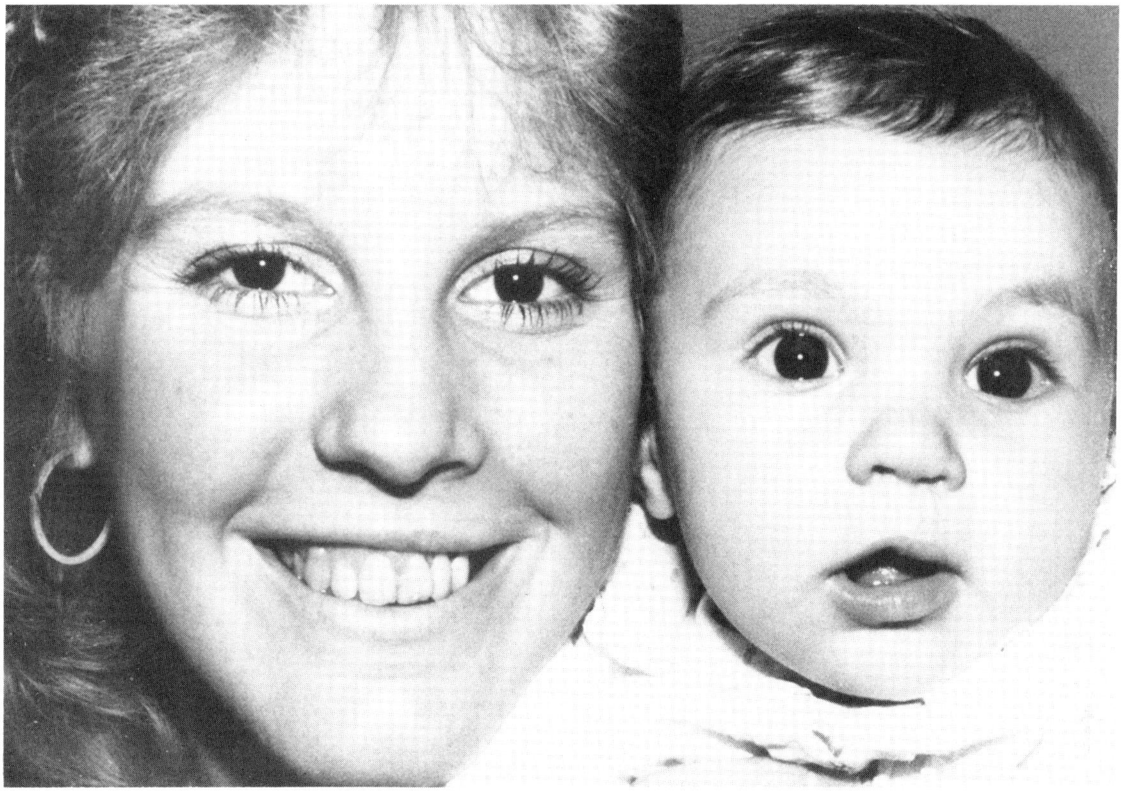

Figure 4-12. Mother and daughter had unilateral cleft lip. Author (FWP) repaired mother's lip in 1955 and daughter's lip in 1985, 30 years later. Modified Hagedorn technique with improvisations used in both (from Furnas DW: Straight-line closure: A preliminary to Millard closure in unilateral cleft lips. *Clin Plast Surg,* 11:721, 1984).

Millard's use of mucosa, with some adaptation, can be applied to all these methods as needed. Since the mucosa is pared away from the cleft borders, superiorly based medial and lateral flaps can be prepared. These flaps can be rotated to augment the alar rim (lateral flap), buccal sulcus (either flap) or aid in the repair of alveolar/palatal defects (medial flap).

The necessity of locating certain landmarks is common to all methods. The philtral ridge, alar base and columnellar base on the normal side all are located easily. This gives the height of the normal philtral ridge and width of the normal nostril.

The junction of philtral column and vermillion border on the left side can be identified in most instances. In difficult cases the midline is estimated and a distance measured equal to the distance to the normal philtral column.

Lateral to the cleft, the point at which the vermillion border will be incised and approximated to the medial side is important. It has been loosely defined as the spot where the white roll of the vermillion border becomes indistinct. More precisely, though perhaps no more accurately, it can be measured from its commisure as the equal of the distance from normal commisure to normal eminence of the Cupid's bow.

The Tennison Repair

Tennison's original method of the triangular flap repair[50] involved using a Z-shaped wire to mark the patient. Each leg of the Z should equal about half of the height of the normal side of the lip, and the distance from one tip to the other should equal the height of the normal side. Medially, two legs only are marked: the first is parallel to the vermillion; the second makes about a 90-degree angle with the apex at the cleft side eminence of Cupid's bow. Laterally, the Z is marked with the lowest leg approximately parallel to the vermillion border and starts at the point where the white roll begins to disappear. Vermillion is incised perpendicular to its border and closure obtained after discarding excess tissue.

The basic principle of the Tennison repair is lengthening of the cleft lip by use of a lateral interposition flap. Minimal tissue is discarded; it is useful for wide clefts. The principle disadvantage is a tendency for subsequent growth to produce an excessively long lip, particularly if the flap is large. The surgeon should take account of this. For this reason, Randall[51] advised a maximum flap width of 4 mm.

Several modifications to this procedure are widely used. Hagerty devised a system of intraoperative measurements to ensure equal philtral lengths of the cleft and noncleft sides.[52] First, a line is marked from the midpoint of Cupid's bow to the base of the columnella. A perpendicular is drawn to this line so that it passes through the apex of Cupid's bow on the medial side of the cleft. Halfway between the midpoint of Cupid's bow and the intersection of the two perpendiculars is a point which determines the medial cutback.

Brauer noted that the height of the lip on the normal side equals the sum of two distances: the imaginary base of the lateral triangular flap and the upper limb of the lateral Z. He also stated that the lateral markings should not fall outside a vertical line from the outer base of the alar to the vermillion.[48]

Randall devised an intricate system of measurement.[53] Essentially he marked the medial side in accordance with Tennison's plan. Next the upper limb on the lateral side of the cleft is marked out so that it is the same length as the upper limb on the medial side. The sides of the laterally based triangular flap are marked to equal the length of lower limb on the medial side of the cleft. Correction is made for the angulation of the base of the triangular flap from the vertical (in the final repair) by measuring from the inferior corner of the flap to a point midway on the opposite side. The markings are then corrected as necessary to obtain the required height on the cleft side.

He also applied a further lateral flap to the base of the columnella to prevent notching of the nostril floor and to add fullness to the columnella, as previously described for other repairs.[54,55]

Cronin[55] started both medial cutback and lateral triangle 1 mm above the vermillion border, crossing the white roll perpendiculary to preserve this feature.

The Tennison repair is simple in principle and simple to execute. The main disadvantages are the unnatural line of the lower portion of the scar, a rigid surgical plan once marked and a tendency for a long lip to become apparent with subsequent growth. The latter defect is more easily prevented than corrected. The repair does not have the same popularity as the Millard; however, the results are probably as good.[57]

The Millard Repair

The Millard repair has created a large body of literature. The principle is, however, simple. The Cupid's bow is rotated down and tissue lateral to the cleft advanced to fill the resulting defect. When well executed, the lower portion of the closure mimics the philtral column.

The rotation incision is marked out on the medial side. Starting at the eminence of Cupid's bow on the cleft side, it curves away from the vermillion border to the columnellar base on the cleft side, across the base of the columnella and stops before crossing the normal philtral column. A backcut is marked downward from this point immediately medial to the normal philtral column. It will not be cut out unless needed. The advancement flap is referred to as the A flap.

A second cut on the medial side is marked along the vermillion border up to the nostril. With the rotation incision, this outlines a triangular flap, the C flap. Lateral to the cleft, the vermillion border is marked from the point which will form the Cupid's bow eminence up into the nostril. The advancement flap (B flap) is then completed by a curve around the alar base. If the lateral portion's height from eminence to mid-alar base is much less than the normal side, this curve may be placed 1-2 mm up the alar base. The distance that the cut continues around the alar base determines the amount of advancement possible. The freed alar base is called the D flap.

The flaps are then interdigitated. Further adjustments can be made by increasing the backcut of the A flap or the cut around the alar base. The flaps can then be sutured in place sequentially. First the C flap is more fully released by incising the membranous septum from the lateral end of the flap up to the nasal tip. The flap can then both rotate into the backcut and provide some columnellar lengthening on the cleft side.

The lateral element is freed from the maxilla and the muscle dissected. The mucosal flaps then can be applied as discussed, and a muscle repair performed as outlined. Millard bases his repair on Fara's description of the anatomy. Finally, the main rotation and advancement flaps are sutured in place.

Additional refinement at the vermillion border can be produced by a laterally based flap about 1 mm thick, 2 mm long and 1.5 mm wide at the base. This is interposed to the medial edge along the vermillion border to mimic the white roll. The nasal floor also may need a small excision from the alar base, lateral to the repair, to give symmetry of the nares.

As Millard acknowledges, a complete cleft usually will require a preliminary lip adhesion to avoid a raised Cupid's bow on the cleft side. With this caveat, the repair can give excellent results, with good aesthetic placement of scars. It remains the most popular method of repair in the United States.

Straight Line Repairs

As the importance of functional muscle repair has been recognized, there has been a resurgence of interest in straight line skin closure. Of itself, a properly performed muscle repair will rotate the lateral element and alar base into better position. The lateral skin edge of the cleft will be advanced toward the medial, though somewhat stretched.

Except in the most trivial incomplete cleft, some technique must still be used to lengthen the lip on the cleft side. However, straight line repairs as performed today still keep the incisions largely in the line of the philtral column and avoid large rotations or interpositions of skin flaps.

As with any repair, the major landmarks must be marked first. After marking the planned incisions for the repair, mucosa and muscle can then be dissected and repaired as already described.

The straight line repair is probably the oldest method of repair (see chapter on history). Within the modern era of anesthesia and asepsis, this technique was popularized by William Rose,[59] using curved incisions, concave toward the cleft on each side. This technique sacrifices unnecessarily large amounts of tissue and, as a result, cannot be used in significant clefts.

Recently Thatte has shown interesting results in both partial and complete clefts using classic straight closure of the pared skin edges after a modern muscle repair.[59] This approach remains too radical for most surgeons to accept at this time.

Pfeifer modified the straight line with a variety of sinuous, gentle curves along each side of the cleft. The approach is applicable to all grades of clefts and is individualized for each patient.[60] It is accompanied by a radical muscle mobilization and repair.

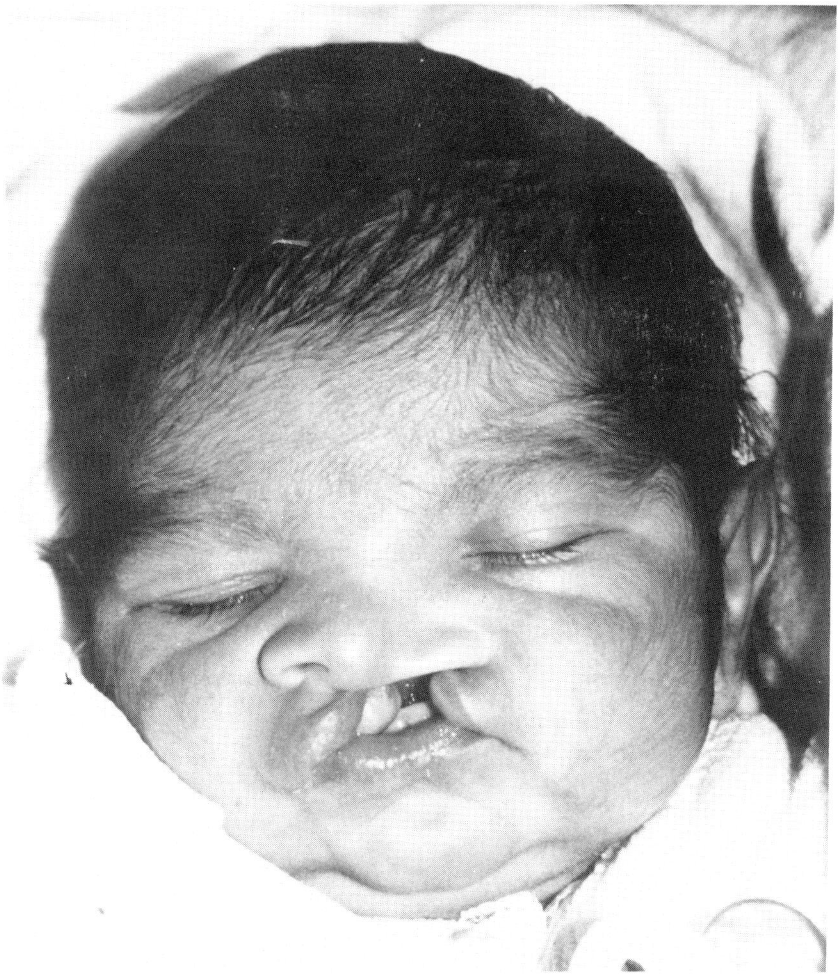

Figure 4-13. Unilateral complete cleft lip (from Kernahan DA, Bauer BS: Functional cleft lip repair: A sequential, layered closure with orbicularis muscle realignment. *Plast Reconstr Surg,* 72:459, 1982).

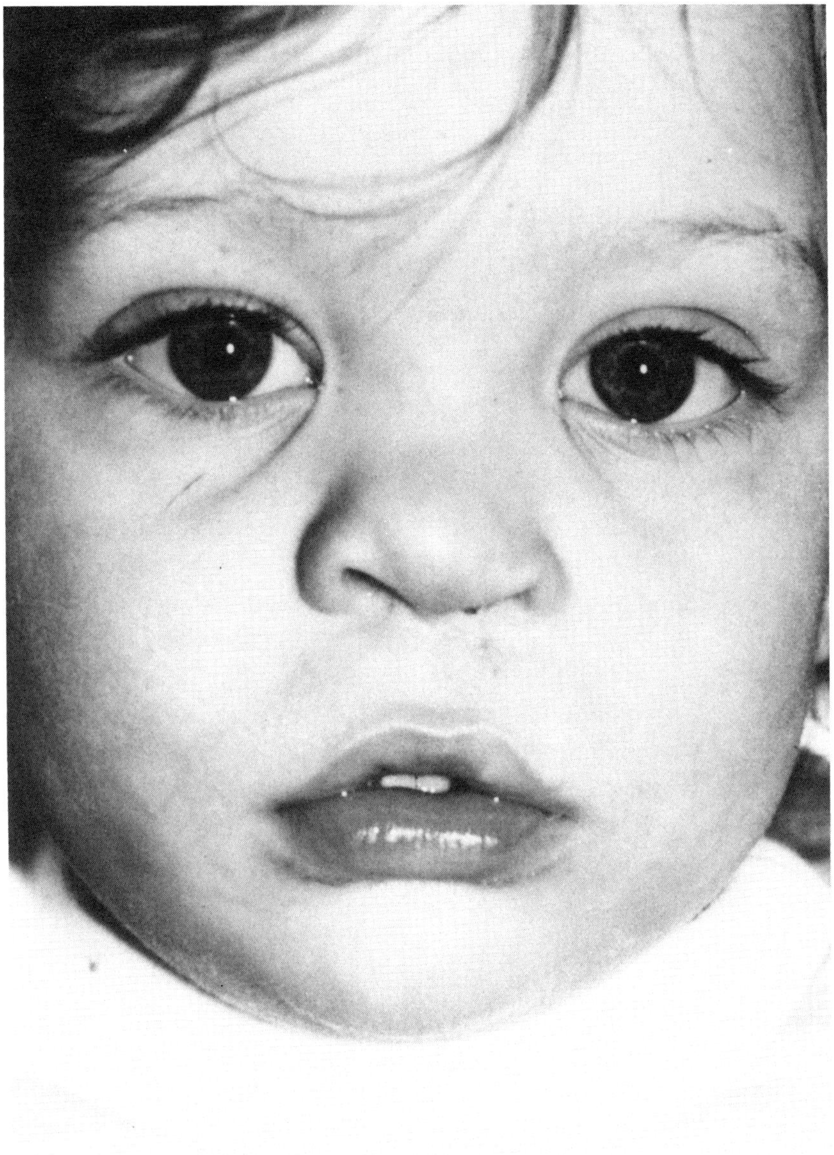

Figure 4-14. Repaired unilateral lip (from Kernahan DA, Bauer BS: Functional cleft lip repair: A sequential, layered closure with orbicularis muscle realignment. *Plast Reconstr Surg,* 72:459, 1982).

The late results are reported as being superior to triangular and quadrilateral flap repair.[61] As with straight line closures in general, poor results tend toward a short lip. This deformity is easier to correct secondarily than the opposite problem. The scar tends to mimic the philtrum nicely, particularly in its lower portion.

Pre- and Postoperative Care of the Cleft Lip Patient

The postoperative care of the patient with a repaired lip is aimed at avoiding disruption of the orbicularis muscle. Feeding is accomplished with a syringe to avoid the stress of sucking. Similarly, pacifiers are forbidden. After two weeks a nipple can be used. On theoretical grounds, a low resistance nipple is preferable for four weeks or more to reduce stress until the muscle repair is strong.

Removal of sutures should be done five to seven days following surgery. Clumsy suture removal can spoil a good repair. Good lighting and magnification both will help. Regular cleansing and application of an antibacterial ointment on the suture line will minimize crusting around the sutures.

Some surgeons prefer to administer sedation or a brief general anesthetic to aid removal of sutures. Assistants to firmly immobilize the patient, combined with a good body wrap, are somtimes a satisfactory way to avoid an extra anesthetic. On occasion the task can be accomplished successfully on the mother's lap during a postprandial sleep.

Management of Secondary Cleft Lip Deformity

The frequency of secondary cleft deformities attests to our present failure to produce uniformly satisfactory, reproducible results from primary repair. Defects can be classified as:

1. Unsatisfactory scarring
2. Inadequate functional muscle across the cleft
3. Irregularity of vermillion or its border
4. Tightness of the lip
5. Discrepancies of the medial and lateral sides following a triangular or quadrilateral flap repair.

Unsatisfactory scarring may result from poor suture technique, excessive wound tension or from the patient's innate tendency toward excessive scar. Analysis of the cause in the individual case and the application of the basic principles of plastic surgery are needed. Dermabrasion is frequently useful if contour irregularity is a problem. Scar excision should be approached with caution.

Correction of underlying excessive tendon due to poor muscle repair may be useful. Because of the initial tension and the amount of tissue excised, W-plasty is usually contraindicated. If the configuration of the undesired scar permits, Pfeifer's wavy line method is a good way to close with less tissue loss after a complete scar excision. Overlapping or imbrication of the dermis after scar excision may lessen tension on the epidermal closure.

Inadequate functional muscle, often evidenced by a lateral bulge of orbicularis upon smiling, requires opening the anterior surface of the repair and dissecting the muscle widely. The muscle is then repaired again in similar fashion to a primary repair. Revision of the mucosal repair also may be necessary.

Vermillion problems may represent a failure of the primary repair to fully correct the cleft. The resulting appearance is that of a forme fruste cleft with an elevated Cupid's bow on the cleft side. The repair must be taken down and repeated. A straight line closure is easily revised with further muscle advancement as needed either with conversion to a Millard skin closure or with any of the straight line methods discussed.

Similarly, the Millard repair is easily revised with a more radical rotation-advancement with a lengthened backcut. Triangular and quadrilateral flaps are less easily converted, usually only with marked tissue loss. A short upper lip is not commonly seen, however, with these repairs. The long lip is discussed below.

Fullness of the vermillion in one area can be excised. Lack of vermillion is a more difficult problem. The primary problem may be a true lack of vermillion or that the primary repair has placed the mucocutaneous junction too low. Vermillion can be advanced from within, followed by a flap of buccal mucosa to the secondary defect. If the deficiency is localized, a simple Z-plasty will suffice.

To elevate the mucocutaneous junction, an ellipse of skin can be excised, parallel to and immediaely above the white roll of the vermillion border. Localized irregularities of the vermillion border can be corrected by interposition flaps of the white roll or by small Z-plasties. A free skin graft also can be used to mimic the white roll.

Tightness of the upper lip due to a general inadequacy of tissue requires a new source of tissue, generally the lower lip. If revision of the muscle repair leaves only a deficiency of skin and mucosa, a sandwich Abbe flap of skin and mucosa may be used. Jackson[62] feels that muscle transfer is never needed if the muscle repair is adequate. The flap should be transferred in the midline and used to mimic the philtral column.

Following triangular or quadrilateral flap repair, the lateral segment may be overly long. Correction requires taking down the original repair and excising wedges from the flaps to reduce their width. This also may be necessary if there is gross irregularity of the vermillion border.

The timing of secondary revisions will, in general, follow the landmarks already mentioned. Severe problems may need attention before school entry to avoid the patient's being teased by other children. More minor problems may be left until growth is complete and the tendency to scar lessened. Additionally, they may be combined with nasal correction at that time.

Summary

The aim of the surgeon must be a perfect primary repair, though this rarely is achieved. The importance of functional muscle repair is becoming increasingly clear.

Although the Millard repair remains the operation of choice for most surgeons in North America, newer variations on the straight line theme are showing promise. The triangular flap is gradually losing ground, not so much because of poor results, but because of reduced flexibility intraoperatively and at secondary revision.

When and where a preliminary lip adhesion or preliminary straight line closure should be employed remains unsolved. Whether intrauterine correction ever will be advantageous is unknown. Though much progress has been made in the last 30 years, most of our questions remain unanswered.

REFERENCES

1. Fraser FC: The genetics of cleft lip and palate. *Am J Hum Genet,* 22:336, 1970.
2. Chung CS, Myrianthopoulos NC: Racial and prenatal factors in major congenital malformations. *Am J Hum Genet,* 20:44, 1968.
3. Fujino H, Tanaka K, Sanui Y: Genetic study of cleft lips and cleft palates based on 2828 Japanese cases. *Kyushu J Med Sci,* 14:317, 1963.
4. Cohen MM: Craniofacial disorders, in Emery AEH, Rimoin DL (eds): *Principles and Practice of Medical Genetics.* Edinburgh, Churchhill Livingstone, 1983.
5. Wilson MEAC: A ten year survey of cleft lip and cleft palate in the south west region. *Brit J Plast Surg,* 25:224, 1972.
6. Fogh-Anderson P: *Inheritance of Harelip and Cleft Palate.* Copenhagen, Munksgaard, 1942.
7. Fogh-Anderson P: Incidence of cleft lip and palate: Constant and increasing. *Acta Chir Scand,* 122:106, 1961.
8. Fogh-Anderson P: Rare clefts of the face. *Acta Chir Scand,* 129:275, 1965.
9. Kawamoto H: The kaleidoscopic world of rare craniofacial clefts: Order out of chaos (Tessler classification). *Clin Plast Surg,* 3:529, 1976.
10. Veau V: *Bec-de-Lievre.* Paris, Masson, 1938.
11. His W: *Unsere Koerperform und des Physiologische Problem inhrer Entstehung.* Leipzig, Verlag Con FC Vogel, 1874.
12. Veau V, Politzer J: Embryologie due bec-de-lievre. *Ann Anat Pathol,* 13:278, 1936.
13. Veau V: *Division Palatine: Anatomie, Chirurgie, Phonetique.* Paris, Masson, 1931.
14. Pansky B: *Review of Medical Embryology.* New York, MacMillan Pub, 1982.
15. Jirasek JE: *Atlas of Human Prenatal Morphogenesis.* Boston, Martinus Nijhoff, 1983.
16. Hamilton WJ, Mossman HW: *Human Embryology,* ed 4. Baltimore, Williams & Wilkins, 1972.
17. Nicolau PJ: The orbicularis oris muscle: A functional approach to its repair in the cleft lip. *Brit J Plast Surg,* 36:141, 1983.
18. Latham RA, Deaton TG: The structural basis of the philtrum and the contour of the vermilion border: A study of the musculature of the upper lip. *J Anat,* 121:151, 1976.
19. Fara M, Chlumska A, Hrivnakova J: Musculus orbicularis oris in incomplete harelip. *Acta Chir Plast,* 7:281, 1965.
20. Fara M: Anatomy and arteriography of cleft lips in stillborn children. *Plast Reconstr Surg,* 42:29, 1968.
21. Kernahan DA: Muscle repair in unilateral cleft lip based on findings on electrical stimulation. *Ann Plast Surg,* 1:48, 1978.
22. Kernahan DA, Dado DV, Bauer BS: The anatomy of the orbicularis oris muscle in unilateral cleft lip based on a three-dimensional histologic reconstruction. *Plast Reconstr Surg,* 73:875, 1984.

23. Nicolau PJ, Dowman IJ, Wickens EH: *The Function of the Orbicularis Oris Muscle in Cleft Lip Patients.* (Unpublished, London, University College, 1981).
24. Nicolau PJ: *Close Range Stereo Photogrammetry in Pre- and Post-Operative Assessment of Cleft Lip Muscles.* London, International Society of Photogrammetry, 1980. (Personal communication)
25. Siegel MI, Mooney MP, Kimes MR, Gest TR: Traction, prenatal development and the labioseptopremaxillary region. *Plast Reconstr Surg,* 76:25, 1985.
26. Isiekwe MC, Sowemimo GO: Cephalometric findings in a normal Nigerian population sample and adult Nigerians with unrepaired clefts. *Cleft Palate J,* 21:323, 1984.
27. Bardach J, Bakowska J, McDermott-Murray J, et al: Lip pressure changes following lip repair in infants with unilateral clefts of the lip and palate. *Plast Reconstr Surg,* 74:476, 1984.
28. Ortiz-Monasterio F, Serrano-Rebeil AR, Barrera GP, et al: A study of untreated adult cleft palate patients. *Plast Reconstr Surg,* 38:36, 1966.
29. Mazaheri M, Harding RL, Cooper JA, et al: Changes in arch form and dimensions of cleft patients. *Am J Orthod,* 60:19, 1971.
30. Bardach J, Mooney MP: The relationship between lip pressure following lip repair and craniofacial growth on beagles. *Plast Reconstr Surg,* 73:544, 1984.
31. Randall P: Cleft lip. *Clin Plast Surg,* 2:215, 1975.
32. Stark RB: Cleft lip—a timetable. *Ann Plast Surg,* 8:107, 1982.
33. Christ JE, Meininger MG: Ultrasound diagnosis of cleft lip and cleft palate before birth. *Plast Reconstr Surg,* 68:854, 1981.
34. Hallock GG: In utero cleft lip repair in A/J mice. *Plast Reconstr Surg,* 75:785, 1985.
35. Musgrave RH, Garrett WS Jr: The unilateral cleft lip, in Converse JM (ed): *Reconstructive Plastic Surgery.* Philadelphia, W B Saunders Co, 1977.
36. Randall P: A lip adhesion operation in cleft palate surgery. *Plast Reconstr Surg,* 35:371, 1965.
37. Millard DR Jr: A preliminary adhesion, in Millard DR Jr (ed): *Cleft Craft: The Evolution of Its Surgery,* Boston, Little Brown, 1976, vol 1: *The Unilateral Deformity.*
38. Furnas DW: Straight-line closure: A preliminary to Millard closure in unilateral cleft lips. *Clin Plast Surg,* 11:701, 1984.
39. Namba K, Abe M: The muscle reconstruction in primary cleft lip repair. *Jpn J Plast Reconstr Surg,* 19:245, 1976.
40. Zimman OA, Robles JM, Lee JC: Muscle reconstruction in unilateral cleft lip. *Ann Plast Surg,* 5:95, 1980.
41. Kernahan DA, Bauer BS: Functional cleft lip repair: A sequential, layered closure with orbicularis muscle realignment. *Plast Reconstr Surg,* 72:459, 1982.
42. Thatte RL, Prasad S: Radical muscle mobilization in the surgical repair of a unilateral cleft lip: A follow up report. *Brit J Plast Surg,* 37:296, 1982.
43. Millard DR: A primary camouflage of the unilateral harelip, in *Transactions of the International Society of Plastic Surgeons, 1st Congress (1955).* Baltimore, Williams & Wilkins, 1957.
44. Millard DR Jr (ed): *Cleft Craft: The Evolution of Its Surgery.* Boston, Little Brown, 1976. vol 1: *The Unilateral Deformity.*
45. Millard DR: Complete unilateral clefts of the lip. *Plast Reconstr Surg,* 25:595, 1960.
46. Hagedorn W: Uber ein Modifikation der Hasenschartenoperation. *Zentralb Chir,* 11:756, 1884.
47. Le Mesurier AB: A method of cutting and suturing the lip in treatment of complete unilateral clefts. *Plast Reconstr Surg,* 4:1, 1949.
48. Brauer RO: A comparison of the Tennison and Le Mesurier lip repairs. *Plast Recontr Surg,* 23:249, 1959.
49. Farkas LG, Lindsay WK: Morphology of the adult face following repair of the unilateral cleft lip and palate in childhood. *Plast Reconstr Surg,* 52:652, 1973.
50. Tennison CW: The repair of cleft by the stencil method. *Plast Reconstr Surg,* 9:115, 1952.

51. Randall P: Cleft lip—triangular flap cheilorraphy, in Grabb WC, Rosenstein SW, Bzoch KR (eds): *Cleft Lip and Palate.* Boston, Little Brown, 1971.
52. Hagerty R: Unilateral cleft lip repair. *Surg Gynecol Obstet,* 106:119, 1958.1
53. Randall P: Primary repair of unilateral clefts. *Plast Reconstr Surg,* 23:331, 1959.
54. Collis MH: The aesthetic treatment of harelip. *Q Dublin J Med Sci,* 45:392, 1868.
55. Brauer RO: A consideration of the LeMesurier technique of single harelip repair with a new concept as to its use in incomplete and secondary harelip repairs. *Plast Reconstr Surg,* 11:275, 1953.
56. Cronin CD: A modification of the Tennison-type lip repair. *Cleft Palate J,* 3:376, 1966.
57. Holtmann B, Wray RC: A randomized comparison of triangular and rotation-advancement unilateral cleft lip repairs. *Plast Reconstr Surg,* 71:172, 1983.
58. Rose W: *On Harelip and Cleft Palate.* London, H K Lewis, 1891.
59. Thatte RL: Radical muscle mobilization in the surgical repair of a unilateral cleft lip. *Brit J Plast Surg,* 35:356, 1982.
60. Pfeifer G: Uber ein entwicklungsgeschichtlicht bergundetes Verfahren des Verschlusses von Lippenspalten. *Dtsch Zahn-, Mund- und Kieferheilkunde,* 54:69, 1970.
61. Gundlach KKH, Schmitz R, Maerker R, Bull HG: Late results following different methods of cleft lip repair. *Cleft Palate J,* 19:167, 1982.
62. Jackson IT, Soutar DS: The sandwich Abbe flap in secondary cleft lip deformity. *Plast Reconstr Surg,* 66:38, 1980.

CHAPTER 5

SURGICAL REPAIR OF CLEFT LIP AND PALATE

PETER JOHNSON and FRANK W. PIRRUCCELLO

. . . The good man does not grieve that other people do not recognize his merits. His only anxiety is lest he should fail to recognize theirs.

. . . Confucius

Introduction

LITTLE FURTHER needs to be written to emphasize the complexity of problems associated with cleft palate. A simple review of the literature demonstrates a vast amount of both clinical and experimental research. It also emphasizes the diversity of opinion present and the importance of a team approach. In this chapter we can try to cover only some of the basic surgical approaches to the cleft palate patient. No one procedure can be applied to all clefts, and most surgeons would agree there is no one best operation. Consistently good results can be obtained only with a knowledge of cleft embryology and anatomy. The cleft repair must optimize speech development, hearing and facial growth.

From the moment of birth the palate is involved with such basic functions as maintenance of airway, swallowing and feeding, as well as preserving middle ear function. If the cleft also involves the primary palate and lip, the child presents with a gross visible deformity. The goal of treatment comprises a "functional" palate closure in such a way as to preserve maxillary growth, to prevent recurrent serous otitis and associated hearing loss and to allow for normal speech development.

Early counseling and staffing with a team approach is paramount to success. Often, though, the initial interview is one-on-one with the plastic surgeon; therefore, a broad background in cleft care is required. Ideally, this meeting should be followed by complete staffing, palate impressions and a comprehensive treatment plan. Early counseling is very important because parents will have feelings that they are somehow guilty or at fault for the deformity. They may ask about specific causes and prevention. These fears are compounded by questions as to what can be done when, and whether it will happen again. The answers to these questions about the goals of normal speech, hearing and appearance that have stimulated the interdisciplinary approach.

Incidence

The overall incidence of facial clefting appears to be 1 in 700.[1,2,3] The incidence varies with race being less common in blacks (1 in 2000) and more common in Orientals (1 in 500).[4,5,11] Racial variation is more marked in cleft lip and palate than in cleft palate alone.

The etiology of cleft palate is unknown, though genetics play an important role (see Chapter 3). This was noted by Woolf et al.,[6] who in their series identified a significant increase in heredity of cleft lip and palate as compared to cleft palate alone. Recent authors indicate that more severe cleft lip and palate shows a greater familial recurrence.[7] Cleft lip and palate is more frequent in females (2:1). Cleft lip and palate on the left is more common (approximately 3:1).[8] There have been more than 150 syndromes associated with clefting,[9,10] and of these patients there is a preponderance of cleft palate. In the absence of specific syndromes, the risk of a second child with cleft palate is 2 percent unless a parent also has a cleft. The latter raises the risk to 15 percent. The risk of a second child with cleft lip and palate is 4 percent and rises to 10 percent if two children are affected. When a parent also is affected with cleft lip and palate, the risk of future children with cleft lip and palate is approximately 16 percent.[12]

Van der Woude's syndrome is an exception to the independence of the group of cleft lip and palate and cleft palate alone. In this group, an autosomal dominant disorder indicated by lip pits or fistulas, a high penetrance of both cleft palate and cleft lip and palate is found.[2]

Despite these genetic factors, the majority of cleft lip and palate and cleft palate patients are isolated cases. Numerous investigators have produced experimenal clefts.[13,14,15] Factors identified in human clefting include aminopterin[16] and thalidomide.[17] Others include tongue position in Pierre Robin syndrome.[18] Many other factors and their interrelationship have yet to be identified.

Anatomy

The anatomy of the soft palate was first described by von Luschka[19] and later by Veau[20] who contrasted normal and cleft anatomy. The hard palate is composed of bony support comprised of the premaxillary and palatine processes of the maxilla, which join the aveolus. The premaxilla contains the central and lateral incisor teeth and ends at the incisive foramen. The majority of the hard palate is comprised of the maxilla with a smaller posterior contribution from the palatine bones. The hamulus extends from the medial pterygoid plate directly posterior to the major and minor palatine foramina.

The major blood supply is via the greater palatine arteries, with some contribution from the lesser palatine arteries, through the greater and lesser palatine foramina respectively. Some contribution also enters from the nasal septal artery through the incisive foramen. Nerves follow arteries through these foramina from the nasal side to supply sensation.

The soft palate is attached to the posterior edge of the palatine bones by the palatine aponeurosis. Soft palate musculature is comprised of the musculus uvulae, which acts to form a posterior convexity of the soft palate in speech,[21] and the levator palati and the tensor palati muscles. The levator palati pulls the palate in a posterior superior direction in addition to giving off fibers to the eustachian tube. Its origin is the undersurface of the petrous portion of the temporal bone and the medial side of the posterior part of the cartilage of the eustachion tube. Its fibers enter the soft palate along the upper border of the superior pharyngeal constrictor. These fibers spread out and decussate with fibers from the opposite side, ending in the palatine aponeurosis. The tensor palati originates from the scaphoid fossa at the base of the medial pterygoid plate and spine of the sphenoid, and from significant attachments to the lateral side of the membranous and cartilagenous portion of the eustachion tube. This muscle courses around the hamulus and attaches to the palatal aponeurosis. It has minimal importance as a tensor of the palatal aponeurosis and is essentially inactive during speech. However, this muscle by its attachments opens the eustachion tube.[22,23] The palatopharyngeous muscle, which forms the posterior tonsilar pillar, originates from the palatine aponeurosis both poster-superior and anter-inferior to the levator and musculus uvulae. It descends along the lateral pharyngeal wall to insert along the lateral and posterior pharyngeal walls. This muscle, though more active in swallowing, pulls the soft palate both backward and downward. It often acts in balance with the levator to cause a more posterior direction of the velum and narrowing of the lateral pharyngeal walls. Whillis[24] and Brown[25] contributed to the understanding of the functional anatomy of the superior constrictor. This muscle supplies fibers to the palatal aponeurosis and forms overlapping slings, referred to as the palatal pharyngeal sphincter. When the constrictor and the levator palati contract together, a circumferential narrowing causes palatal occlusion of the nasopharynx in speech.

The anatomy of palatal clefting can be understood with a brief review of embryology. The most important changes in facial development occur during the 4th to 8th weeks, while palatal development continues until the 12th week. At the 4th week the oral depression or stomodeum opens with breakdown of the buccopharyngeal membrane. Further facial development begins as proliferation of mesenchyme forming the frontonasal and maxillary processes. From the frontonasal process a medial nasal process grows more rapidly, eventually giving rise to the central upper lip, alveolus and palate anterior to the incisive foramen known as the primary palate.[26] Theories developed by Veau[27] and later by Stark[28] suggest these processes are formed by mesodermal penetration. A lack or disruption of mesodermal penetration results in clefting in the primary palate.

The secondary site develops later at 8-12 weeks after lip formation has occurred. As the neck begins to extend the tongue moves downward. Palatal fusion begins at the incisive foramen and proceed anterior to posterior. Clefting of the secondary palate results from lack of fusion because of either mechanical interference by the tongue or a failure of mesoderm to migrate far enough into the palatal shelves to allow fusion to take place.[26,29]

Clefts follow the lines of fusion on either side of the primary palate, and the midline of the secondary palate. The alveolar clefts lie between the lateral incisor teeth and the canine teeth. Anatomical characteristics identified by Veau[23] and later by Kriens[30,31] and Dickson[20,21] identify the forward and transverse displacement of the muscular insertions of both the tensor and the levator palati and the altered palatal aponeurosis. Also of note, synergistically woven portions of the levator palati and the palatalpharyngeous muscle form Veau's cleft muscle, apparent on clinical examination.

Classification

As described above, the incisive foramen separates clefts of the primary and secondary palate. Clefts may be complete or incomplete. The most rudimentary cleft is a submucous cleft of the palate, often associated with a bifid uvula. The purpose of classification is accurate recording and grouping according to the anatomical configuration. A familiar classification is that of Veau,[23] though it fails to be inclusive. The most useful classification currently is that of Kernahan and Stark.[32] Clefts are divided as involving the primary palate, the secondary palate or both. They may be complete, incomplete, unilateral or bilateral. A secondary cleft may be submucous. This system has since been adapated graphically[33] and modified by Millard.[34]

History of Repair

Over time the emphasis in palatal repair gradually has evolved from simply closing a defect to restoring function of malpositioned and deficient parts. Soft palate closure or veloplasty was performed as early as 1817 by von Graefe[35] in Germany and extended to hard palate closure by Dieffenbach.[36] The von Langenbeck procedure, consisting of bipedal flaps, was introduced in 1861.[37] In 1984 Brophy[43] developed a system of applying maxillary compression for cleft closure. It was in 1927 that Veau[38] showed that children with clefts closed after age two had much poorer speech than those whose clefts had been repaired earlier. The new concern for improved speech resulted in the development of pushbach procedures by both Veau, who was unsatisfied with speech results following contemporary methods of repair, and by Kilner[39] and Wardell,[40] and later by Peet[41] as a variation of the V-Y technique. A more radical complete U-shaped retroposition was introduced by Dorrance[42] in the United States.

Many of these techniques tended to cause terrible maxillary deformity, particularly Brophy's technique as noted by Gillies.[44] Gillies introduced closure of the soft palate, primary veloplasty and delayed hard palate closure until four to five years of age. Graber[45] in 1949 reported a study confirming facial growth deformity as a result of palate surgery.

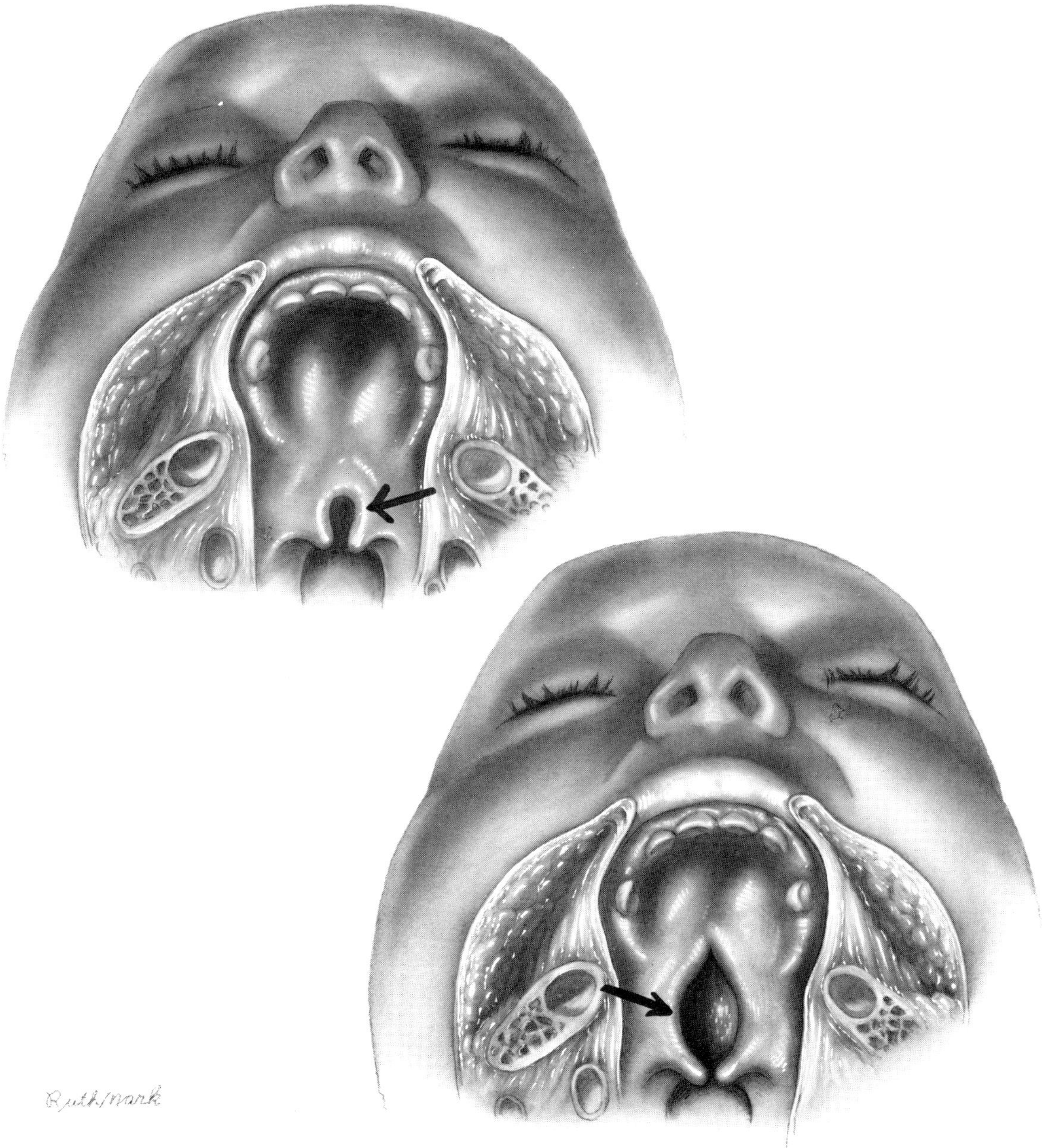

Figure 5-1. Four kinds of cleft palate.

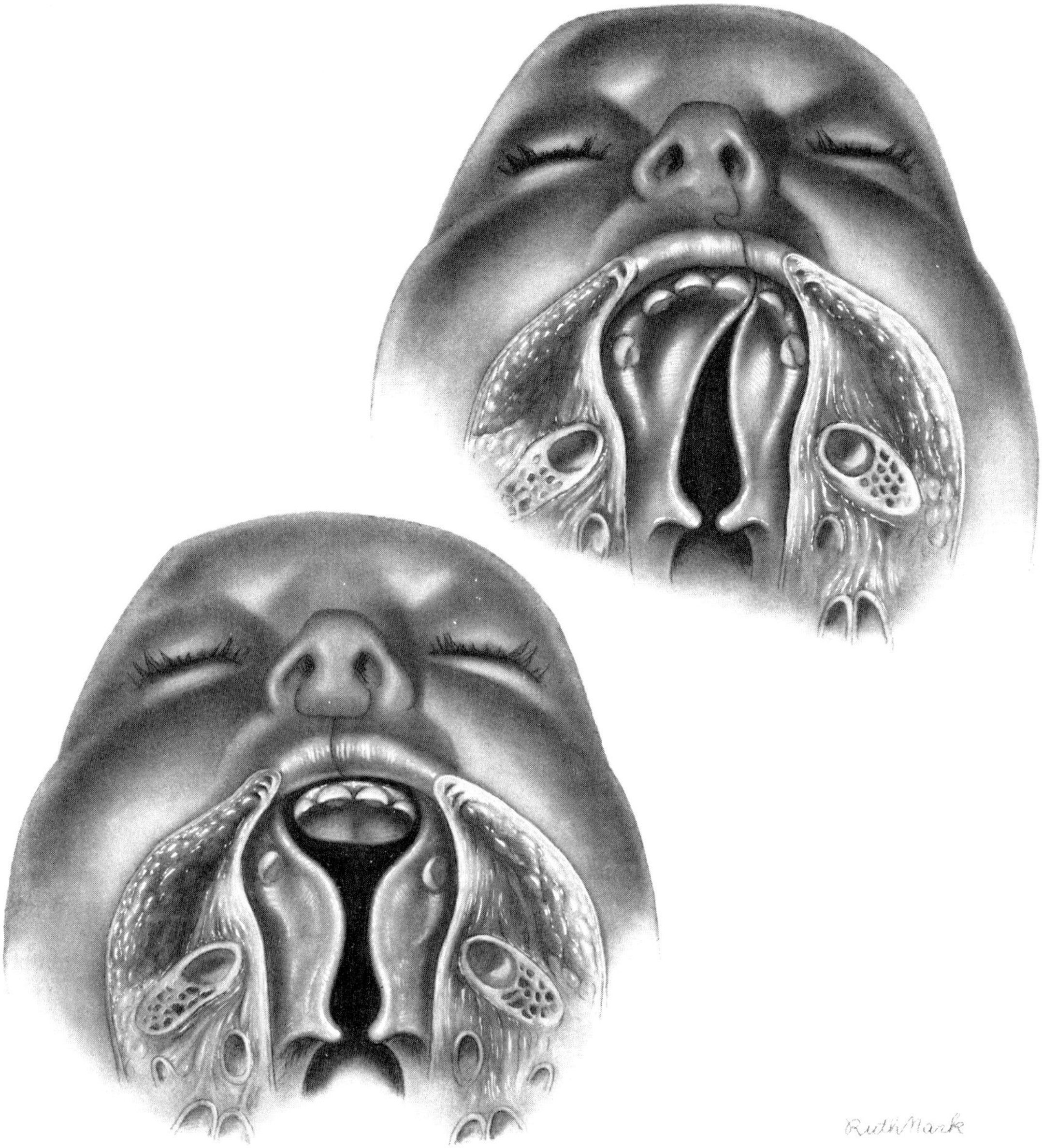

Figure 5-1. (Continued)

The timing and technique of palatal closure and its effect on both speech and subsequent maxillary growth have set the stage for controversies still unsettled. Because of surgical effects on maxillary growth, Schwechendiek,[46] Slaughter and Pruzansky[47] continued primary veloplasty and later hard palate repair, hoping to preserve a favorable outcome on speech. Current trends, as will be discussed later, move toward earlier complete palatal repair.

Evaluation

Complete evaluation is performed with special attention to associated anomalies, which may be as frequent as 30 percent. Consideration also is given to early management of feeding difficulties and middle ear disease. A Brecht-type feeder or soft plastic bottle is useful and easily managed by parents. Because of lack of suction force and increased air swallowing in cleft palate infants, feeding is accomplished best by controlled flow with the infant at 45°. A premature infant nipple, cleft palate nipple or standard nipple using a crosscut at the top all have given good results.

Middle ear disease is found in almost all infants with cleft palate.[48] Skolnik[49] has reported an incidence of conductive hearing loss of 6 percent in infants under one year and up to 67 percent in the 5 to 13-year-old group. Ear examination can be performed at the time of lip repair, usually at 8-10 weeks of age. With isolated cleft palate, early ear examination and tube placement are performed if necessary prior to palatoplasty. Repeated examination of the ears should be performed with each anesthetic for lip or palate repair and revision.

Timing of Surgery

In timing and planning surgical repair, speech development must be balanced against effects on maxillary growth. Clearly, too radical a procedure interrupts maxillary blood supply and interferes with growth. Late closure preserves maxillary growth to the detriment of speech development.

Since Veau's analysis of closure at two years of age, most agree that palatal closure before this time is essential. Our knowledge of speech development has prompted a continuing trend toward earlier closure[50,51]—in some centers closure is performed as early as three to six months.[52] There also appears to be evidence that soft palate repair and later palatoplasty, though resulting in decreased crossbite, yields poorer speech results than complete palate repair prior to one year of age.[53,54,55] For these reasons many surgeons perform complete palate repair at nine months to one year of age. At this time, the best operation for palate closure is unknown. The anatomy often can determine the best approach for repair. Presurgical maxillary orthopedics is commonly used before lip repair with palate repair to prevent maxillary collapse. In 1949 Graber[45] reported a study confirming facial growth deformity as a result of palate surgery.

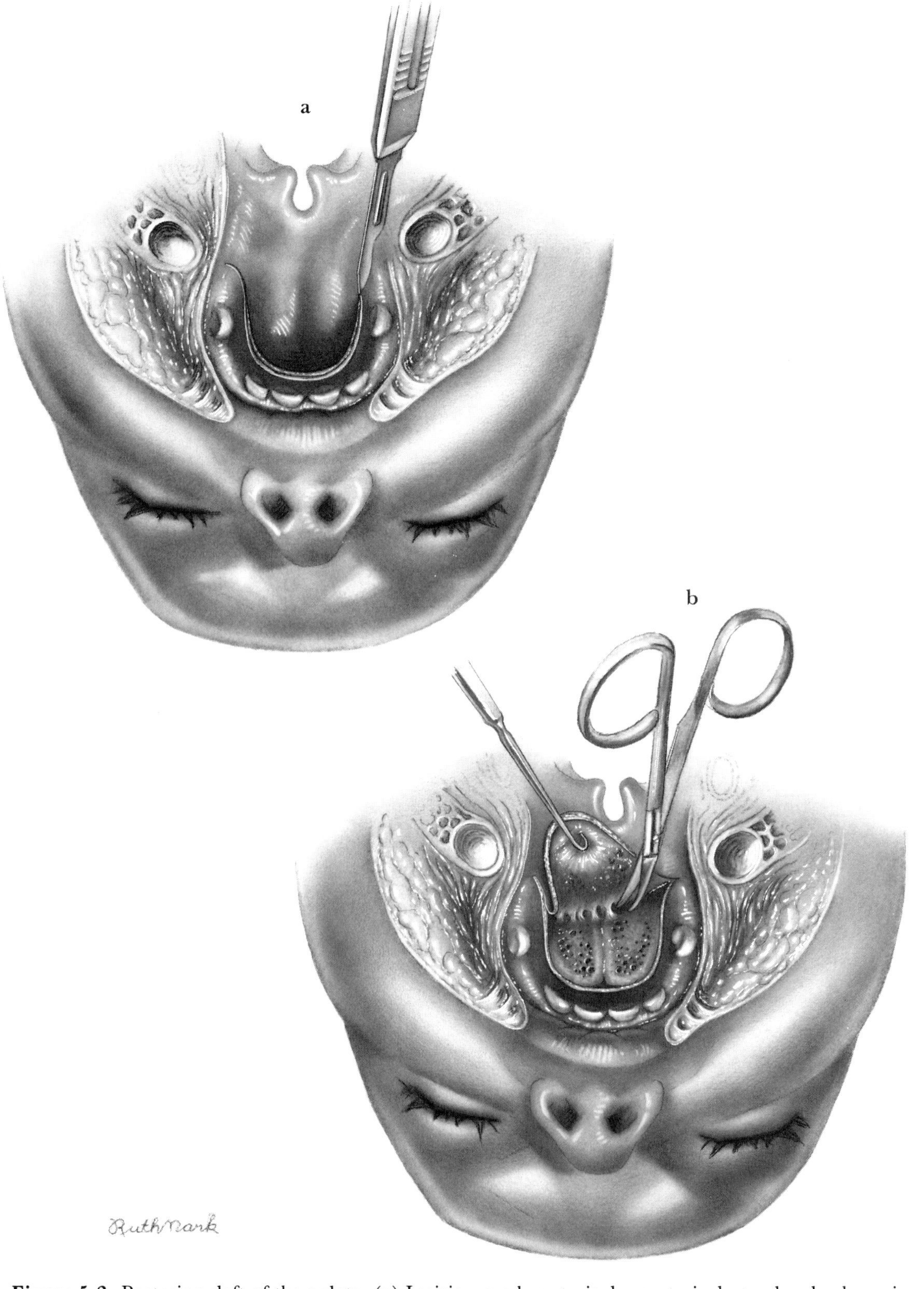

Figure 5-2. Posterior cleft of the palate. (a) Incision made anteriorly, posteriorly to alveolar bone in preparation for a pushback operation. (b) The mucoperiosteum is dissected from the underlying bone.

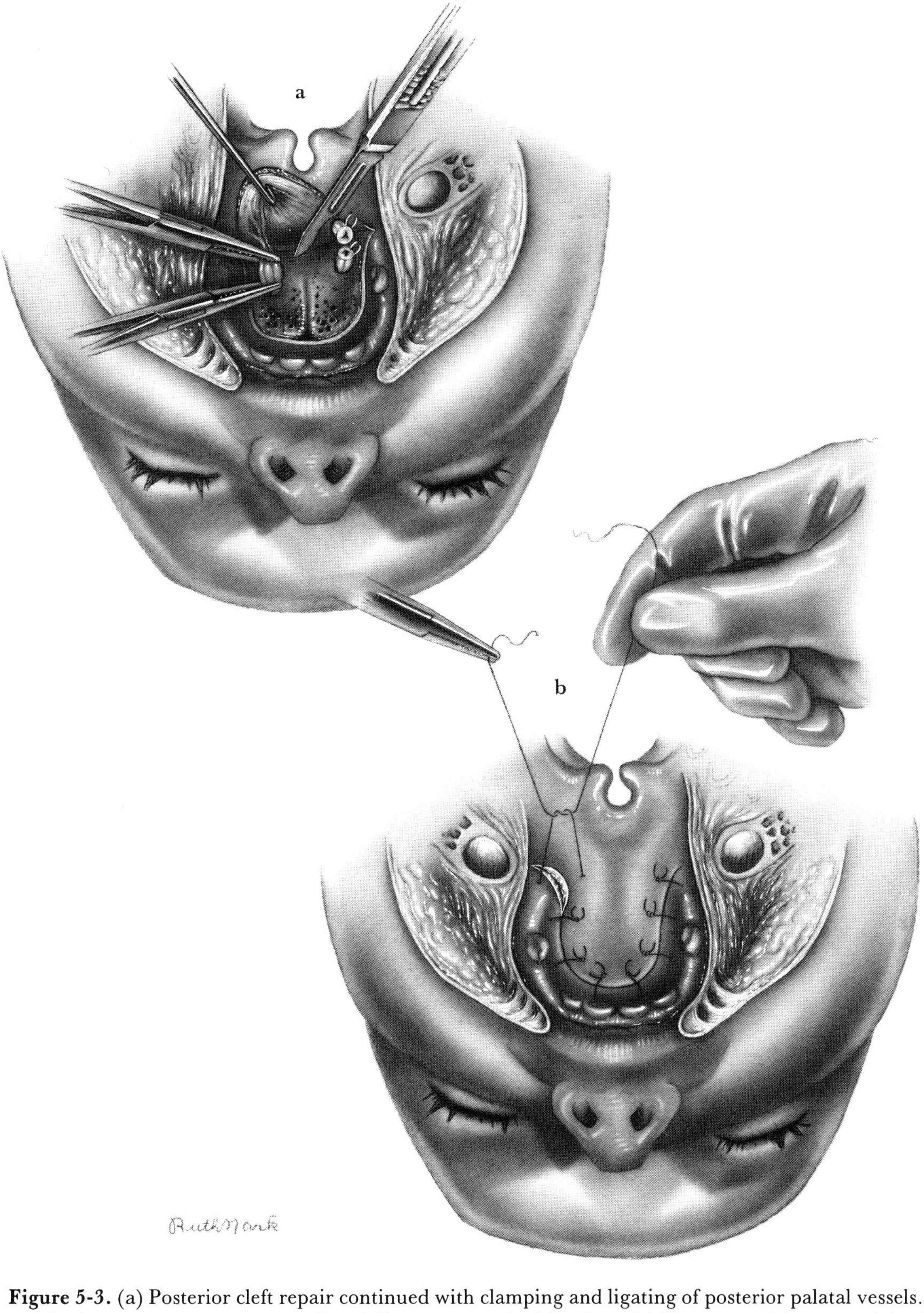

Figure 5-3. (a) Posterior cleft repair continued with clamping and ligating of posterior palatal vessels. A delaying procedure to enhance blood flow to the end of the flap. (b) Flap sutured into its original position to assure adequate blood supply.

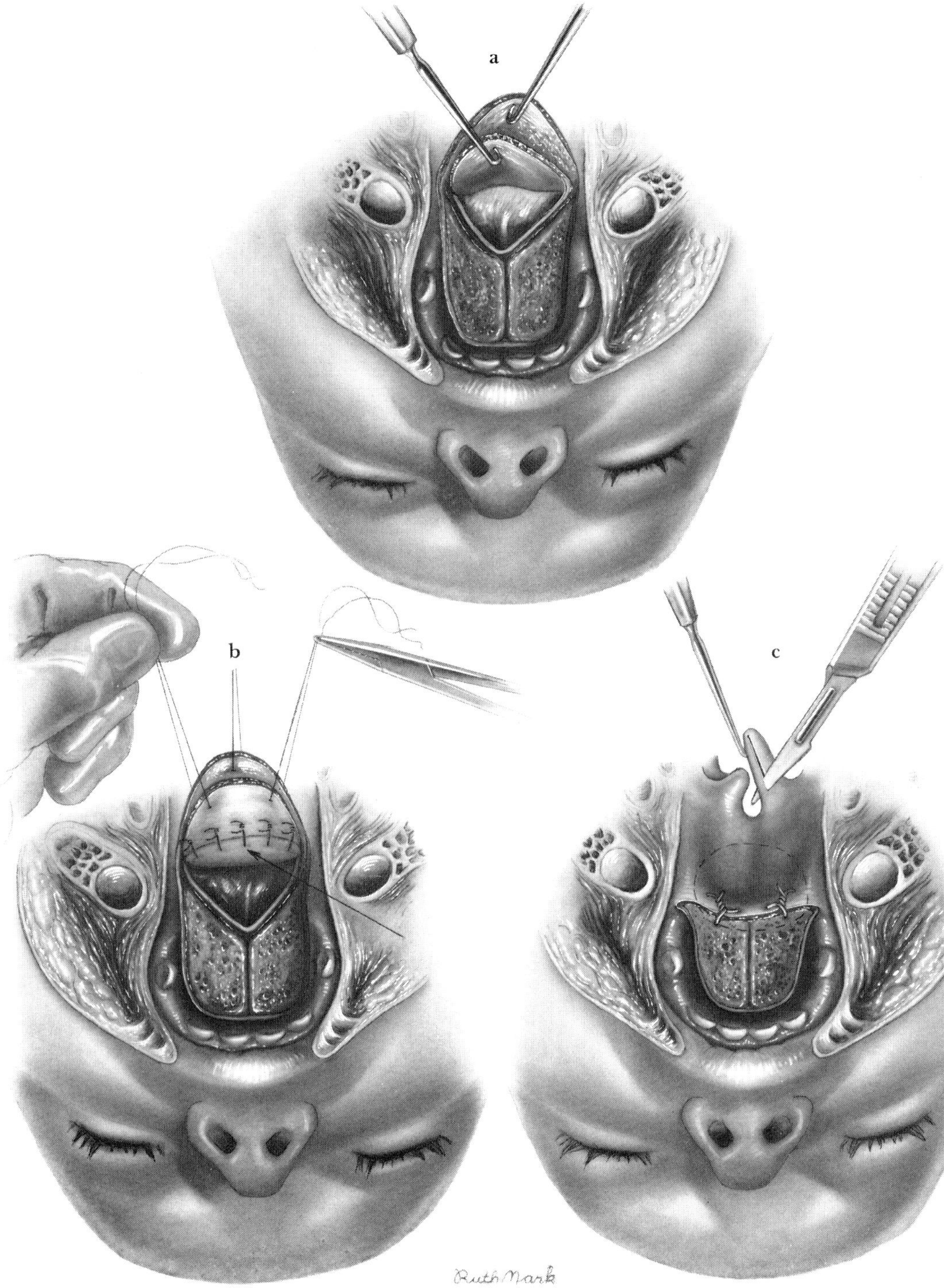

Figure 5-4. (a) Further repair of posterior cleft. Soft palate retracted demonstrating opening into pharynx. (b) Split thickness skin graft placed over superior surface of denuded pushed back palate. This minimizes scar tissue correction of the soft palate. (c) Palate secured onto the posterior surface hard palate into a new "pushed-back" position. Graft outline can be seen. Stainless steel wire used to achieve attachments to bone.

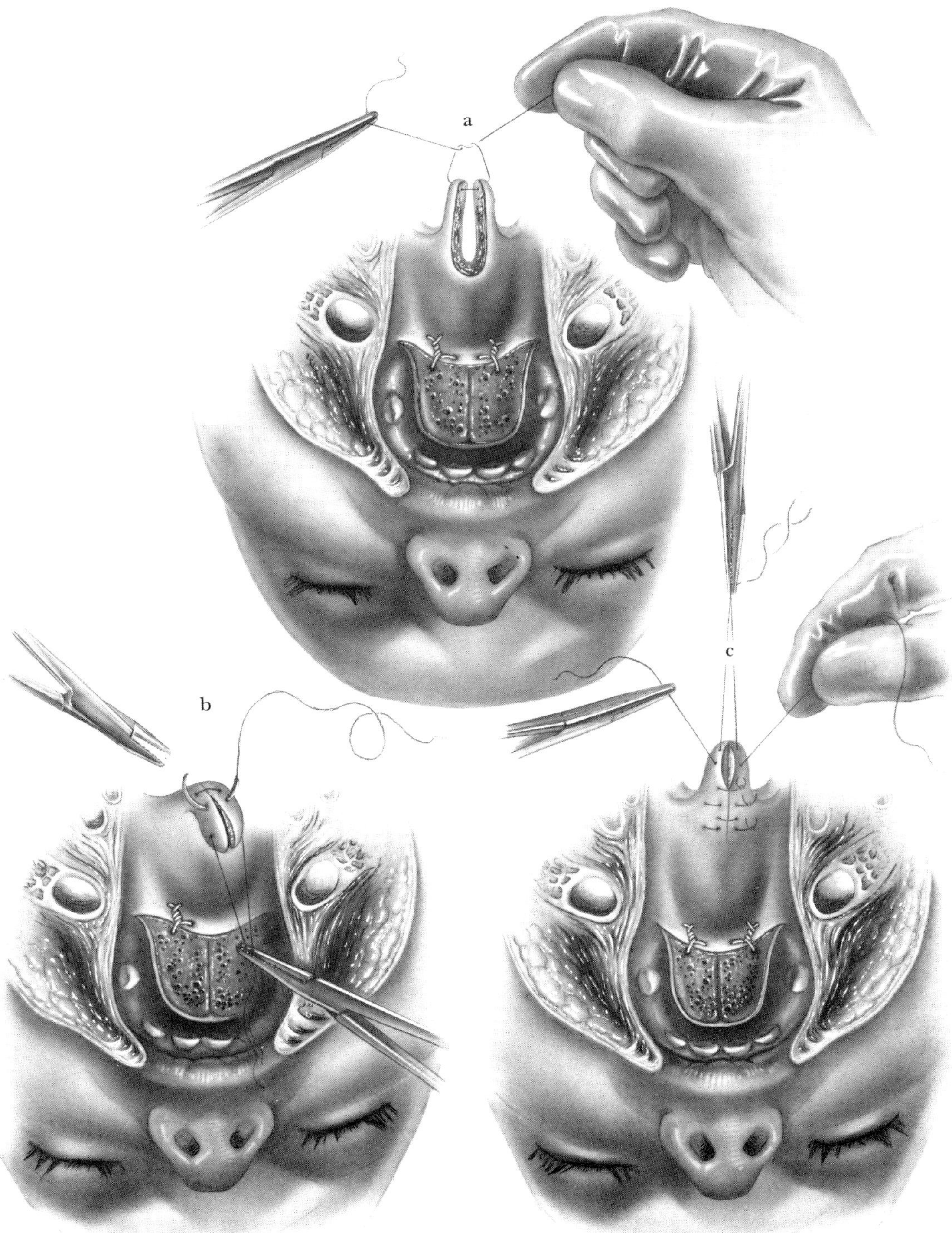

Figure 5-5. (a) Completion of procedure with approximation of soft palate. (b) Nasal surface of palate is closed with simple uninterrupted sutures. (c) Mattress sutures used to close cleft palate on the oral side.

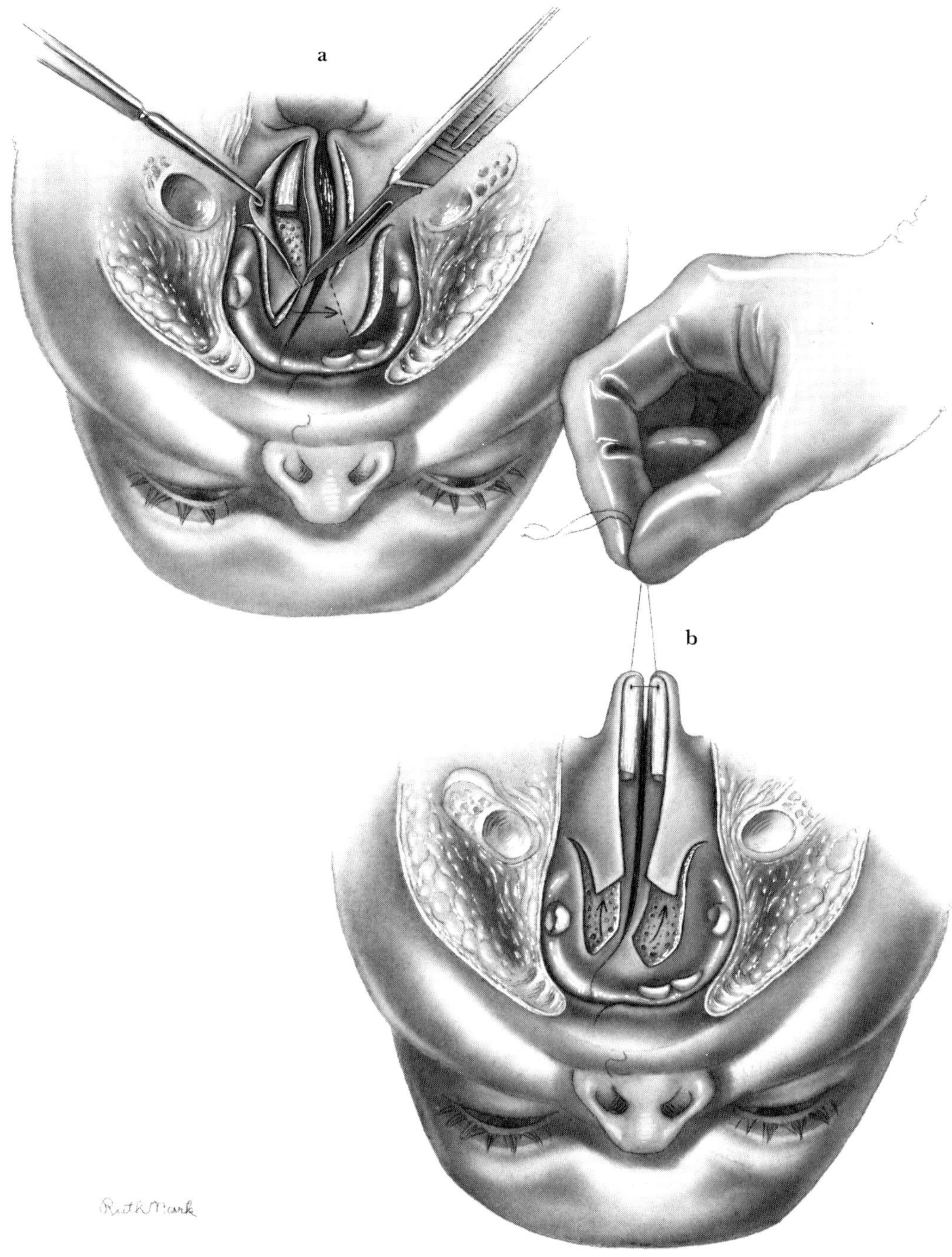

Figure 5-6. (a) Ganzer incisions which allow for anterior freedom of the palatal flaps. (b) Diagramatic illustrations after suture had been placed through the uvula in the approximation of the soft palate. The palate is lengthened.

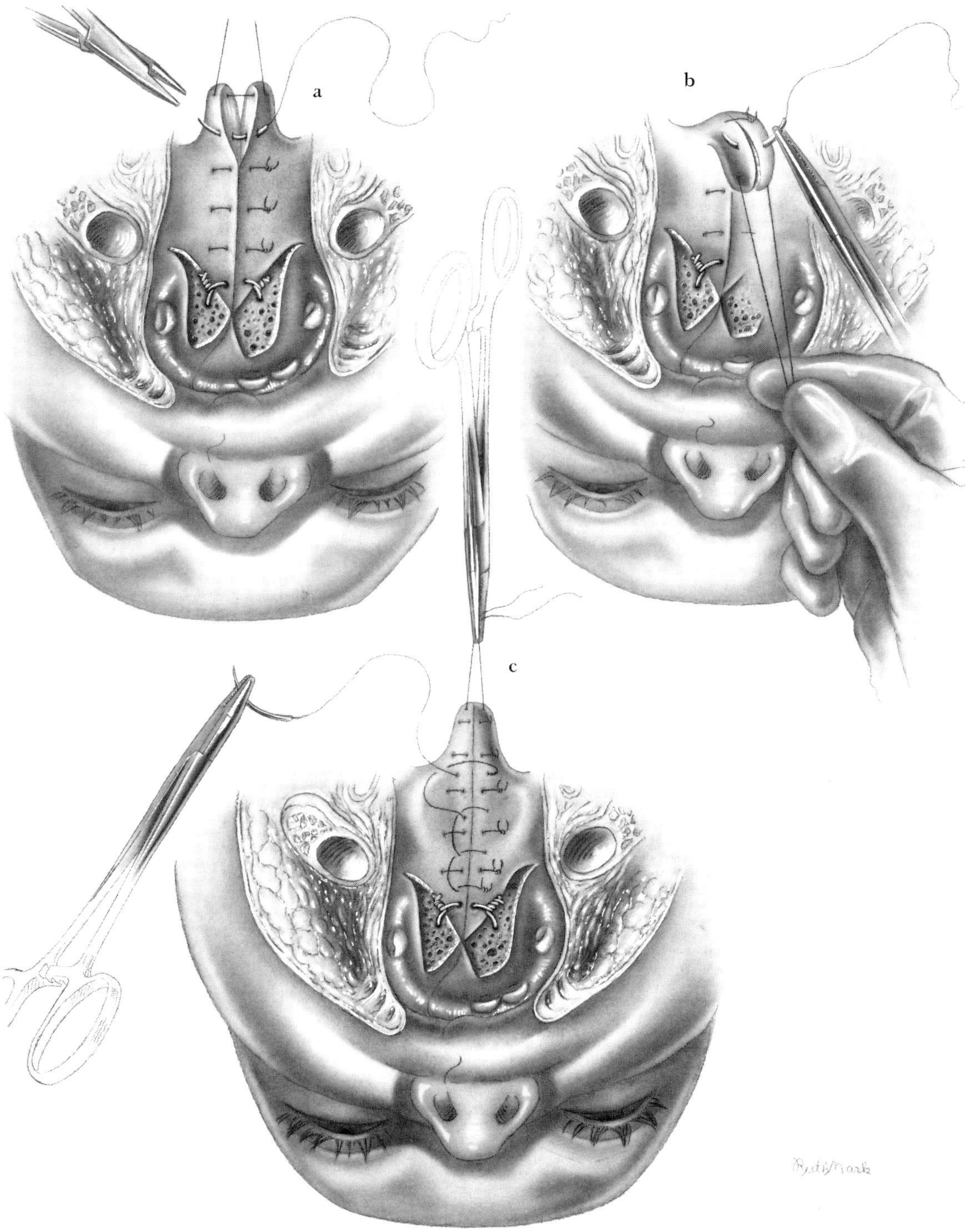

Figure 5-7. (a) Five stainless steel sutures secure the anterior palate to the maxillary bone. (b) Nasal portion of palate is approximated. Suture used for retractor. (c) Closure completed with a running suture to assure proper seal.

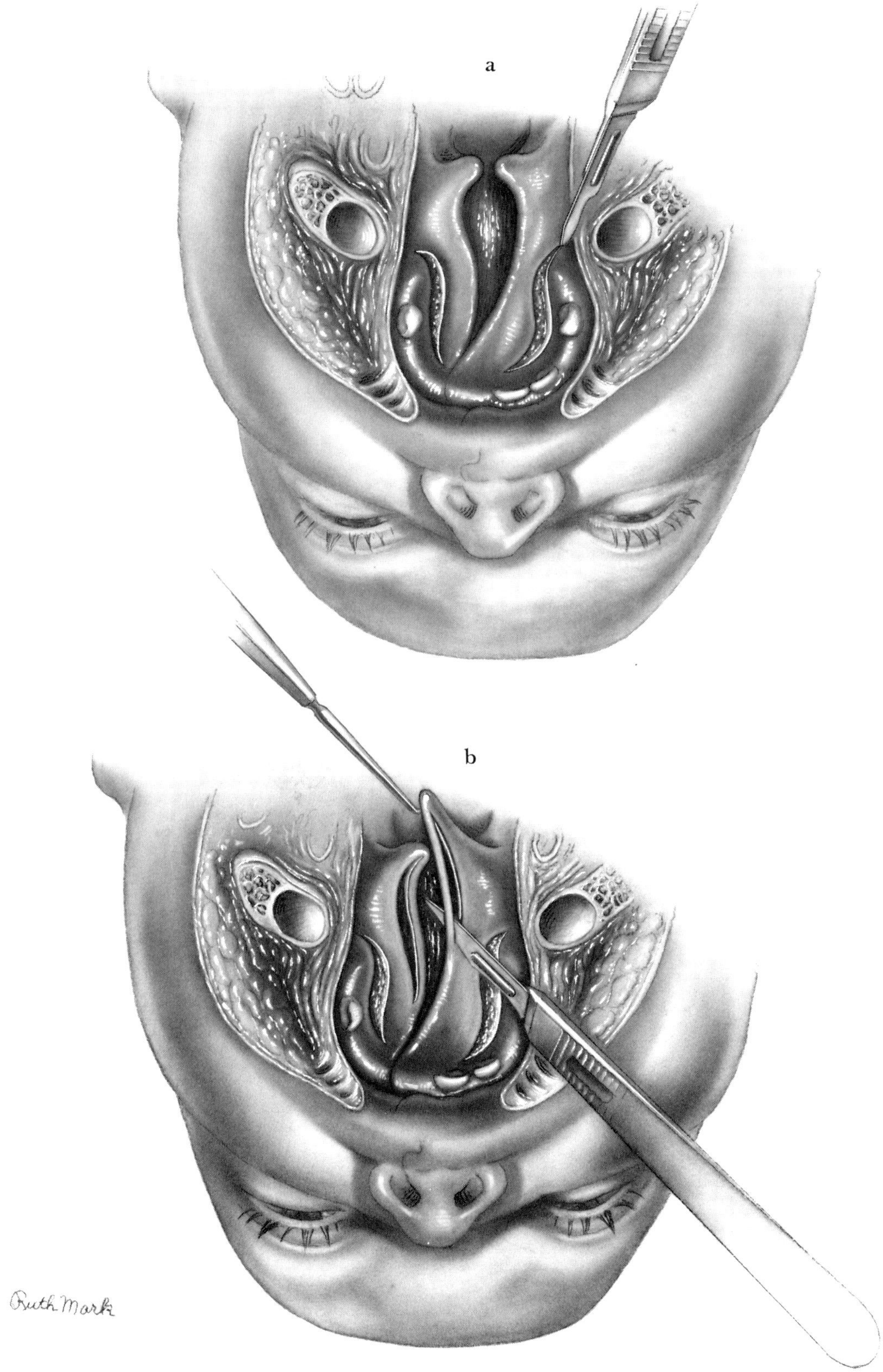

Figure 5-8. Closure of unilateral complete cleft palate. (a) Relaxing incisions made along the inguinal portion of the alveolar bone. The mucoperiosteum is easily raised from the underlying bone by means of a periosteal elevator. (b) The edges of the cleft are trimmed through its full thickness. Usually a right-angle knife is necessary to trim the attachments of the cleft margins.

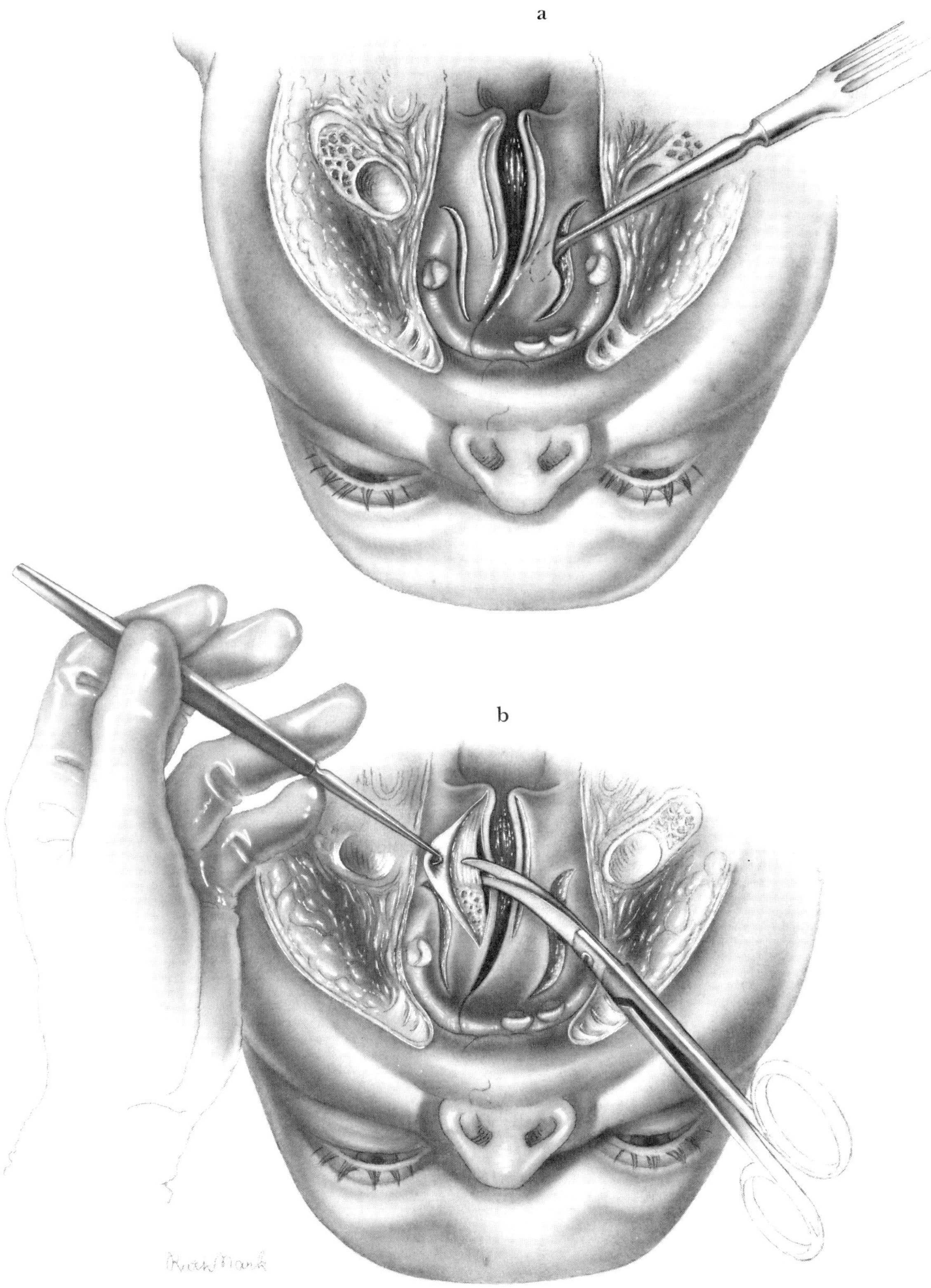

Figure 5-9. (a) Periosteal elevator used to elevate the mucoperiosteum through the relaxing incision. (b) Palatal aponeurosis is trimmed back, freeing the soft palate from its attachments to the posterior border of the hard palate.

Operative Considerations

Patients presenting for surgery must be free of any present or impending upper respiratory infection, which can be difficult in winter months. Presurgical maxillary orthopedics, if used, should be discontinued one to two weeks before surgery because of increased irritation of mucosal surfaces. In palate repair crossmatched blood is routine; so is penicillin surgical prophylaxis starting the morning of surgery. Blood replacement is given after more than 15 percent of the total blood volume is lost.

In the postoperative period a tongue stitch is temporarily placed for traction in case of airway difficulty and removed the morning following surgery. Arm restraints are kept in place one and a half weeks. Clear liquids are allowed when the infant is fully awake; the diet is advanced to blenderized food, given only through a Brecht- or syringe-type feeder for two to three weeks. Patients are discharged on the second or third postoperative day if they are feeling well.

Alveolar Cleft

Alveolar clefts are associated with cleft lip. Because of a lack of orbicularis pull, the alveolus is rotated upward and anteriorly, which often makes tension-free lip repair difficult. A nasal labial fistula, if persistent, can be troublesome during eating. If possible it is desirable to close the fistula at the time of lip repair. Both single layer closure and buccal flaps have been used.[56] In wide clefts or marked alveolar displacement, further alveolar dissection must be weighed against interruption of growth. Alternately, a maxillary appliance placed prior to lip repair will prevent maxillary collapse and may improve feeding. Following lip repair, muscle pull in the restored orbicularis improves alveolar displacement by a moulding effect and alveolar cleft can then be closed with the palate repair. With successful maxillary orthopedics, correct alveolar alignment can be achieved with a normal maxillary relationship. At this point alveolar bone grafting has been applied for stabilization and fistula closure.

Bone Grafting

Stabilization of the alveolar cleft by bone grafting was introduced in the 1950s[57,58] to reduce orthodontic problems and maxillary collapse. Reports of poor stabilization and growth[59,60,61] have caused most centers to abandon early bone grafting procedure, though surgical techniques and timing have varied widely. Skoog[62] developed a periosteoplasty, but this procedure currently is not applied widely. Early bone grafting has been performed by Rosenstein et al.[63] with a 15-year follow-up showing good stabilization and preservation of maxillary growth. They used an onlay technique with split rib and minimal dissection at six months of age. These results are encouraging though the technique is not accepted widely at the present time.

Late bone grafting has been useful in most cases to stabilize the premaxilla, to improve support and eruption of teeth and to improve appearance in the complete unilateral cleft. Grafting can correct the hypoplastic maxilla and nasal sill on the cleft side.[64] Traditional bone graft donor sites are used, such as rib and iliac crest; in some centers calvarial bone grafts have given promising results.[65]

Von Langenbeck Operations

The von Langenbeck palate repair, introduced in 1861, is a useful operation, widely performed and strongly advocated by some centers. It is particularly well applied to narrow clefts and those that do not involve the alveolus. The repair leaves smaller raw areas laterally than a pushback type of palatoplasty and has been felt to cause less interference with forward maxillary growth. Studies by Bishara directly comparing cephalometric evaluations of both the von Langenbeck and the Wardill-Kilner types of palatoplasties have not supported this contention.[66] The von Langenbeck palatoplasty is begun after careful infiltration of the hard and soft palatal mucosa with .5 percent Lidocaine with epinephrine 1:200,000. A sufficient period of time is allowed to elapse for full development of the vascular constrictive effect of the epinephrine. The free margins of the cleft are then incised sharply. A small strip of mucosa is removed in the region of the uvula. This assures that the repaired uvula will not be bifid. Lateral releasing incisions are then made medial to the alveolar processes and posteriorly around the maxillary tuberosity. The anterior extent should be behind the incisive foramen. Bipedal mucoperiosteal flaps which will contain their greater palatine blood supply are then developed. Next the soft palatal musculature is dissected sharply from both nasal and oral mucosal surfaces. Particular attention should be made to freeing attachments of the palatal musculature and aponeurosis from the bony palatal edge. Hamular infracture is advocated by some to relieve tension for soft palatal repair. Infracture is not routine; it is preferable in most cases to limit dissection and scarring behind the maxillary tuberosity. Closure of the soft palate is meticulously performed; this is the functional portion of the repair. Closure is performed in three layers. First the nasal layer is closed with interrupted 4-9 chromic sutures. Soft palatal muscular bundles which have been freed carefully from the bony palatal edge are redirected medially in a proper orientation. Muscle repair is performed end-to-end with a nonabsorbable suture such as 5-0 clear nylon. Hard palate closure is completed in two layers. Nasal mucosa is freed from the palatal shelves and complete closure of the nasal layer is performed with chromic suture. The oral mucosa is closed with interrupted 4-0 chromic vertical mattress suture. Finally, the uvula is repaired with an absorbable 6-0 suture. Gellfoam can be placed within the raw areas laterally to aid in the hemostasis.

Speech results with the von Langenbeck repair have been good and this method is used widely. Results have been reported to be better with the pushback type procedures though the von Langenbeck repair also has its strong advocates.[67,68] Emphasis should be given to meticulous soft palatal release and dissection. The cornerstone to a functional repair involves soft palatal repair or intravelor veloplasty as referred to by Kreins.[37]

Wardill-Kilner Pushback

The Wardill-Kilner pushback type of procedure was developed in response to the initial high incidence of velopharyngeal incompetence following simple palatal repairs without attention to the ordinarily short velum in the cleft patient. This technique uses the principle of V-Y advancement to produce soft palatal lengthening and prevent tethering to the hard palate repair. The procedure can be modified to close clefts through the alveolus or bilateral clefts as a three-flap or four-flap modification respectively.

Again infiltration with .5 percent Lidocaine with epinephrine 1:200,000 is used. After satisfactory take of the epinephrine, incisions are begun much like a von Langenbeck-type repair. The free margins of the cleft are opened sharply and a mucosal strip is removed only in the region of the uvula to prevent a bifid deformity from recurring. Lateral releasing incisions are then made from the canine back along the alveolus posteriorly around the maxillary tuberosity, as illustrated. A backcut is made at approximately 90° to the alveolus, directed toward the apex of the cleft. In the four-flap modification this cut is placed somewhat more posteriorly between two-thirds and the anterior third. Care must be taken with the lateral incision to preserve blood supply from the alveolus to the anterior flap. Mucoperiosteal flaps are developed based on the greater palatine artery blood supply. The palatal vessels are identified easily in these mucoperiosteal flaps. The vessels are stretched from the greater palatine foramen by blunt dissection. All soft tissue attachments are carefully released to allow maximum relaxation and tension-free closure. Soft palatal dissection is begun as in the von Langenbeck-type repair. Soft palatal mucosa, both nasally and orally, is meticulously dissected from the soft palatal musculature. Muscle attachments are freed from the posterior bony edge of the hard palate. The nasal mucosa can be lengthened by incorporation of a Z-plasty if needed.[69] Cronin also has described the technique of elevating mucosa on the nasal side, allowing for further soft palatal lengthening. Nasal mucosa is closed as before with interrupted 4-0 chromic sutures. The soft palatal musculature is rotated medially and approximated end-to-end with a nonabsorbable suture. The delicate uvula is repaired with a 6-0 absorbable suture. A V-Y pushback is performed on the oral side; it lengthens and prevents tension on the soft palatal repair, as illustrated. Repair proceeds posteriorly to anteriorly with interrupted 4-0 chromic vertical mattress sutures. The repair should be closed *without tension.*

A four-flap modification can be used in clefts through the alveolus not closed at the time of lip repair; or it can be used in the case of bilateral clefts, as illustrated. This procedure becomes technically more difficult because the blood supply to the anterior alveolar flaps must be preserved. A two-layer closure is important insurance against fistula formation, though in the four-flap modification, as in all bilateral cleft repairs, the rate of fistula formation is much higher. Failure of the four-flap procedure has resulted in particularly large anterior fistulas which may be difficult to deal with in a secondary repair. Therefore, the utmost care, technique and dissection are emphasized.

Island Pushback

The island pushback, as developed by Millard,[70] adds tissue on the nasal surface where it is lacking. It takes tissue as a vascular island from the oral side, which is an area of relative excess. The procedure in essence produces more lining on the nasal side, as Cronin advocated in his repair, to produce maximum lengthening of the soft palate. As illustrated, the mucoperiosteum of the hard palate is elevated on the greater palatine blood supply. Mucosa of the most anterior portion of the palate can be dissected as individual flaps based solely on these pedicles. They can be turned to provide nasal and oral lining as needed. This procedure produces a large raw area on the oral palatal side. Island pushback currently is advocated by Millard at three to five years of age after lip repair and primary veloplasty. Speech results with the island flap have not been encouraging.[71,72] The results with primary veloplasty also are disappointing, as previously noted.

Secondary Procedures

Secondary procedures are required for palatal fistulas and velopharyngeal incompetence. Scarring and inelasticity of tissue make fistula repair a difficult problem. Emphasis is placed on excision of mucosa within the fistulous tract and on complete relaxation and tension-free closure. No attempt at closure should be made for at least six months after palatoplasty. Closure is often delayed until age five.

The incidence of velpharyngeal incompetence varies according to the severity of the cleft and type of repair. In the English language, competence is required for all sounds except /m/, /n/ and /ng/. Fricatives are most sensitive and require a turbulant air flow. Marked incompetence usually can be demonstrated by age three to five and tends to worsen with age due to growth of the pharynx and adenoid involution.[73] Refinements in demonstrating velopharyngeal incompetence include videofluoroscopic examination[74] and, more recently, direct nasoendoscopic techniques.[75]

Three basic approaches are used to correct velopharyngeal incompetence. The first method commonly used is the pharyngeal flap. Different groups advocate superiorly and inferiorly based flaps though few differences have been shown between the two.[76] It is easier to raise a long flap with a superior base. The technique is as illustrated. A longitudinal incision is made in the posterior pharyngeal wall down to prevertebral fascia encompassing a little mucosa, and muscle is elevated and divided as far down the oralpharynx as possible. The posterior pharyngeal wall is closed primarily. The free edge of the soft palate is then incised, the nasal mucosa is raised and the pharyngeal flap is elevated and inset with silk mattress sutures. The lateral openings into the nasopharynx are kept approximately one centimeter in size.

A second approach is that of constructing a dynamic sphincter from palatal pharyngeal muscle flaps.[73] Initial results show improvement in hypernasality in only 50

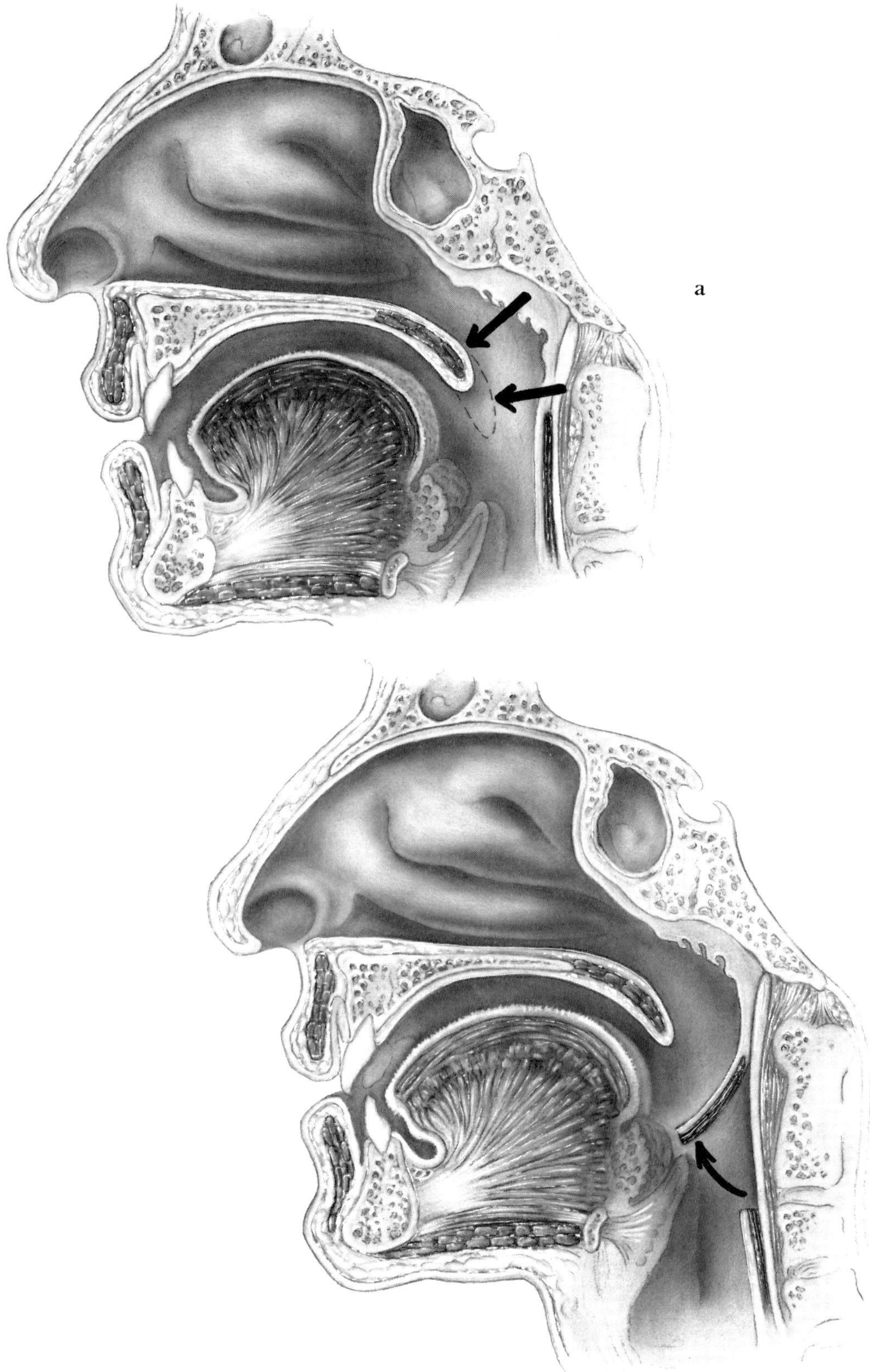

Figure 5-10. (a) Sagittal view of the palate, with ideal position of palate shown in outline. (b) Pharyngeal flap outlined over posterior pharyngeal wall. Dissection carried to prevertebral fascia, on the superiorly based flap.

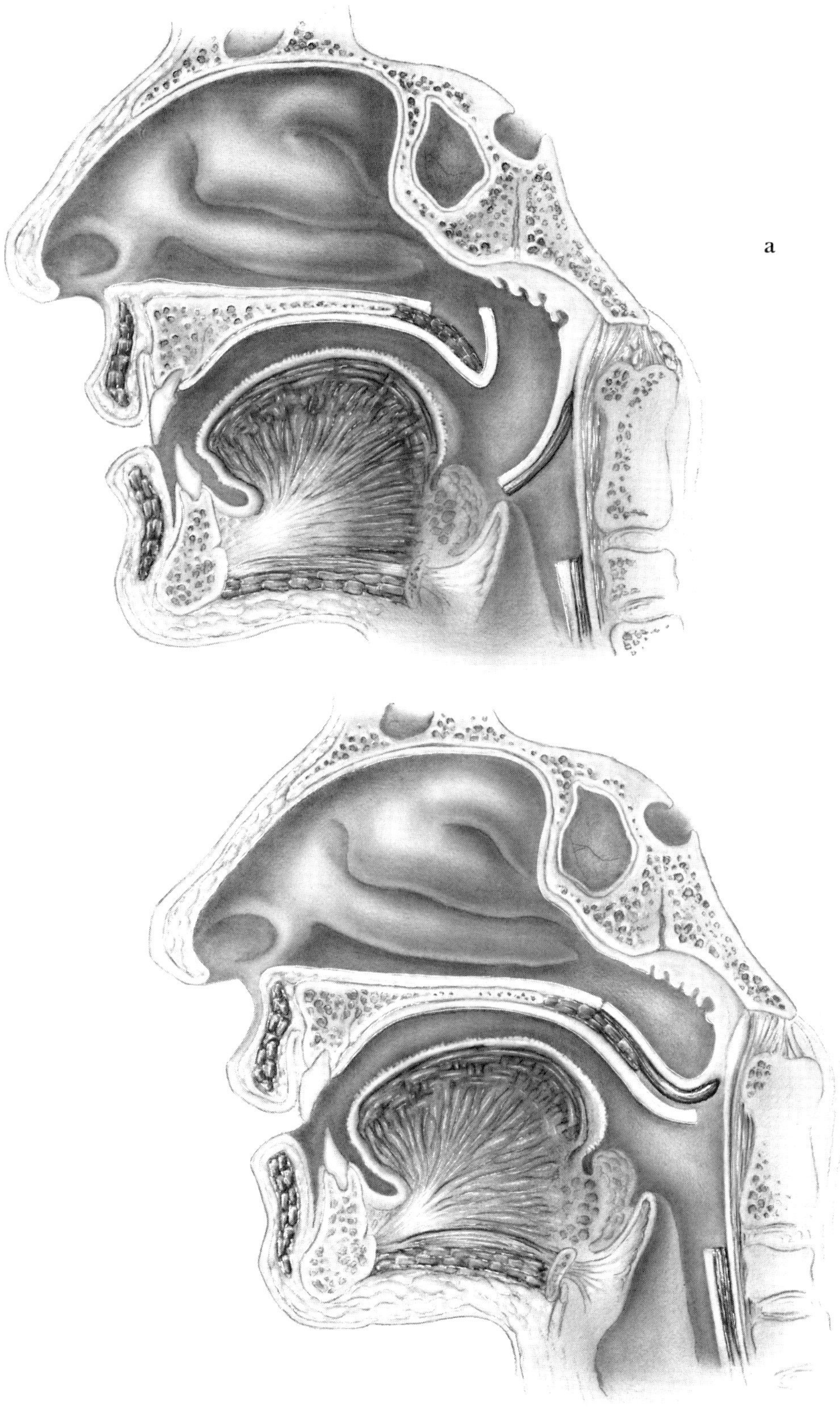

a

b

Figure 5-11. (a) Pharyngeal flap is migrated from the posterior pharyngeal wall. Flap is raised from the soft palate to overlap and cover the denuded areas. (b) Flap completed. Excepting lateral opening to allow for drainage and passage of air, the pharynx is closed.

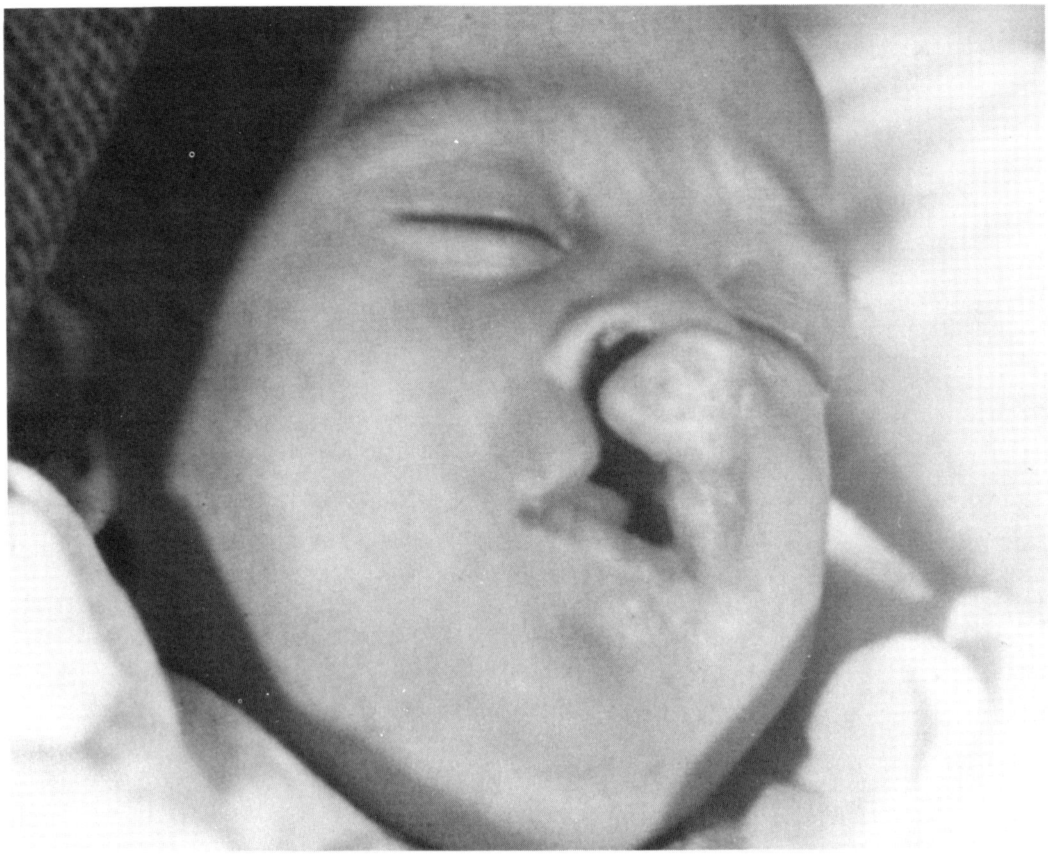

Figure 5-12. Unoperated complete severe bilateral cleft of lip with protruding premaxillary bone containing philtrum and 2 mm columnella. Many surgeons feel that the premaxilla should not be tampered with until the permanent incisors have erupted. They include bone grafting which should be delayed until orthodontic treatment has produced adequate expansion of the maxillary arch.

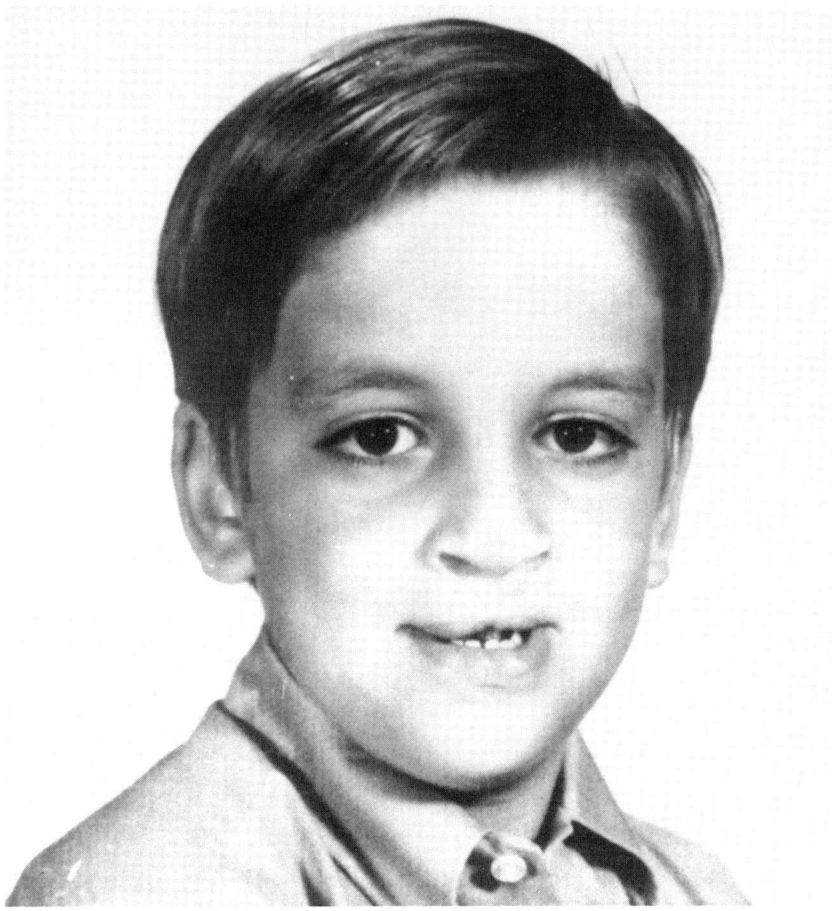

Figure 5-13. Repaired bilateral cleft of lip done in two stages. The pressure inherent in the lip closure has gradually moved the premaxilla back into a better position. The palate was closed by a Ganzer-von Langenbeck-Wardill procedure. A pharyngeal flap was later done to correct air leakage. The principle failures are short columnella, which keeps the tip of the nose tethered to the lip, and a deficiency of tissue in the center of the lip.

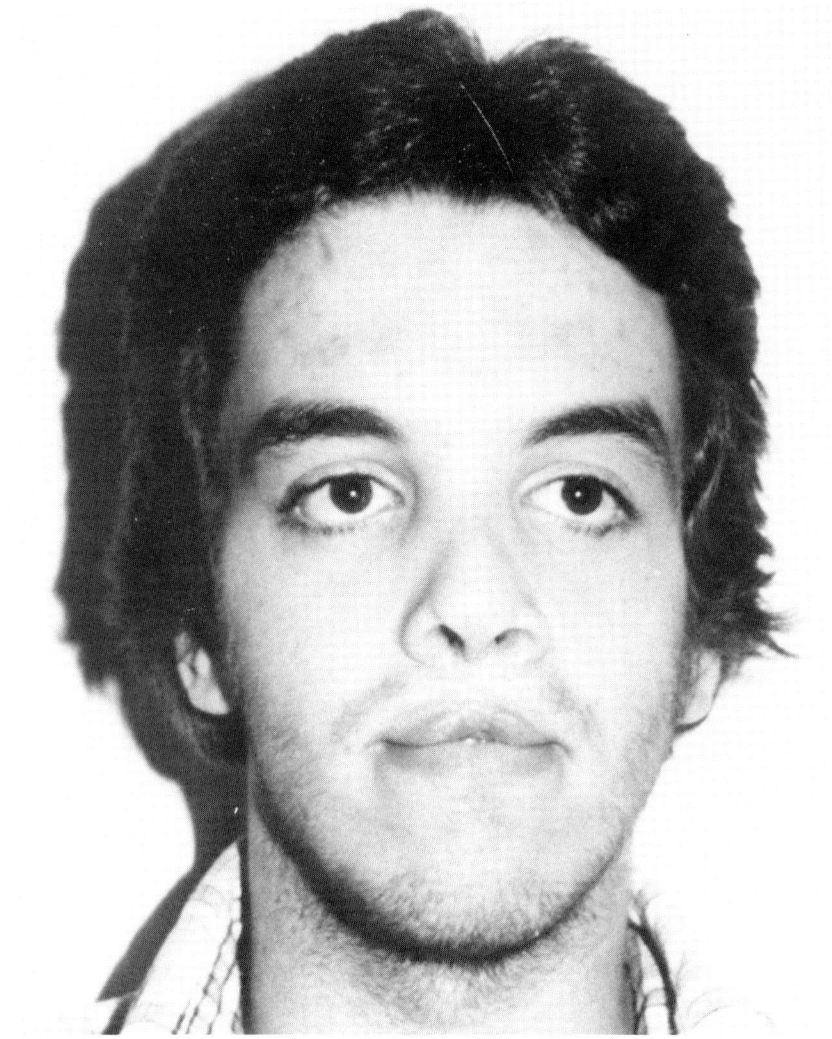

Figure 5-14. The nasal tip was freed from its attachments to the upper lip and a composite graft containing skin and cartilage grafted as a free unit from the auricle to the columnella. A rhinoplasty was carried out to create more roll to the nostrils and to reduce the thickness of the nose and to improve breathing. A deficiency in tissue persists in the upper lip with a relative fullness of the lower lip.

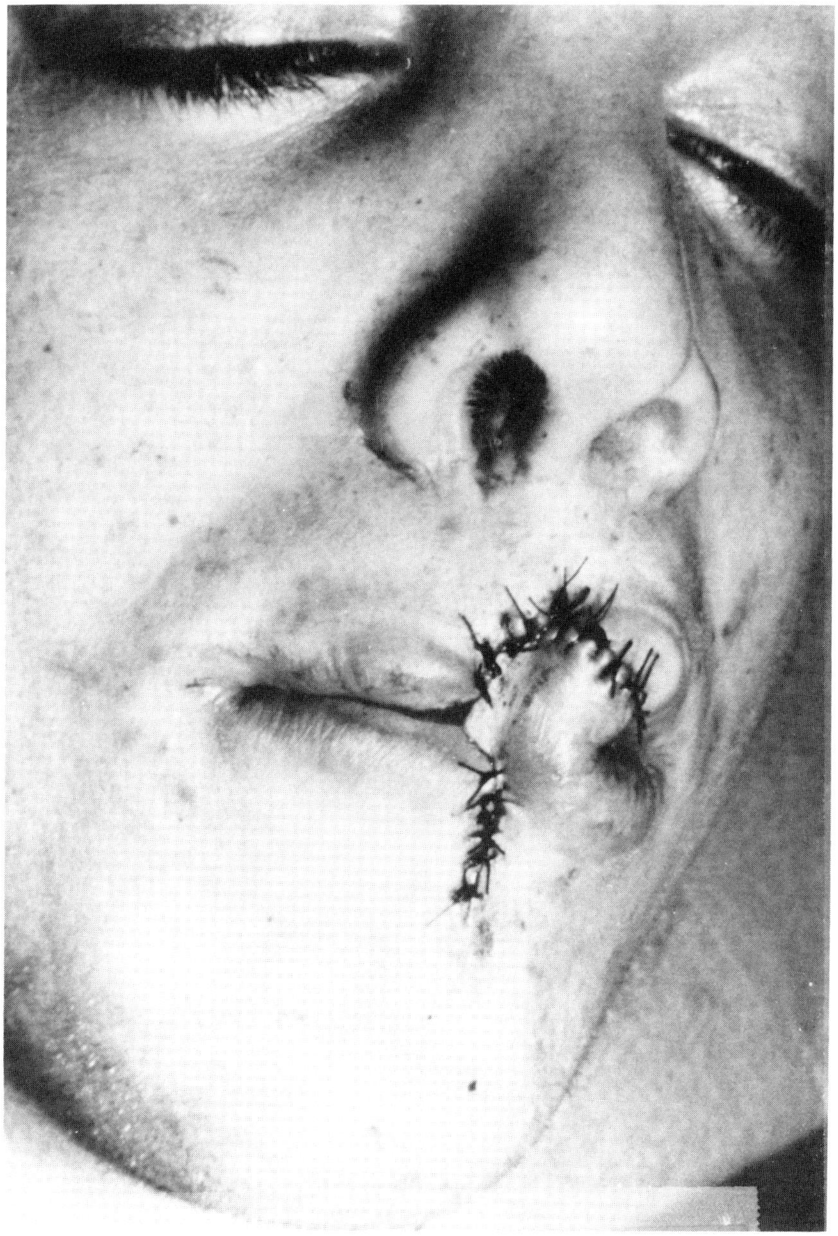

Figure 5-15. A lip switch-Estlander-Abbe-Stein derivative was used to supply tissue to the upper lip and to reduce the relative fullness of the lower lip.

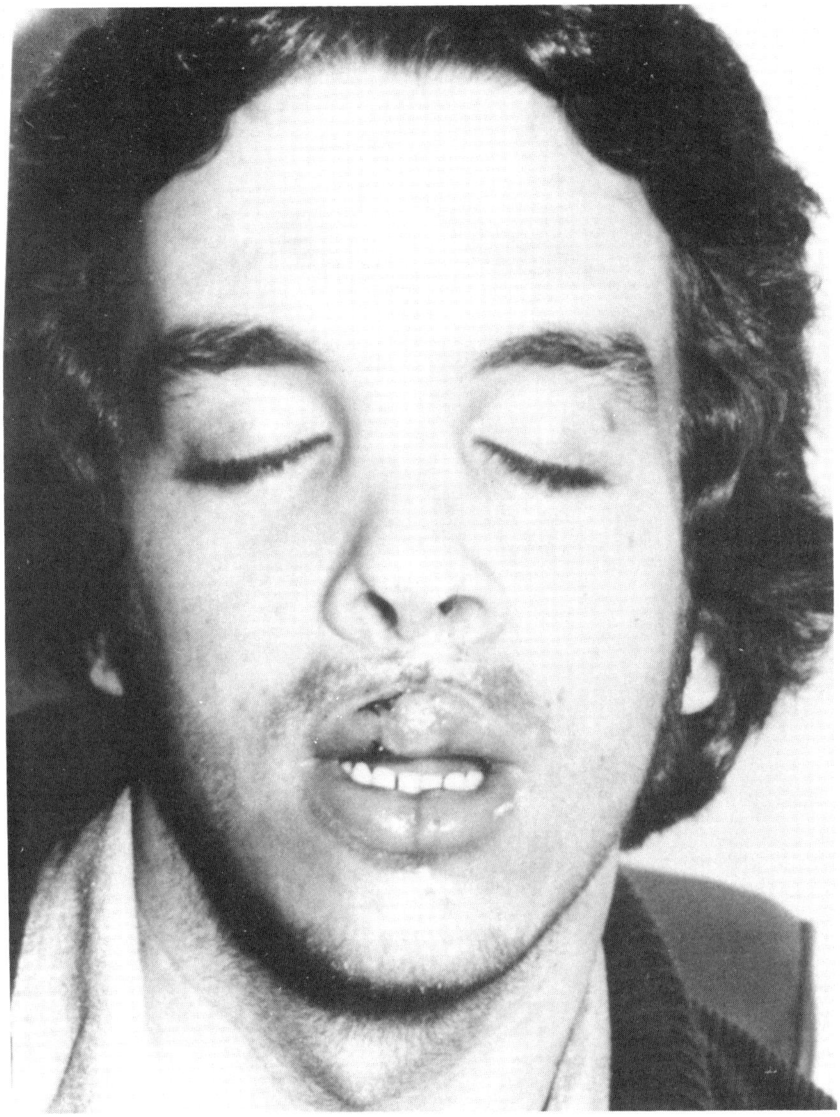

Figure 5-16. Tissue restored to upper lip after switch flap is severed.

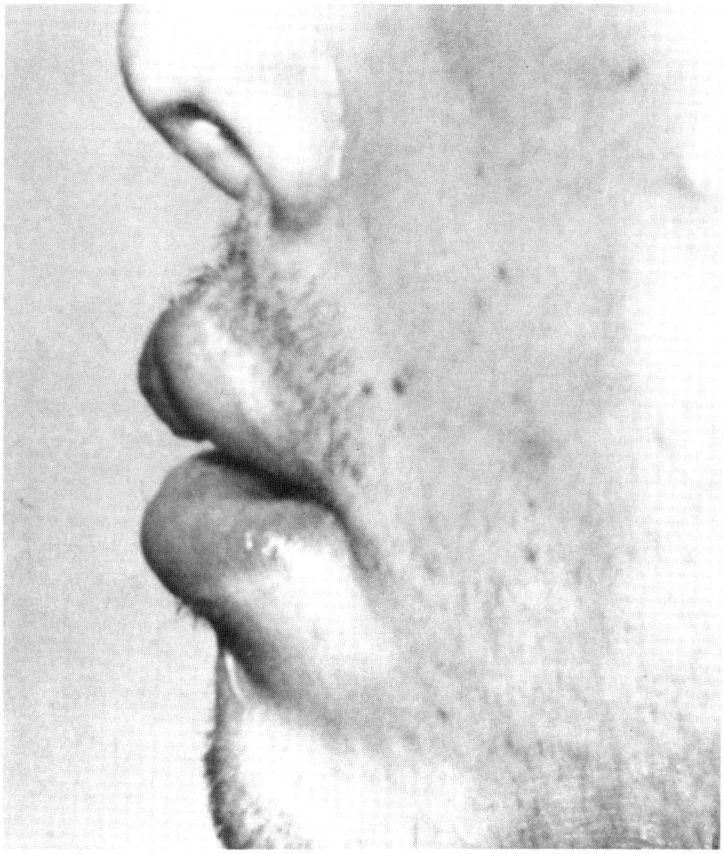

Figure 5-17. Profile view reveals a good looking balance on the protrusion of the upper and lower lip. The orthodontist and prosthodontist deserve most of the credit. Composite graft of the columnella is readily seen: it forms most of the columnella.

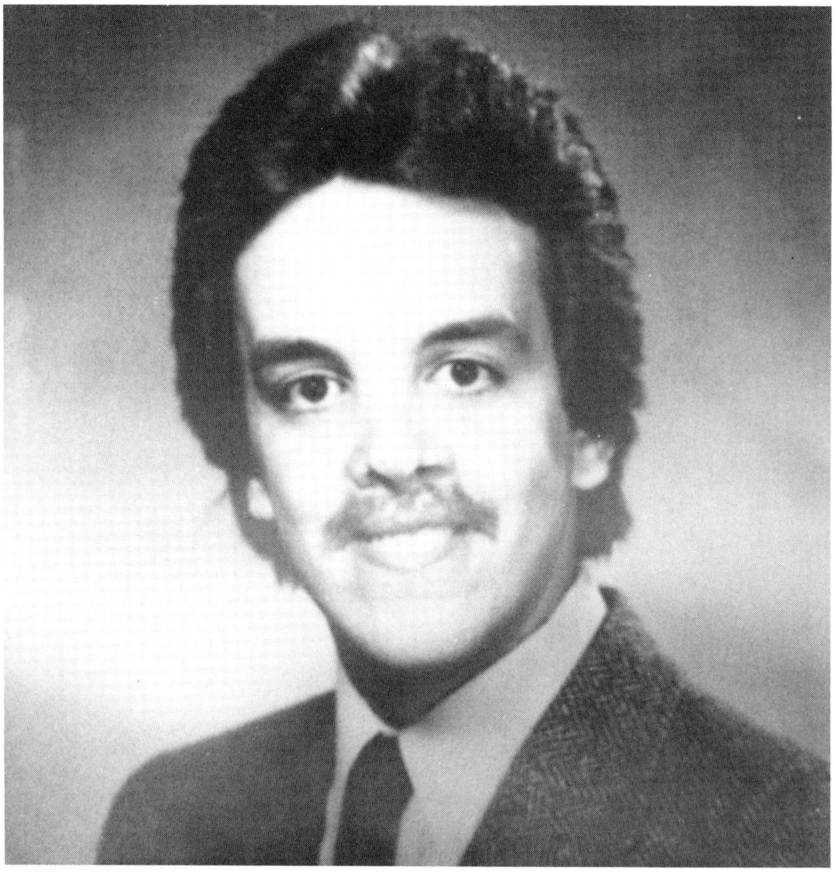

Figure 5-18. Recent photo of this patient at age 23 years reveals a result that is aesthetically and psychologically acceptable to the patient. He has finished college, has a job and has a girlfriend.

percent of cases.[77] Recent improvements in the technique have made this procedure successful in 93 percent of cases,[78] so that it may be an alternative to the standard pharyngeal flap procedure.

The third approach is that of palatal lengthening used to correct velopharyngeal insufficiency. Specifically, the island flap has been used to correct mild nasal escape depending on the length of the velum.[70] As previously mentioned, disappointing speech results are causing this technique to lose favor. With improved diagnostic techniques, velopharyngeal surgery may be tailored further to the patient's specific anatomic and functional problems.[79]

To conclude, a variety of modalities are used to provide reconstruction of the face.

REFERENCES

1. Fogh-Andersen P: *Inheritance of Hare Lip Cleft Palate.* Nyt Nordisk Forlag, Copenhagen, 1942.
2. Fogh-Andersen P: Genetic and non-genetic factors in the etiology of facial clefts. *Scan J Plast Reconstr Surg,* 1:22, 1967.
3. Ivy RH: Modern concepts of cleft lip and cleft palate management. *Plast Reconstr Surg,* 9:121, 1952.
4. Fogh-Andersen P: Incidence of cleft lip and palate: Constant or increasing? *Acta Chir Scand,* 122:106, 1961.
5. Sesgin MZ, Stark RB: The incidence of congenital defects. *Plast Reconstr Surg,* 27:262, 1961.
6. Woolf CM, Woolf RM, Broadbent TR: Genetic and non-genetic variables related to cleft lip and palate. *Plast Reconstr Surg,* 32:65, 1986.
7. Fraser FC: Etiology of cleft lip and palate. *Am J Hum Genet,* 22:125, 1970.
8. Fraser FC: Etiology of cleft lip and palate, in Grabbe WC, Rosenstein SW, Bzoch KR (eds): *Cleft Lip and Palate.* Boston, Little Brown, 1971.
9. Gorlin RJ, Cervenka J, Pruzansky S: Facial clefting and its syndromes. *Birth Defects Original Article Series,* 7, 1971.
10. Gorlin RJ, Pindborg JJ, Cohen MM: *Syndromes of the Head and Neck,* ed 2. New York, McGraw-Hill, 1976.
11. Ivy RH: The influence of race on the incidence of certain congenital anomalies, notably cleft lip and palate. *Plast Reconstr Surg,* 30:581, 1962.
12. Curtis E, Fraser FC, Warburton D: Congenital cleft lip and palate: Risk figures for counseling. *Am J Dis Child,* 102:853, 1961.
13. Cohlan SQ: Excessive intake of vitamin A as a cause of congenital anomalies in the rat. *Science,* 117:535, 1953.
14. Kalter H, Warkany J: Experimental production of congenital malformations in strains of inbred mice by maternal treatment with hypervitaminosis A. *Am J Pathol,* 38:1, 1961.
15. Walker BE: The association of mucopolysaccharides with morphogenesis of the palate and other structures in mouse embryos. *J Embryol Exp Morphol,* 9:22, 1961.
16. Warkany J, Beaudry PH, Bornstein S: Attempted abortion with aminopterin. *Am J Dis Child,* 97:274, 1959.
17. Fogh-Andersen P: Thalidamide and congenital cleft deformities. *Acta Chir Scand,* 131:197, 1966.
18. Randall P: The Robin anonmalad: Micrognathia and glossoptosis with airway obstruction, in Converse JM (ed): *Reconstructive Plastic Surgery,* ed 2. Philadelphia, W B Saunders Co, 1977.
19. von Luschka H: *Die Anat des Menschlichen,* vol 1, part 1, Tubingen, Halses, 1870.

20. Veau V: *Division Palatine: Anatomie, Chirurgie, Phonetique.* Paris, Masson, 1931.
21. Pigott RW: The nasendoscopic appearance of the normal palatopharyngeal valve. *Plast Reconstr Surg,* 43:19, 1969.
22. Dickson DR: Anatomy of the normal velopharyngeal mechanism. *Clin Plast Surg,* 2:235, 1975.
23. Dickson DR, Dickson WM: Velopharyngeal anatomy. *J Speech Hear Res,* 15:372, 1972.
24. Whillis J: A note on the muscles of the palate and the superior constrictor. *J Anat,* 65:92, 1931.
25. Browne D: The orthopedic operation for cleft palate. *Br Med J,* 2:1093, 1935.
26. Patten BM: Embryology of the palate and maxillofacial region, in Grabbe WC, Rosenstein SE, Bzoch KR (eds): *Cleft Lip and Palate.* Boston, Little Brown, 1971.
27. Veau V: *Bec-de-Lievre.* Paris, Masson, 1938.
28. Stark RB: Embryology of cleft lip and palate, in Converse JM (ed): *Reconstructive Plastic Surgery.* Philadelphia, W B Saunders Co, 1977.
29. Poswillo D: The pathogenesis of submucous cleft lip and palate. *Scand J Plast Surg,* 8:34, 1974.
30. Kriens O: An anatomical approach to veloplasty. *Plast Reconstr Surg,* 43:29, 1969.
31. Kriens O: Fundamental anatomic findings for an intravelar veloplasty. *Cleft Palate J,* 7:27, 1970.
32. Kernahan DA, Stark RB: A new classification for cleft lip and cleft palate. *Plast Reconstr Surg,* 22:435, 1958.
33. Kernahan DA: The striped Y—a symbolic classification for cleft lips and palate. *Plast Reconstr Surg,* 47:469, 1971.
34. Millard DR Jr (ed): *Cleft Craft: The Evolution of Its Surgery.* Boston, Little Brown, 1976, vol 1: *The Unilateral Deformity.*
35. von Graefe CF, Kurze Nachrichter und Auszuge. *J Pract Arznek Wundarzke,* 44:116, 1817.
36. Deffenbach JF: Uber das Gaumensegel des Menschen und der Saeugenthiere. *Litt Ann Gilk,* 4:298, 1826.
37. von Langenbeck BRK: Operation der angleborenen totalen Spaltung des harten Gaumens nach einer neuer Methode. *Dtsch Klin,* 13:231, 1861.
38. Veau V: The treatment of cleft palate by operation. *Proc Roy Soc Med,* 20:127, 1926-7.
39. Kilner TP: Cleft lip and palate repair technique, in Maingot R (ed): *Postgraduate Surgery,* vol 3. London, Medical Pub, 1931.
40. Wardill WFM: Cleft palate. *Br J Surg,* 16:127, 1928.
41. Peet E: The Oxford techniques of cleft palate repair. *Plast Reconstr Surg,* 28:282, 1961.
42. Dorrance GM: Lengthening of the soft palate in cleft operations. *Ann Surg,* 32:208, 1925.
43. Brophy TW: A new operation for cleft palate. *Boston Med Surg J,* 2:656, 1896.
44. Gillies HD, Fry K: A new principle in the surgical treatment of congenital cleft palate and its mechanical counterpart. *B Med J,* 1:335, 1921.
45. Graber TM: Craniofacial morphology in cleft palate and cleft lip deformities. *Surg Gynecol Obstet,* 88:359, 1949.
46. Schweckendieck W: The primary veloplasty: Long-term results without maxillary deformity. *Cleft Palate J,* 15:268, 1978.
47. Slaughter WB, Pruzansky S: The rationale for velar closure as a primary procedure in the repair of cleft palate defects. *Plast Reconstr Surg,* 13:341, 1954.
48. Paradise JL, Bluestone CD: On the universality of otitis media in fifty infants with cleft palate. *Pediatrics,* 44:35, 1969.
49. Skolnik E: Otologic evaluation in cleft palate patients. *Laryngoscope,* 68:1908, 1958.
50. Kaplan EN: Early primary palate repair. Read before the American Cleft Palate Educational Foundation Symposium, Northwestern University, Chicago, 1977.
51. Dorf DS, Curtin JW: Early cleft palate repair and speech outcome. *Plast Reconstr Surg,* 70:74, 1982.

52. Randall P, LaRossa DD, Fakhraee SM, Cohen MA: Cleft palate closure at 3 to 7 months of age: A preliminay report. *Plast Reconstr Surg,* 71:624, 1983.
53. Robertson NRE, Jolleys A: The timing of hard palate repair. *Scand J Plast Reconstr Surg,* 8:49, 1974.
54. Jackson IT, McLennan G, Scheker LR: Primary veloplasty or primary palatoplasty: Some preliminary findings. *Plast Reconstr Surg,* 72:153, 1983.
55. Bardach J, Morris HL, Olin WH: Late results of primary veloplasty: The Marburg project. *Plast Reconstr Surg,* 73:207, 1984.
56. Muir IFK: Repair of the cleft alveolus. *Br J Plast Surg,* 29:30, 1966.
57. Nordin KE, Johensen B: *Frie Knochen-Transplantation bie Defekten in Alveolarkam nach Kieferortopadischer Enetelluling der Maxilla bei Lippen-Kiefer-Gaumenspalten,* vol 1. Stuttgart, Thieme, 1955.
58. Schmid E, Die Annaherung der Kieferstumpfe: Ihre Schdelidren Folgen und Vermeidung. *Fortschr Keifer-Ges Chir,* 1:37, 1955.
59. Jolleys A, Robertson NRE: A study of the effects of early bone grafting in complete clefts of lip and palate—5 year study. *Br J Plast Surg,* 25:229, 1972.
60. Lynch JB, Wisner HK, Evans RM, et al: Cephalometric study of maxillary growth five years after alveolar bone grafting of cleft palate infants. *Plast Reconstr Surg,* 46:564, 1970.
61. Nylen B, Korlof B, Arnander C, et al: Primary early bone grafting in complete clefts of the lip and palate: A follow-up study of 53 cases. *Scand J Plast Reconstr Surg,* 8:79, 1974.
62. Skoog T: The use of periosteal flaps in the repair of the primary palate. *Cleft Palate J,* 2:332, 1965.
63. Rosenstein SW, Monroe CW, Kernahan DA, et al: The case for early bone grafting in cleft lip and palate. *Plast Reconstr Surg,* 70:297, 1982.
64. Millard DR: Early correction of the unilateral cleft lip nose. *Plast Reconstr Surg,* 70:64, 1982.
65. Wolfe SA, Berkowitz S: The use of cranial bone grafts in the closure of alveolar and anterior palatal clefts. *Plast Reconstr Surg,* 72:659, 1983.
66. Bishara SE, Enemark H, Tharp RF: Cephalometric comparisons of the results of the Wardill-Kilner and von Langenbeck palatoplasties. *Cleft Palate J,* 13:319, 1976.
67. Musgrave RH, McWilliams BJ, Matthews HP: A review of the results of two different surgical procedures for the repair of clefts of the soft palate only. *Cleft Palate J,* 12:281, 1975.
68. Krause CJ, Tharp RF, Morris HL: A comparative study of the results of the von Langenbeck and V-Y push-back palatoplasties. *Cleft Palate J,* 12:11, 1976.
69. Stark DB: Nasal lining in partial cleft palate repair. *Plast Reconstr Surg,* 32:75, 1963.
70. Millard DR Jr (ed): *Cleft Craft: The Evolution of Its Surgery.* Boston, Little Brown, 1980, vol 3: *Alveolar & Palatal Deformities.*
71. Lewin M, Heller JC, Kojak DJ: Speech results after Millard island flap repair in cleft palate and other velopharyngeal insufficiencies. *Cleft Palate J,* 12:263, 1975.
72. Luce EA, McClinton M, Hoopes JE: Long-term results of the island flap palatal push-back. *Plast Reconstr Surg,* 58:332, 1976.
73. Orticochea M: Construction of a dynamic muscle sphincter in cleft palates. *Plast Reconstr Surg,* 41:323, 1968.
74. Skolnick ML: Videofluoroscopic examination of the velopharyngeal portal during phonation in lateral and base projections: A new technique for studying the mechanism of closure. *Cleft Palate J,* 7:803, 1970.
75. David DJ, White J, Sprod R, Bagnall A: Nasendoscopy: Significant refinements of a direct-viewing technique of the velopharyngeal sphincter. *Plast Reconstr Surg,* 70:423, 1982.
76. Whitaker LA, Randall P, Winchester R, Graham WP: A prospective and randomized series comparing superiorly and inferiorly based posterior pharyngeal flaps. *Cleft Palate J,* 9:304, 1972.

77. Jackson IT, Silverton JS: The sphincter pharyngoplasty as a secondary procedure in cleft palates. *Plast Reconstr Surg,* 59:518, 1977.
78. Riski JE, Serafin D, Riefkohl R, et al: A rationale for modifying the site of insertion of the orticochea pharyngoplasty. *Plast Reconstr Surg,* 73:882, 1984.
79. Jackson IT: A rationale for modifying the site of insertion of the orticochea pharyngoplasty: Discussion. *Plast Reconstr Surg,* 73:891, 1984.

CHAPTER 6

ALVEOLAR CLEFT MANAGEMENT

ROGER H. KALLAL and JOHN TANNER

> . . . *There were few things that the master practiced: he took nothing for granted; he was never over positive, never obstinate, never egotistic.*
>
> . . . *Confucius*

THE FIRST recorded closure of a cleft palate was in 1776 by the French dentist, LeMonnier. Dieffenbach[1] moved bilaterally fractured palatal shelves medially toward the palatal midline. With this technique the posterior palatal muscle attachments remain intact; the nasal blood supply to the palate is not violated, and the palatal vault continuity is restored. In 1861 von Langenbeck described the use of two palatal releasing incisions and the reflection of mucoperiosteal flaps for midline approximation.[2] This resulted in tissue breakdown. Lexer[3] and Drachter[4] are credited with the first attempts at alveolar bone grafting in a growing patient. Cleft palate repair techniques continued to develop with the work of Beck and Jesser,[5] Wardill,[6] Veau,[7] Kilner[8] and Axhausen.[9] They felt the future of cleft palate repair was by osteoplasty or induction of bone formation in the defects. The use of iliac bone grafts between maxillary segments to prevent collapse and contracture into the cleft area was demonstrated by Schmid[10] and Clausen.[11] Primary osteoplasty was first presented by Schruddle and Stellmach in 1958 by combining the surgical closure of the cleft lip and alveolar defect with bone grafting during infancy.[12] When bony clefts were repaired subsequent to soft tissue closure, it was termed secondary osteoplasty. Nylen[13] further subdivided secondary repair into early bone grafting (after eruption of deciduous teeth) and late secondary osteoplasty (grafting after complete eruption of permanent dentition). The debate between the two groups has continued for many years and will be discussed.

Alveolar Deformities and Problems

Alveolar clefts are the result of the failure of fusion between the maxillary lateral palatal process and the premaxilla. The defect can be in the form of a unilateral or bilateral cleft and in conjunction with posterior palate defects. Unilateral clefts are more frequently found on the left and seem to be more prevalent in males.[14,15] A multitude of complications are associated with these anomalies.[16,17,18] The most obvious problem is the bony defect and maxillary segment instability. It results in periodontal deficits and poor bone support of the surrounding dentition. Often a decrease in maxillary development is seen secondary to growth disturbances initiated by previous operations. Positional changes of the mandible can produce an acceptable facial balance in many cases.[19] Poor alar base support can cause nasal asymmetry and poor facial contours. A displaced alveolar ridge toward the palate with tooth malalignment can arise from the scar tissue of early operations. Malocculsions of this type frequently are seen and increase in severity with the size of the cleft. Buccal crossbites are twice as common (32%) as in noncleft lip and palate patients and anterior crossbites are 6-12.5 times more frequent in the cleft patient.[20] The instability of the cleft segments and malposition compromise orthodontic and prosthetic rehabilitation. An oronasal fistula creates a problem that results in free passage of material between the oral cavity and nose. It is often accompanied by nasal crusting and food retention in the mucosal recess. This retention coupled with malalignment of the dentition results in poor oral hygiene. The fistula also produces hypernasal speech and swallowing difficulties that often can be improved with an obturator.

Dental abnormalities are also common.[21] Early loss of deciduous teeth and congenitally missing and altered eruption patterns often are seen. There is an increase in occurrence of supernumerary teeth and dental aplasia, especially in the deciduous dentition.[22,23] As the cleft sizes increase, the frequency of supernumerary teeth declines. The opposite is true for aplasia and the occurrence of fissural teeth; they increase with the severity of the cleft. Overall dental development is slower and eruption delayed.[24,25]

Objectives

The treatment objectives of alveolar cleft repair are both functional and aesthetic.[26,27,28,29] A major concern is to restore the osseous contour of the arch. This will prevent arch collapse and increase stability of the dento-osseous segment. In a bilateral cleft it will stabilize the premaxilla. A decrease in relapse potential also is achieved by disruption of scar beds from the previous operations.[30] In augmentation of the alveolar ridge the bony deficiency is eliminated and will improve the prosthetic result.

Increasing the viable alveolar ridge will improve the periodontal health of the surrounding teeth and therefore decrease tooth loss. The new supporting bone will allow for spontaneous eruption of developing canines and orthodontic movement of surrounding teeth. The repair also will provide the needed support for effective oronasal fistula closure. Aesthetics are improved by providing a nasal floor and increased alveolar base support. In addition, the upper lip is elevated, resulting in an improved cosmetic appearance.

Timing

There are two schools of thought regarding the timing of cleft repair. They are divided into primary osteoplasty and secondary osteoplasty.[13] True primary grafting of the alveolar cleft is performed in combination with soft tissue closure of the cleft lip in infancy. Secondary osteoplasty is divided into early and late repair. Early secondary grafting is delayed until eruption of the deciduous teeth. The bone is placed in a soft tissue bed that was prepared at the time of lip repair, usually before the second year of life. The growth problems associated with primary and early secondary grafting will be discussed later. Late secondary or tertiary osteoplasty[31] delays bone grafting until after eruption of the permanent teeth. In this technique lip repair is performed in the first few months of life. This philosophy has become the preferred modern-day procedure.

Cleft palate operations should be designed to have the least harmful effect on midface growth. Interference and surgical stimulation of active growth centers will retard development. Grafting of alveolar defects appears to have negligible effect on maxillary growth (transversely and anterio-posteriorly) after 7 to 8 years of age.[32,33,34,35] The maxillary first molar usually has erupted by that time. Most writers on the subject agree that the grafting should be performed prior to the eruption of the maxillary canine, when the root is one-quarter to one-half formed.[17,21,27,36] This corresponds to 9 to 12 years of age. When grafting is performed prior to eruption of the maxillary canine, the tooth may erupt spontaneously into the reconstructed cleft area and provide additional alveolar height by physiologic osteogenesis. When autogenous iliac grafts were used by El Deeb et al,[21] 27 percent of the developing canines erupted spontaneously and the remainder were moved into position with surgical uncovering or a combination of surgical exposure and orthodontics. Others have had similar impressive results.[18]

Treatment

Primary Repair. Cleft palate operations are designed to have the least possible adverse effect on midface growth. Since primary osteoplasty, or early bone grafting, was presented it has had many followers.[37-45] These authors advocate soft tissue repair of the cleft lip, bone grafting of the cleft palate and palatoplasty in the first year of life. They feel that early grafting of the arch provides maxillary fixation and prevents arch collapse, allows tooth migration into the graft and facilitates unit growth of the maxilla.[26] They also suggest that feeding, speech and psychologic development are improved by early bone grafting. Unfortunately most of the studies are marred by short followup and poor design. They concentrate on bone graft consolidation and crossbite frequency rather than on long-term effect on maxillary growth.

A new principle of primary cleft repair known as periostealplasty was presented by Skoog in 1965[46] He recommended the reflection of periosteal flaps to achieve periosteal continuity on both sides of the cleft. Skoog felt that the periosteum has sufficient osteogenic potential to provide osseous bridging, prevent maxillary collapse and improve symmetry. This procedure usually is performed between 3 to 6 months of age. The nasal floor is first reconstructed by subperiosteal reflection and suturing of the cleft mucosa. A rotational subperiosteal flap is then obtained from the lateral aspect of the maxilla, extending below the infraorbital foramen. This flap is transposed 180° to the bony cleft. The periosteum to periosteum approximation over the cleft is designed to provide for new bone formation.

Skoog[47,48] subsequently modified his approach to "boneless bone grafting" by recommending the use of Surgicel (oxidized regenerated cellulose) as a scaffold between periosteal layers. The Surgicel maintained a hematoma in the cleft area, provided a matrix and allowed molding postoperatively. He theorized that the hematoma in contact with osteogenic tissue was a perfect environment for osseous formation.

Unfortunately Skoog's results were not reproduced with a high degree of success. Bony production was incomplete and normal anatomy rarely was restored. Rintala et al.[49] used the same "boneless bone grafting" technique with free periosteal flaps. He obtained bony bridging in 54 percent, diffuse bridging in 32 percent and no bone formation in 24 percent of cases. Surgicel, in his experiment, did not improve the results. Engdahl[50] agreed that periosteum was vital for osseous regeneration but illustrated slower and reduced bone production when Surgicel was used compared to periosteum filled only with blood.

Secondary Bone Grafting. Growth retardation of the maxilla has been an unfortunate complication of early cleft procedures. The degree of deformity has been attributed to local manipulation of growth areas, postoperative decrease in circulation, palatal scarring, tension of the upper lip and bony diffusion of the palate. These factors result in a decrease in sutural growth with an increased incidence of lateral and anterior crossbites.[20,28,51,52]

Cephalometric analysis by Mastre et al.[53] and Ortiz-Monasterio et al.[54,55] found there was no difference in growth between unoperated alveolar cleft patients and noncleft patients. The growth may be even greater in patients with an unrepaired cleft lip. This is possibly a result of decreased lip tension of the maxilla. Growth potential may be the same, but cleft lip and palate patients are highly susceptible to extrinsic influences.

Most investigators have recommended abandoning early cleft repair.[26,27,51,55-64] Maxillary retrusion was not the only reason for the decrease in primary osteoplasty. Some authors have raised additional objections to early bone grafting: It is difficult to predict an infant's future deformity or need for orthodontics; extensive surgery can be too time-consuming for an infant; maxillary constriction and retrusion may result from incompatible growth potential of the graft when compared to the surrounding bone; and, infants may require additional bone grafting for stabilization of the arch. When patients have osseous defects of the cleft, even after primary repair, they most likely also will have a deformed maxillary ridge, maleruption of teeth into the cleft, persistent oronasal fistula and a retrognathic maxilla.[65]

Secondary osteoplasty, as mentioned, usually is performed when the root of the unerupted maxillary canine on the cleft side is one-quarter to one-half formed. This usually corresponds to an age of 9 to 12 years. The soft tissue repair of lip is done in the first few months of infancy.

Bone Grafting. The objectives of bone grafting of the alveolar cleft include the following: to stabilize the maxillary arch as a functional unit, to provide a viable bony structure for eruption and orthodontic movement, to close oronasal fistula, to improve prosthetic and facial aesthetics by furnishing osseous bulk and to improve the patient's psychological outlook.

Many bone grafting techniques and graft materials have been used. Rib, tibia and iliac bones have been the major sources. Rib usage has had a reported success rate of 34-81 percent.[26,62] This source is prone to infection and sequestration as a result of delayed and poor revascularization.[66] Ribs are primarily cortical bone and have little osteogenic potential. A true alveolar process is not formed and loss of bone height by resorption is extensive.[67] Teeth are unable to erupt through this graft and do not respond well to orthodontic forces[27,68] due to the excess cortical bone formed.[69] Rib graft harvesting also is associated with an increased morbidity (i.e., pneumothorax) over other donor sites.

Osteogenic propensity of cancellous bone is well documented.[70-74] Autogenous cancellous bone and marrow are capable of complete regeneration of an alveolar defect.[27] The iliac crest is an excellent source of this bone.

An autogenous cancellous bone and marrow graft heals initially by osteogenesis, then by resorption. Cortical bone (rib and block grafts) resorb, then produce bone by osteogenesis after a cavity has been formed.[75] Particulate grafts are preferred over one-piece cortical blocks. They regenerate faster and more completely over small defects.[27,72] Trapping of large nonviable areas that are seen with block grafts is avoided.

These grafts appear to accompany residual growth of the alveolar process and are stimulated with the eruption of a developing canine.[35] Burwell has shown that a combination of marrow and fresh cancellous bone have more osteogenic potential than either used separately.[71] The autogenic bone acts as a calcified matrix which increases the osteogenic potential. Cancellous bone tissue (fresh, frozen or freeze-dried) has the capacity to induce osteogenesis in marrow.

Osteoblasts within the marrow are derived from reticuloendothelial and endothelial origin. The success of the graft depends on the number of viable cells that survive the grafting procedure to form new bone. Marx et al.[76] recommend storing the bone harvest in normal saline or D5W. This will provide a working time of approximately four hours with 95-100 percent survival. Autologous serum, distilled water and variations in toxicity have been shown to decrease the viability of marrow cells.

The success of iliac bone grafting has been quite good. Recent studies have had a greater than 96 percent success rate.[18,63,77] The bone graft produces a stable, organized osseous bridge in three to six months.

Heterogenous and allogenic bone are also potential sources of graft material. The most notable heterograft is chemically treated calf bone, or Boplant. It produces poor results and is unable to stimulate osteogenesis.[78] Allogenic bone is obtained by cadaver harvest and then either cooled, frozen or freeze-dried. There are large areas of acellular matrix, so it is less antigenic than fresh allograft. Allogenic bone also is resorbed faster since it is not treated chemically. This bone does not have osteogenic potential. Urist,[79] however, identified an acid insoluable protein called bone morphogenetic protein (BMP) which mediates bone induction. It also induces mesenchymal cells of cancellous and marrow bone and fibroblasts of the recipient bed to differentiate into osetoblast. The latter are capable of stimulating bone formation. Higher levels of protein are found in cortical bone. Decalcified allogenic bone also has increased BMP when compared to a nondecalcified source.[80]

Allogenic graft material has several advantages.[81,82,83] Morbidity is decreased by avoiding an additional operation (iliac crest harvest), which is especially important in children. A large amount of bone is readily available when needed for extensive procedures (grafting of a LeFort I maxillary advancement in the cleft palate patient), thereby decreasing the amount of autologous bone needed. Histologically, it is similar to fresh allografts[84,85] and is immunologically compatible. There are several disadvantages. The possibility of transfer of infection or pathogenic agents is present but extremely remote due to the extensive screening and preparation of the donor source. There is a delayed rate of incorporation of allogenic bone compared to autogenous sources. This may require a longer period of immobilization postoperatively. Improved results are seen when mixed with fresh autogenous cancellous bone. Surface decalcified freeze-dried allogenic bone, as mentioned, has increased BMP levels when compared to freeze-dried only variety.[80] It appears to be more effective in grafting procedures. Recent studies show nondecalcified allografts have produced only a 30 percent bony retention,[86,87] while nearly 100 percent retention is seen with an autogenous cancellous marrow graft. Osteogenic potential of completely demineralized bone appears to be greater with less rejection when compared to partially demineralized allogenic grafts.[88]

In spite of the initial delay in bone formation with allogenic grafts when compared to autogenous sources histologically, after six weeks there is no difference in the rate.[86] Evidence of the inflammatory response is similar to the autografts with excellent host acceptance. Unfortunately the allografts do not appear to respond to passive eruption of teeth, and orthodontic or maxillary growth forces.[86,87] compared to the osteogenic potential of various grafting materials. Boyne found that most bone was formed with combinations of autogenous marrow and cancellous bone followed by autogenous marrow and cortical bone, and finally by autogenous marrow alone. Surface decalcified allograft with autogenous marrow was next, and the least amount of bone formation was seen with freeze-dried allogenic bone and autogenous marrow combination. Use of surface decalcified allogenic bone may be indicated when large quantities of grafting material are required and a limited source is available. However, for most alveolar cleft procedures autogenous marrow and cancellous bone are preferred.

Bone Substitutes. Many sources of nonbiologic bone substitutes have been used in grafting procedures.[88,89] Metals such as gold foil[90] and tantalum plate[91] have several disadvantages. These materials do not promote tissue adherency, corrode in a biologic environment, do not promote osteogenesis and have a tendency for fatigue failure. Surgicel, as mentioned earlier, and gelatin sponges also have been used, but they have not been shown to promote bone formation.

Silastic and proplast implants have been used in cleft augmentation.[92] They are encapsulated in fibrous tissue and lack bony support. Tooth eruption is not possible through these substances. They can, however, provide excellent contour restoration in the cleft area and improve the aesthetics of a prosthetic result. Bone resorption is seen occasionally below the graft as a result of the increased pressure and tension of the implant on the surrounding osseous structure.

Ceramics appear to provide the greatest potential of nonbiologic materials in cleft repair. They are extremely biocompatible and have high compression strength. Their specific gravities, coefficients of friction and surface characteristics are similar to bone.[93] Disadvantages include brittleness and poor tensile and flexural strength.[93] Fibrous and osteoid tissue is deposited on the surface of ceramics, forming an adherence between the host and implant.[95]

There are two categories of ceramics: soluable and insoluable. The most commonly used nonresorbable ceramic is hydroxylapatite. It is a nonporous calcium phosphate, polycrystalline ceramic with properties similar to enamel and cortical bone.[96] Normal bone healing and calcification is seen around the implant without fibrous capsule interference. Denissen[97] suggests a possible chemical bond occurs between hydroxylapatite and bone. Hydroxylapatite can be used alone or as a marrow extender in the repair of alveolar defects.[87] In the growing child eruption of maxillary canine into the cleft side repaired with hydroxylapatite (or in combination with marrow) has not been observed. This ceramic is extremely useful where tooth eruption and postoperative orthodontic movement are not a concern. The material's excellent biocapability and stability when placed subperioesteally make it an ideal adjunct for minor defects after tooth alignment and improving gingival contours for prosthetic rehabilitation.

Soluable ceramics are capable of augmenting bony defects and theoretically allow new bone formation on the lattice provided by the implant. Variable results have been achieved with plaster of paris. Researchers claim that the rate of absorption coincides with the rate of new bone deposition.[98] This material's high soluability rate limits its ability to function as a scaffold for bone formation. The rapid resorption and inherent weakness of the material results in frequent fragmentation.[99] This provides only transient support of surrounding structures.

Promising results have been obtained with another soluable ceramic, B tricalcium phosphate. Forbes[100] implanted this substance in artificially created clefts of secondary palates in beagles. The ceramic does not induce bone formation but elicits an exaggerated repair response from fibroblasts and osteoblasts, resulting in active bone formation. This possibly is mediated by macrophages which are attracted to the area. The macrophages ingest the ceramic and then may stimulate osteoid formation by osteoblasts adjacent to the tricalcium phosphate particles. This ceramic gradually is resorbed and then replaced with bone. The substance tends to break and migrate as a result of its low flexural strength and brittleness. These properties prevent adequate fixation and stabilization of the material.

Diagnosis and Treatment Planning

Extensive presurgical treatment planning is essential for successful alveolar cleft repair. A complete medical history, thorough clinical examination, mounted study casts, facial photographs and radiographic examination (panorex, anterioposterior, lateral cephalometric and periapical views) are required. With this data preoperative cephalometric soft tissue and dental analysis as well as postoperative predictions can be made.

A coordinated pretreatment evaluation should be made by a Cleft Palate Team, including an orthodontist, speech pathologist, otolaryngologist, prosthodontist, general dentist, psychologist and plastic and maxillofacial surgeons. This joint analysis will improve preoperative judgment regarding speech, hearing, dento-skeletal compensations and abnormalities. A prediction of the changes in these areas and their effects postoperatively are discussed with the patient.

Other factors also must be considered: the type (unilateral or bilateral) and extent (alveolar only or with palatal involvement) of the cleft, the amount of scar tissue (from previous operations), the presence of a fistula (oronasal) and the need for a pharyngeal flap. All of these concerns affect the surgical treatment. An assessment of existing dental malocclusion is made and the relationship to maxillary and mandibular skeletal abnormalities is defined. A combined maxillary and/or mandibular repositioning at the time of cleft repair may be required. Consideration of all of the mentioned variables is essential in formulating a treatment plan that will provide the patient with a stable, functional and aesthetic result.

Midface hypoplasia from impeded growth as a result of surgical scarring can be corrected partially by early maxillary orthopedics.[101] Frequently surgery is required to improve their transverse and anterior deficiencies. Orthodontic therapy usually is limited in repositioning malopposed segments. There are many advantages in the use of surgery to resolve these problems.[102] Treatment time is shortened and surgical expansion is more stable than with orthodontic techniques (especially when bone grafting is used). Improved occlusal harmony from surgical repositioning of the maxilla also will increase skeletal stability postoperatively as a result of dental interdigitation. Surgical segmental movement can improve the alar base and check support and restore arch form.

Alveolar cleft repair should be performed between the ages of 9 and 12. At this time the maxillary canine is one-quarter to one-half formed. Osteotomies should be delayed until growth is complete except when dramatic functional and psychological indications are present. The patient then should be warned of possible need for an additional operation when growth is complete. Boys, among cleft lip and palate patients, are at a greater risk of continued growth.[103] Continued forward growth of the mandible is the usual reason for unacceptable results. Females at 17 and males at 18 years of age usually have completed mandibular and maxillary growth; osteotomy should be deferred until this time. This rough age restriction should be correlated with serial cephalometric radiographs to confirm cessation of facial growth.

Maxillary advancement and segmental osteotomies have been described by other authors.[102,104,105] When performing these procedures in a combined manner, several requirements should be considered.[30,106] The incision should be designed to maintain blood supply; oral and nasal lining should be provided early in the procedure to improve healing and avoid oronasal contamination; segments must be mobilized adequately with passive repositioning; scar tissue must be excised to improve stability postoperatively; appropriate bone grafts are placed to assure stability; fragments must be fixated adequately; and, rotational or sliding flaps (from the gingiva, lips or tongue) are used as needed for closure without tension.

Postoperative stability is a prime consideration. Scar tissue from earlier operations causes vascular compromise and decreases mobility in the area. This results in production of counteractive forces of relapse. It is therefore vital to disrupt the scar beds with excision or rotational flaps. Establishing proper occlusal interdigitation also will improve stability, especially when a good canine relationship is obtained.

Bone grafting of maxillary advancement in the cleft patient is essential.[106] The graft material should be placed in the pterygomaxillary area, lateral osteotomy and cleft sites. Without grafting relapse has been reported to be between 31-68 percent. When bone grafts are utilized the figure decreases to 0-5 percent.[106] When bone grafts are used in maxillary advancement procedures it is not necessary to overcorrect the maxillary segment. In order to establish a good osseous union, skeletal fixation should be maintained for a period of four to eight weeks.[107]

Surgical management must coordinate with orthodontic treatment. Presurgical orthodontics should be aimed at improving alignment of the malopposed dentition. This will improve the hygiene and increase surgical access to the cleft area. Care should be taken not to destroy supporting bone of the teeth adjacent to the cleft by orthodontic treatment. The ability orthodontically to expand the palate in a cleft patient is severely compromised by the presence of scar tissue. Relapse is certain to occur. Orthodontic and prosthetic refinement of occlusion can begin six to eight weeks postoperatively.[108] Orthodontic movement at this time will be accelerated secondary to the postoperative increase in osteogenic potential of the surgically involved bone. Further reconstructive work should be delayed at least one year postoperatively. This will allow for complete resolution of edema from the secondary cleft repair.[107]

Technique

Once the patient is developmentally and orthodontically ready, the procedure is performed. The technique for secondary cleft repair is basically the same when done as a simple graft and oronasal fistula closure or when done in combination with maxillary repositioning.

Immediately preoperatively the patient is placed on intravenous antibiotics and steroid therapy. A first generation cephalosporin is preferred with iliac crest bone grafts to cover for possible skin and oral pathogens. Steroids have been found to significantly decrease postoperative swelling.[109] When not contraindicated, Solumedrol is given postoperatively for a period of 36 hours followed by an IM injection of a long-acting steroid (Depomedrol).

Systemic antihistamines have been recommended over topical vasoconstrictors (i.e., topical cocaine) for intubating purposes.[108] It is felt that use of topical agents such as cocaine could possibly compromise the vasculature of the nasal mucosa and therefore endanger the success of the repair.

Proper incision and flap design are essential for a good result. A properly developed mucoperiosteal flap will cover the cleft without tension. When possible, attached gingiva should cover the alveolar crest region. This will have the added benefit of providing attached gingiva to the maxillary ridge and erupting canine, if present.[35]

The initial incision is made at the cleft margin, outlining the labial and palatal extent of the defect. Unwanted scar and soft tissue is excised but mucoperiosteum is maintained in the area. A subperiosteal dissection is then performed on the lining of the nasal side of the cleft. The mucoperiosteal flaps are then raised the full length of the cleft superiorly (cephalod), providing tissue for the closure of the floor of the nose. Watertight approximation is obtained by interrupted horizontal mattress sutures with 4-0 Vicryl. This closure of the oronasal fistula will prevent contamination of the bone grafts by nasal secretions and certain graft failure.

A sulcular incision is carried out anteriorly and posteriorly to the cleft around the necks of the maxillary teeth on the facial and palatal aspects extending to the molar teeth. The oral mucoperiosteum at the margin of the cleft is then elevated to create an adequate flap for relaxed tissue closure. The width of the cleft is evaluated preoperatively by radiographs and clinical exam. The soft tissue required for closure of the defect is divided equally between both sides with an extra 2 mm added to allow for closure.[29] The undermined oral mucoperiosteum then can be advanced toward the midline, providing attached gingiva over the cleft area.

Often the defect is too large to be covered adequately with a sliding thickness flap, even with vertical facial and lateral palatal relaxing incisions. In cases of extensive clefts a pedicled mucosal flap can be used. Vestibular mucosa can be rotated 90°; or a trapezoidal lip flap taken superior to the cleft can be advanced. Proper flap design is required to assure sufficient blood supply to maintain the viability of the pedicle and graft below. The base of the flap should be at least one third of the length[29] to provide adequate arterial blood flow. Supraperiosteal releasing incisions can be used to decrease tissue tension that may occur with pedicle advancements.

Tongue flaps also can be used[110] as a highly vascular tissue source for fistula closure. A secondary tongue releasing procedure is required with this procedure, but the technique may be indicated in cases of combined cleft repair and maxillary osteotomies when vascular compromise is a greater risk.

Mucosal flaps do not provide attached gingiva, and they often cause a decrease in vestibular depth as a result of scar contracture. Vestibuloplasty with free gingival grafts (i.e., palatal grafts) to the alveolar ridge may be needed at a later time. All secondary procedures should be delayed until at least eight weeks after the alveolar cleft repair.[29]

Prior to closure of the oral mucoperiosteal flaps a cancellous bone and marrow graft is placed into the cleft. The bone is obtained from the iliac crest. An estimate of the amount of bone required is made by preoperative radiographs. The harvest should be performed concurrently with the development of the mucoperiosteal flaps via a two-team approach. This will minimize procedure time and length of time the bone must be stored prior to placement.

The prepared cleft bed is slightly overfilled with cancellous bone and marrow graft. This will improve bone contours and assure adequate height following postoperative resorption. The defect should not be filled to such an extent that tension-free tissue closure is not possible.

Once the bone graft has been placed in the alveolar graft, watertight closure is again obtained with multiple interrupted 4-0 Vicryl sutures. As previously stressed, to improve blood supply and graft viability the closure should be done without tension.

Bilateral alveolar clefts are complicated by the compromised blood supply to the premaxilla. Depending on the extent of the defect, the area receives its main blood flow from the nasal septum and the soft tissue in the vestibule of the upper lip. Incisions are made at the cleft margins as in a unilateral case. The mucoperiosteum of the alveolar defects are reflected to provide tissue for the nasal floor and fistula closure. The oral mucoperiosteal flap is developed posterior to the defect only. Reflection of the limited tissue from the frequently mobile premaxilla will damage the blood supply and may adversely affect the viability of the area. This restriction will necessitate greater development of the flap distal to the clefts and the increased use of releasing incisions.

Often the premaxilla is malpositioned and protruding in bilateral cleft situations. It should be repositioned and stabilized into a harmonious relation to the remaining dentition prior to bone grafting. This is accomplished by disimpacting the premaxilla from the vomer and nasal septum with removal of sufficient bone to allow for passive repositioning in a retruded position.

Postoperative stabilization is then obtained by maxillary splints and/or orthodontic archwire. Splints should remain in place for several weeks to allow a bony bridge to form at the graft site. Long-term retention is essential for a stable result. This also can be provided by orthodontic or prosthetic appliances.

The patient is placed on a liquid diet for several days to decrease masticatory trauma to the surgical area and to allow for healing. Advancement to a soft diet is done gradually and then maintained for several weeks. Healing also is improved with continuous emphasis on vigorous oral hygiene postoperatively. Salt water rinses are instituted for the first day following the operation.

As a result of the frequent dental and skeletal dysplasia (anteriorposterior, transverse and vertical malpositions) of these patients, a combined alveolar cleft repair and maxillary repositioning often is performed. Collapse of the maxillary arch and maxillary hypoplasia are the most common abnormalities.

Indications and technique for Le Fort I osteomies have been well documented,[111] as well as in combination with alveolar cleft repair.[29,102,104,107,108] When planning an incision and flap design for a combined procedure, consideration of the presence of oronasal fistula, scar tissue and blood supply is crucial. Scar tissue from previous operations has decreased vascularity and therefore limits the amount of oxygen delivered to the surgical area. The scar tissue also initiates a potent relapse force. To improve maxillary mobility, release of scar contractures should be included. The standard maxillary osteotomy incision is placed high in the vestibule. This may need to be altered to accomodate fistula closure. Including a sulcular incision and flap development around the teeth in the cleft area may be necessary. Palatal releasing and horizontal incisions anterior to the cleft should be used sparingly in order to preserve blood flow to areas that already have a tenuous supply.

When a horizontal vestibular incision is not possible, vertical incisions can be placed at the alveolar defect site and tuberosity on the cleft side. Osteotomy cuts are made through a tissue tunnel that is created by developing a subperiosteal communication between the two incisions. Sectioning of the anterior and lateral wall can be performed as well separation of the pterygoid plates from the maxillary tuberosity with a curved osteome.

Osteotomies of the medial wall of the maxilla can be performed if needed with an osteome directed to the bony areas through the lateral and anterior maxillary osteotomy site. Prior to down fracture, the mucoperiosteum lining the lateral nasal wall should be reflected. This will provide tissue for the future nasal floor and prevent tearing of tissue on disimpaction.

When the segment(s) has been mobilized adequately and the lateral nasal and septal mucoperiosteum have been sutured to form the nasal floor, an occlusal splint should be inserted. Once the teeth have been positioned into the desired occlusion and secured into the splint, the segment(s) is skeletally fixed with intraosseous wiring. Le Fort I osteotomies require intermaxillary fixation and skeletal suspension to assure stability. Bone grafting to the pterygomaxillary and lateral osteotomy sites is essential for all maxillary advancement procedures in cleft palate patients. Without grafting, significant relapse is certain (greater than 30%).[106]

The cancellous bone and marrow graft is placed in the prepared defect bed and palatal suturing is performed prior to placement of intermaxillary fixation wires. When fixation is secured the final bone is placed and the facial mucoperiosteal flaps are suture closed. Intermaxillary fixation is maintained for an average of four to six weeks. Stabilization of the maxillary arch will then require extended retention devices to prevent segmental collapse until a true bony union has formed.

Postoperative Complications

A close monitoring of the patient postoperatively is required for observation of possible complications.[13,27,36,77] Wound dehiscence often is seen with partial loss of the graft. This can be decreased by reflecting an adequate mucoperiosteal flap to close the defect without tension. Venous congestion and resulting edema may contribute to the dehiscence. Palatal splints and daily milking of the pedicle toward its base also may help the problem. When a dehiscence does occur, frequent irrigation, curettage of loose bone and meticulous oral hygiene should be stressed. If an infection is present with the dehiscence, antibiotic therapy also should be initiated. Infection can be avoided by controlling gingivitis and caries and stressing oral hygiene preoperatively.

Nasal hemorrhage can be avoided by careful contralateral nasal intubation. The surgeon can assist the anesthesiologist intraorally by guiding the endotracheal tube through the pharyngeal flaps, if present. Oral intubation is preferred in bilateral cleft patients. Pressure, nasal packs, cauterization or arterial ligation may be required when bleeding does occur.

A mucous discharge indicates failure of the nasal closure and possible recurrence of the nasal fistula. The frequency of the complication can be decreased by a avoiding postoperative nasal suctioning and nose blowing. Ample humidification to keep the nasal mucosa moist and nasal decongestants are recommended. When breakdown occurs, frequent normal saline irrigation and antibiotics should be started. Hall and Posnick[77] have reported a 2 percent recurrence rate of oronasal fistulas following repair of alveolar clefts by secondary bone grafts.

Loss of vestibular sulcus height from scar contraction may cause tension on the nasal philtrum. This can be treated when healing is complete with a vestibuloplasty procedure.

Instability can be controlled postoperatively with adequate orthodontic or prosthetic treatment. The mobility will improve if bony union is good. The use of long-term lingual wire retention or a prosthesis usually is required.

Occasionally laterally femoral cutaneous sensory nerve paresthesia and hematoma formation are seen at the iliac crest bone graft donor site. Nerve damage can be prevented by knowledge of surgical anatomy and careful dissection. Hematomas can be avoided with meticulous control of hemostasis, use of hemostatic agent (Gelfoam) in the donor site and adequate pressure dressing postoperatively. Potential iliac developmental disturbance can be prevented by avoiding the iliac crest in children. This area contains the epiphyses of the developing bone.[122] Iliac fracture and peritoneal perforation are additional complications that are possible, but with careful surgical technique they are rarely encountered. Harvest from the medial table of the iliac crest is the preferred source of antogenous marrow and cancellous bone.

REFERENCES

1. Diffenbach JF: Über des garamensegal des menchen und der saugetheire. *Lit Ann Ges Heilk,* 4:289, 1826.

2. von Langenbeck BRK: Operation der Anglebornen Totalen Spaltung des Harten Gaumens nach einer Neuer Methode. *Dtsche Klin,* 13:231, 1861.
3. Lexer E: Die Verwendung de freinen Knochenplatik nebst Versuchen üb Glenkeversteifung und Gelenktransplantation. *Langenbecks Arch Klin Chir,* 86:939, 1908.
4. Drachter R: Die Gaumenspalte und deren operative Berhandlung. *Dtsche Chir,* 131:1, 1914.
5. Beck C, Jesser J: Plastic surgery of the face. *Int J Orthod Oral Surg,* 7:81, 1921.
6. Wardill WFM: Cleft palate. *Br J Surg,* 16:127, 1928.
7. Veau V: *Division Palatine: Anatomie, Chirurgie, Phonetique.* Paris, Masson, 1931.
8. Kilner TP: Cleft lip and palate repair technique. *St Thomas Hosp Rep,* 2:122, 1937.
9. Axhausen G: *Technik und Ergebisse der Spalplastiken.* Munchen, Hanser, 1952.
10. Schmid E: Ännaherung der Kieferstumpfe bei Lippen-Kiefer-Gaumenspalten: ihre schadlichen folgen and Vermeidung. *Fortschr Kiefer Geischtschir,* 1:37, 1955.
11. Clausen H: Über die Korrektur angleborner Kiefer-spalten durch auf baunde Kieferkammplastik nach Schmid. *Dtsch Zahnarzteblatt,* 9:592, 1955.
12. Schruddle J, Stellmach R: Die primäre Osteoplastik der Defeckte des Kieferbogens bie Lippen-Kiefer-Gaumenspalten am Sauglinge. *Zentrable Chir,* 83:894, 1958.
13. Nylen B: Surgery of the alveolar cleft. *Plast Reconstr Surg,* 37:42, 1966.
14. Mirsa FM, Ray RK, Kapoor DN: Dental abnormalities in cases of cleft lip and palate. *J Indiana Dent Assoc,* 44:1, 1972.
15. Zilberman Y: Observations on the dentition and face in clefts of the alveolar process. *Cleft Palate J,* 10:230, 1973.
16. Boyne PJ, Sands NR: Combined orthodontic-surgical management of residual palate-alveolar cleft defects. *Am J Orthod,* 70:20, 1976.
17. Waite DE, Kersten RB: Residual and alveolar palatal clefts, in Bell WH, Profitt WR, White RP (eds): *Surgical Correction of Dentofacial Deformities.* Philadelphia, WB Saunders Co, 1980, pp 1329-1367.
18. Troxell JB, Fonseca RJ, Osborn DB: A retrospective of alveolar cleft grafting. *J Oral Maxillofacial Surg,* 40:721, 1982.
19. Shibasaki Y, Ross RB: Facial growth in children with isolated cleft palate, in *2nd Hamburg International Symposium.* New York, Grune & Stratton Inc, 1966.
20. Hellquist R, Ponten B, Skoog T: The influence of cleft length and palatoplasty on the dental arch and the deciduous occlusion in cases of clefts of the secondary palate. *Scand J Plast Reconstr Surg,* 12:45, 1978.
21. El Deeb M, Messer LB, Lehnert MW, et al: Canine eruption into grafted bone in maxillary alveolar cleft defects. *Cleft Palate J,* 19:9, 1982.
22. Bohn A: Dental anomalies in harelip and cleft palate. *Acta Odontol Scand,* 21:suppl 38:1, 1963.
23. Ranta R: The development of permanent teeth in children with complete cleft lip and palate. *Proc Finn Dent Soc,* 68:suppl 3, 1972.
24. Fishman LS: Factors related to tooth number, eruption, time and tooth position in cleft palate individuals. *J Dent Child,* 37:303, 1970.
25. Ranta R: Eruption of premolars and canine and factors affecting it in unilateral cleft lip and palate cases: An orthopantomographic study. *Suom Hammaslaakitoim,* 67:350, 1971.
26. Epstein LI, Davis BW, Thompson LW: Delayed bone grafting in cleft palate patients. *Plast Reconstr Surg,* 46:363, 1970.
27. Boyne PJ, Sands NR: Secondary bone grafting of residual alveolar and palatal clefts. *J Oral Surg,* 30:87, 1972.
28. Freide H, Johansen B: A follow-up study of the facial skeleton in adolescence. *J Maxillofacial Surg,* 5:267, 1977.
29. Epker BN, Wolford LM: *Dentofacial Deformities.* St. Louis, C V Mosby Co, 1980.
30. Kinnebrew MC, Kent JN: Late definitive correction of the orofacial cleft. *Am J Orthod,* 84:104, 1983.

31. Pickrell K, Quinn G, Massengill R: Primary bone grafting of the maxilla in cleft of the lip and palate: A four year study. *Plast Reconstr Surg,* 41:438, 1968.
32. Lebret L: Growth change of the palate. *J Dent Res,* 41:1391, 1962.
33. Bjork A, Skieller V: Growth in width of the maxilla studied by implant method. *Scand J Plast Reconstr Surg,* 8:26, 1974.
34. Bjork A, Skieller V: Growth in the maxilla in three dimensions as revealed radiographically by implant method. *Br J Orthod,* 4:52, 1977.
35. Abyholm FE, Bergland O, Semb G: Secondary bone grafting of alveolar grafts. *Scand J Plast Reconstr Surg,* 15:127, 1981.
36. Broude DJ, Waite DE: Secondary closure of alveolar defects. *J Oral Surg,* 37:289, 1974.
37. Backdahl M, Nordin KE: Replacement of maxillary bone defect in cleft palate. *Acta Chir Scand,* 122:133, 1961.
38. Georgiade NC, Pickrell KL, Quinn GW: Varying concepts in bone grafting of alveolar palate defects. *Cleft Palate J,* 1:42, 1964.
39. Lynch JB, Lewis SR, Blocker TG: Maxillary bone grafts in cleft palate patients. *Plast Reconstr Surg,* 37:91, 1966.
40. Monroe CW, Griffith HB, Rosenstein SW, Jacobson BN: The correction and preservation of arch form in complete clefts of the palate and alveolar ridge. *J Plast Reconstr Surg,* 41:108, 1968.
41. Robinson F, Wood B: Primary bone grafting in the treatment of cleft lip and palate with special reference to alveolar collapse. *Br J Plast Surg,* 22:336, 1969.
42. Nylen B, Korloff B, Arnander C, et al: Primary early bone grafting in complete clefts of the lip and palate: A follow-up study of 53 cases. *J Plast Reconstr Surg,* 8:79, 1974.
43. Schmid E, Widmeier W, Reichert H, Stein K: The development of cleft upper jaw following primary osteoplasty and orthodontic treatment. *Maxillofacial Surg J,* 2:92, 1974.
44. Rosenstein SW, Jacobson BN, Monroe DA, et al: A series of cleft lip and palate children five years after undergoing orthopedic bone grafting procedures. *Angle Orthod,* 42:1, 1972.
45. Rosenstein SJ, Monroe CW, Kernahan DA, et al: The case for early bone grafting in cleft lip and cleft palate. *Plast Reconstr Surg,* 70:297, 1982.
46. Skoog T: The use of periosteal flaps in the repair of clefts of the primary palate. *Cleft Palate J,* 2:323, 1965.
47. Skoog T: The use of periosteum and Surgicel for bone restoration in congenital clefts of the maxilla. *Scand J Plast Reconstr Surg,* 1:113, 1967.
48. Skoog T: Repair of unilateral cleft lip deformity: Maxilla, nose and lip. *Scand J Plast Reconstr Surg,* 3:109, 1969.
49. Rintala A, Solivio A, Ranta R, et al: On the bone forming capacity of periosteal flap in surgery for cleft lip and palate. *Scand J Plast Reconstr Surg,* 8:58, 1974.
50. Engdahl E: Bone regeneration in maxillary defects. *Scand J Plast Reconstr Surg,* 6(Suppl 8):1, 1972.
51. Slaughter WB, Brodie AG: Facial clefts and their surgical management of recent research. *Plast Reconstr Surg,* 4:3, 1949.
52. Moffet BC: A research perspective on craniofacial morphogenesis. *Acta Morphol Neerl Scnd,* 10:91, 1972.
53. Mestre JC, DeJesus S, Subtelny JD: Unoperated oral clefts at maturation. *Angle Orthod,* 30:78, 1960.
54. Ortiz-Monasterio F, Rebeil As, Valderramo M, Cruz R: Cephalometric measurements of adult patients with nonoperated cleft palates. *Plast Reconstr Surg,* 35:276, 1972.
55. Ortiz-Monasterio F, Olmedo A, Trigos I, et al: Final results from delayed treatment of patients with cleft of the lip and palate. *Scand J Plast Reconstr Surg,* 8:109, 1974.
56. Graber TM: A cephalometric analysis of development pattern of facial morphology of cleft palate. *Angle Orthod,* 19:91, 1941.

57. Graber TM: The congenital cleft palate deformity. *J Am Dent Assoc,* 48:375, 1954.
58. Pruzansky S: Pre-surgical orthopedics and bone grafting for infants with cleft lip and palate: A dissent. *Cleft Palate J,* 1:164, 1964.
59. Stenström SJ, Thilander BL: Facial skeleton growth after bone grafting to surgically created premaxillary suture defects: An experimental study on the guinea pig. *Plast Reconstr Surg,* 40:1, 1967.
60. Robertson NRE, Jolleys A: Effects of early bone grafting in complete clefts of the lip and palate. *Plast Reconstr Surg,* 42:414, 1968.
61. Rehrman AH, Koberg WR, Koch H: Long term post-operative results of primary and secondary bone grafting in complete clefts of the lip and palate. *Cleft Palate J,* 7:206, 1970.
62. Hogeman KE, Jacobson S, Sarnas KV: Secondary bone grafting in cleft palate: A follow-up of 145 patients. *Cleft Palate J,* 9:39, 1972.
63. Johanson B, Ohlsson A, Friede H, Ahlgren J: A follow-up study of cleft lip and palate patients treated with orthodontics, secondary bone grafting and prosthetic rehabilitation. *Scand J Plast Reconstr Surg,* 8:121, 1974.
64. Peat JH: Early orthodontic treatment for complete clefts. *Am J Orthod,* 65:28, 1974.
65. Schuchardt K: Treatment of patients with cleft of the lip, alveolus, and palate. *2nd Hamburg International Symposium.* New York, Grune & Stratton Inc, 1966.
66. Zeiss IM, Nisbet NW, Heslop BF: Studies on transference of bone: Vascularization of autologous and homogenous implants of cortical bone in rats. *Br J Exp Pathol,* 41:345, 1960.
67. Pickrell K, Quinn G, Massengill R: Primary early bone grafting in complete cleft of the lip and palate: A follow-up study of 53 cases. *Scand J Plast Reconstr Surg,* 8:79, 1968.
68. Spriestersbach DC, Dickson DR, Fraser FC, et al: Clinical research in cleft lip and cleft palate: The state of the art. *Cleft Palate J,* 10:113, 1973.
69. Longacre JJ: Treatment of patients with clefts of the lip, alveolus, and palate. *2nd Hamburg International Symposium.* New York, Grune & Stratton, 1966.
70. Mowlem R: Bone grafting. *Br J Plast Surg,* 16:295, 1963.
71. Burwell RG: Studies in transplantation of bone. *J Bone Joint Surg,* 48:532, 1966.
72. Boyne PJ: Restoration of osseous defects in maxillofacial casualties. *J Am Dent Assoc,* 78:767, 1969.
73. Boyne PJ: Autogenous bone and marrow transplants. *Clin Orthop,* 73:199, 1970.
74. Ames JR, Ryan DE, Maki KA: The autogenous particulate cancellous bone marrow graft in alveolar clefts. *Oral Surg,* 51:588, 1981.
75. Albrektsson T: Repair of bone grafts: A vital microscopic and histological investigation in the rabbit. *Scand J Plast Reconstr Surg,* 14:1, 1980.
76. Marx RE, Snyder RM, Kline SN: Cellular survival of human marrow during placement of marrow cancellous bone grafts. *J Oral Surg,* 37:712, 1979.
77. Hall HD, Posnik JC: Early results of secondary bone grafts in 106 alveolar clefts. *J Oral Maxillofacial Surg,* 41:289, 1983.
78. Bell WH: Use of heterogenous bone in oral surgery. *J Oral Surg,* 19:459, 1961.
79. Urist MR: *Isolation and Characterization of Bone Morphogenetic Protein in Bone Grafting: Biology and Application.* Read before the Plastic Surgery Research Foundation of San Diego and The Bone and Joint Disease Foundation Course, Dec 4-6, 1981.
80. Kaban LB, Milliken JB, Glowacki J: Treatment of jaw defects with demineralized bone implants. *J Oral Maxillofacial Surg,* 40:263, 1982.
81. Boyne PJ: Review of the literature on cryopreservations of bone. *Cryobiology,* 4:341, 1968.
82. Epker BN, Wolford LM: *Dentofacial Deformities.* St. Louis, C V Mosby Co, 1980, pp 332; 371.
83. Osbon DB, Lilly GE, Thompson CW, Jost T: Bone grafts with surface decalcified allogenic and particulate autologous bone: Report of cases. *J Oral Surg,* 35:276, 1972.
84. Pike RL, Boyne PJ: Composite autogenous marrow and surface decalcified implants in mandibular defects. *J Oral Surg,* 31:905, 1973.

85. Langer F, Czitrom A, Pritzker KP, Gross AE: The immunogenicity of fresh and frozen allogenic bone. *J Bone Joint Surg,* 57A:216, 1975.
86. Boyne PJ: Implants and transplants: Review of recent research in this area of oral surgery. *J Am Dent Assoc,* 87:1074, 1973.
87. Marx RE, Millir RI, Ehler WJ, et al: A comparison of particulate allogenic and particulate autogenous bone grafts into maxillary alveolar clefts in dogs. *J Oral Maxillofacial Surg,* 42:3, 1984.
88. Narang R, Wells H, Laskin DM: Experimental osteogenesis with demineralized allogenic bone matrix in extraskeletal sites. *J Oral Maxillofacial Surg,* 40:133, 1982.
89. Weinberg S, Moncarz V: Response of oral tissue to implants totally covered by mucous membrane. *Oral Surg Rev,* 5:68, 1974.
90. Goldman EH, Stratigos GT, Arthur AL: Treatment of antraoral fistula by gold foil closure: Report of case. *J Oral Surg,* 27:875, 1969.
91. Budge CT: Closure of antraoral opening by use of Tantalum plate. *J Oral Surg,* 10:320, 1952.
92. Kent JM, Homsy CA, Hinds EC: Proplast in dental facial reconstruction. *Oral Surg,* 39:347, 1975.
93. Bhaskar SN, Brady JM, Getter L, et al: Biodegradable ceramic implant in bone. *Oral Surg,* 32:336, 1971.
94. Kingery WD, Bowen HK, Uhlman DR: *Introduction to Ceramics.* New York, John Wiley & Sons, 1976, p 4.
95. Smith L: Ceramic-plastic material as a bone substitute. *Arch Surg,* 87:653, 1968.
96. McConnell D: *Apatite.* New York, Springer-Verlag, 1973.
97. Denissen HW, de Groot K, Makkes P, et al: Tissue response to dense apatite implants in rats. *J Biomed Mater Res,* 14:713, 1980.
98. Peltier LF: The use of plaster of paris to fill defects in bone. *Clin Orthop,* 21:1, 1960.
99. Driskell TD, O'Hara MJ, Grade GA: *Management of Hard Tissue Avulsive Wounds and Management of Orofacial Fractures.* Report No 2, US Army Medical Research and Development Command. Contract No DAD A17-69-C-9118, 1971, pp 1-139.
100. Forbes DP: *Repair of Surgical Clefts of the Secondary Palate with Beta Tricalcium Phosphate Ceramic in Beagles,* thesis, Northwestern University, Chicago, 1981.
101. Holtz MM, Gnoinski WM: Effects of early maxillary orthopedics in coordination with delayed surgery for cleft lip and palate. *Maxillofacial Surg,* 7:201, 1979.
102. Tideman H, Stoelinga P, Gallia L: Le Forte I advancement with segmental palatal osteotomies in patients with cleft palates. *J Oral Surg,* 38:196, 1980.
103. Freihofer JP: Results of osteotomies of the facial skeleton in adolescence. *J Maxillofacial Surg,* 5:267, 1977.
104. Henderson D, Jackson IT: Combined cleft lip revision, anterior fistula closure and maxillary osteotomy: A one stage procedure. *Br J Oral Surg,* 13:333, 1975.
105. Epker BN, Freidlander G, Wolford LM, West RA: The use of freeze dried bone in middle-third face advancements. *Oral Surg,* 42:278, 1976.
106. Aroujo A, Schendel SA, Wolford LM, Epker BN: Total maxillary advancement with and without bone grafting. *J Oral Surg,* 36:849, 1978.
107. Braun TW, Sotereanos GC: Orthognathic surgical reconstruction of cleft palate deformities in adolescents. *J Oral Surg,* 39:255, 1981.
108. Braun TW, Sotereanos GC: Orthognathic and secondary cleft reconstruction of adolescent patients with cleft palate. *J Oral Surg,* 38:425, 1980.
109. Schaberg SJ, Stuller CB, Edwards SM: Effects of methylprednisolone on swelling after orthognathic surgery. *J Oral Maxillofacial Surg,* 42:256, 1974.
110. Kinnebrew MC, Malloy RB: Posterior based, lateral lingual flaps for alveolar cleft bone graft coverage. *J Oral Maxillofacial Surg,* 41:555, 1983.

111. Epker BN, Fish LC, Paulus PJ: Surgical-orthodontic correction of maxillary deficiency. *Oral Surg,* 46:171, 1978.
112. Crockford DA, Converse JM: The ilium as a source of bone grafts in children. *Plast Reconstr Surg,* 50:270, 1972.

CHAPTER 7

ROLE OF THE PEDIATRIC DENTIST IN CLEFT PALATE REHABILITATION

R. WILLIAM CORNELL

Confucius said, "Never do to others what you would not like them to do to you," one single saying that could be acted upon every day. . .

. . . Confucius

POSSIBLY the greatest challenge in treating children is knowing that what is done today will have a lasting effect upon their lives. It is both challenging and satisfying to render dental care to the patient with cleft palate. The pedodontist and general dentist have a responsibility to this patient to maintain the teeth and supporting structures in optimum health. It is extremely gratifying to know that the treatment provided will result in a healthy, aesthetic, functioning and stable dentition.[1]

All too frequently the role played by the pedodontist in cleft palate rehabilitation is overshadowed by the more dramatic phases of treatment.[2] However, the restoration of a malformed central incisor or painful carious molar can be equally important to the patient. Unless the patient has good dental and periodontal health, the efforts of the surgeon, speech therapist and orthodontist are in jeopardy. It would be very difficult to determine which aspect of the total treatment is the most important to the patient, as each specialist is dependent on the other for an optimal result.[3]

Treatment of the cleft palate patient is a process which begins at birth and continues throughout the life of the patient. Because of the diverse medical, dental and socioeconomic needs of these patients, their management involves many disciplines working together in a coordinated effort. No one practitioner is qualified to undertake complete and total treatment alone. It is imperative that each specialist involved in treatment planning be conversant with the problems, approaches and possibilities of the other members of the treatment team. Each must be willing, within reasonable limits, to compromise his particular treatment philosophy if best interests of the patient are to be fulfilled. No one phase of treatment, no matter how specialized and technical, should be instituted without the consultation and approval of the cleft palate team involved.[4]

The Cleft Palate Team at Northwestern University's Cleft Lip and Palate Institute is composed of the following consultants: a pedodontist, orthodontist, prosthodontist (director), plastic surgeon, speech therapist, otolaryngologist, audiologist and social worker (team coordinator). The Cleft Palate Institute is one of the more than 200 treatment centers listed in the American Cleft Palate Association Directory. Interested dentists should become familiar with the cleft palate team(s) in their areas and assure that their cleft palate patients receive the benefits of this approach.

A major advantage of the team approach is that each specialist has an opportunity to examine the patient on a regular basis. Histories, examination reports and records (dental radiographs, etc.) are secured and reviewed by the consultants. Together the team members assess the patient in a manner that each specialist mutually enhances the others in developing a comprehensive plan of rehabilitation.

At the initial staffing the pedodontist fills out a Dental Consultation Report (Fig. 7-1) which reviews the surgical, medical and dental status and includes a complete clinical examination with recommendations. Each specialist in turn examines the patient and completes a written report to be reviewed with the other members of the team. The coordinator then presents the recommendations to the family and arrangements are made for their implementation. The consultant may or may not be the provider who performs the services recommended for the patient, so the team coordinator must see that the individuals responsible for the patient's care are notified and recommendations are carried through.

Both the consultant of the cleft palate team and the pedodontist or general dentist treating the patient play an important role in cleft palate rehabilitation. The pediatrician's responsibility is to maintain the general health status of the child. The pedodontist's role is analogous to this in that it becomes his responsibility to maintain a superior state of dental health throughout the critical period from birth to early teens when the major portion of the cleft palate treatment is undertaken. The well trained pedodontist has the necessary background to make him conversant with the other dental disciplines such as orthodontics, prosthodontics and restorative dentistry.[4] The problems of the cleft lip and palate patient are fertile ground for the interest and activities of pedodontists, since the entire anatomy and function of the oral cavity and perioral structures of the child are involved in the defect. Clefts of the lip and palate affect eating, speaking, hearing, facial growth, dental occlusion and psychosocial development. The pedodontist, orthodontist and prosthodontist have major roles in the restoration of form and function in the cleft palate.[5]

Clinical Aspects of Cleft Lip and Palate Patients

Cleft lips and palates are best described with reference to their embryologic development[6] (Fig. 7-2). During normal fetal development in the first trimester there

DENTAL CONSULTATION REPORT

NAME________________________ BD________________ DATE__________

Type of Problem: VP Insuff_______ VP Incomp_______ VP Inadq._______ Other_______
Type of Cleft: Veau I____ II____ III____ IV____ Submucous____ Other____
Surgical Repair Status: Lip: Op____ Unopp____ Palate: Op____ Unopp____ Pharyngeal Flap____
Medical Status:____
Dental Status:____

CLINICAL EXAM

Soft Tissue:

Lip____ Frenum____ Palate____ Gingiva____ Buccal Mucosa____ Floor of Mouth____ Pharynx____
Tongue____ Tonsils____

Hygiene:

____ Good ____ Fair ____ Poor ____ Plaque ____ Calculus

Occlusion:

Molar R____ L____ Overjet____
Canine R____ L____ Overbite____
Cross Bites Posterior R____ L____ Anterior____
Alignment Normal____ Crowding____ Spacing____

Teeth:

1	2	3	4	5	6	7	8	9	10	11	12	13	14	15	16
			a	b	c	d	e	f	g	h	i	j			
			t	s	r	q	p	o	n	m	l	k			
32	31	30	29	28	27	26	25	24	23	22	21	20	19	18	17

Caries:________________ Hypoplasias:________________

Radiographic Findings:____
____

RECOMMENDATIONS:

Examination________________ Radiographs________________
Oral Hygiene Instructions__________ Prophylaxis__________ Fluoride__________
Restorative Tx__________ Ortho Tx__________ Extractions__________
Pulp Tx________________ Other________________
COMMENTS:____
____
____
____
____
____
____
____
____
____

____
Staff Consultant

Figure 7-1. Dental Consultation Report used by Northwestern University's Cleft Lip and Palate Institute.

is fusion of the median nasal process with the maxillary process to form the premaxilla, the corresponding segments of the alveolar process (gum pad) and finally the labial tuberculum of the upper lip. Because embryonic growth and fusion of tissue anterior to the incisive foramen precedes the formation of the more posterior palatal structures, the anterior tissue is defined chronologically as the primary palate and the posterior tissue as the secondary palate. The lateral palatal processes fuse posteriorly from the incisive foramen in the midline to form the secondary palate. The palatal processes also fuse superiorly with the nasal septum and anteriorly with the premaxilla. The fusion process begins in the vicinity of the future incisive foramen and proceeds anteriorly and posteriorly from that point. These events occur between the 8th and 10th uterine weeks.[7]

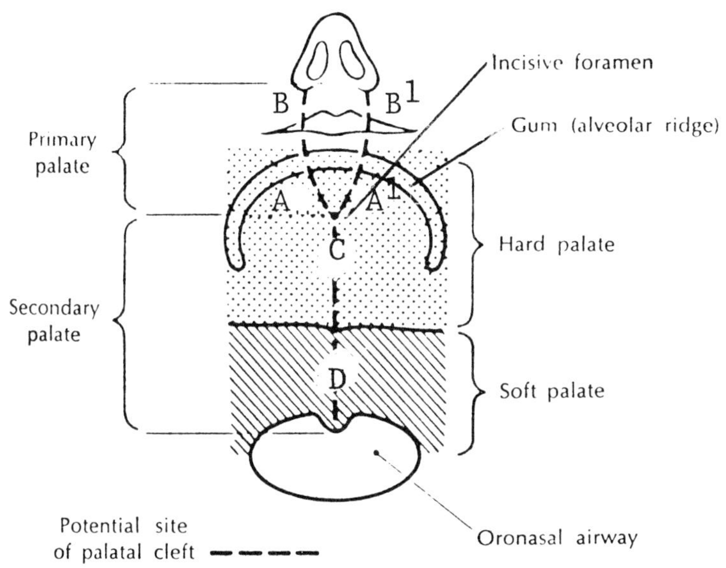

Figure 7-2. The incisive foramen divides the anomalies of cleft lip from cleft palate. Fissures anterior to the foramen (A and/or B or A[1] and/or B[1] are termed primary palatal clefts and may involve the anterior hard palate, alveolar ridge, lip and base of the nose. Those clefts posterior to the foramen (C and/or D) are termed secondary and may include defects of the soft palate and posterior hard palate.

Types of Clefts

Clefts of the primary palate can be unilateral ($A+B$ or A_1+B_1) or bilateral ($A+B$ and A_1+B_1), complete ($A+B$ or A_1+B_1) or incomplete (B or B_1). An incomplete cleft of the primary palate involves the lip only. A complete primary cleft is a fissure which divides the entire lip and involves the base of the nose, the alveolar ridge and the hard palate up to the incisive foramen. Clefts of the secondary palate (those posterior to the incisive foramen) also can be complete or incomplete ($D+C$ or D). An incomplete defect is a posterior fissure which does not communicate with the incisive foramen. It is basically a soft palate deformity but may involve a portion of the hard palate or just the uvula. A complete secondary palatal cleft connects with the incisive foramen and includes all of the soft and most of the hard palate.

Primary and secondary palatal clefts may appear in various combinations.[6] A complete unilateral cleft lip and palate ($B+A+C+D$ or B_1+A_1+C+D), the most common type of cleft, occurs about 50 percent of the time.[9] The unilateral cleft of the lip and palate extends from the soft palate to the incisive foramen, and then passes to either the right or left of the premaxillary segment. It passes through the alveolus and extends through the lip to the base of the nose. Collapse of the lateral border of the nose (ala) on the side of the cleft is due to the lack of continuity of the nostril and inadequate support of the lip.[8]

A complete bilateral cleft lip and palate ($B+B_1+A+A_1+C+D$) is the most severe type of cleft. The palatal cleft extends from the soft palate to the area of the incisive foramen; it then passes to both sides of the primary palate, leaving it isolated at the end of the nasal septum. The resultant deformities require skilled dental treatment.

Role of the Pedondontist

The pedodontist is expected to: (1) See that the developing jaws and dentition are guided into as normal an occlusion as possible, (2) educate the parent and child in dental preventive procedures, and (3) maintain the primary and young permanent dentition in optimum health. To accomplish these goals the pediatric dentist will need to work closely with the other dentists on the cleft palate team. The orthodontist usually is involved early to optimize the patient's occlusion. Later the prosthodontist replaces missing teeth and corrects anatomical deficiencies involving the hard and soft palate. The pedodontist must be attuned to the multiple needs of the young cleft lip and palate child and be ready to meet these needs with knowledge, skill and ingenuity.

The first challenge to the infant with a cleft is eating. Because of the continuity between oral and nasal cavities, food may be forced into the nasal cavity out through the nose. This necessitates long and frequent feedings which are time consuming for the parent and could, as teeth erupt, result in nursing bottle-like caries.[5] Another early problem is the medial collapse of the maxillary segments in unilateral and bilateral complete clefts after lip closure.

Several authors have suggested that an intraoral orthopedic appliance should be placed prior to lip surgery and maintained until the palate is closed.[10-14] It is their opinion that the action of the repaired taut lip will "bend" the segments of the maxillary arch into a more favorable alignment with an orthopedic prosthesis in place.[12] The appliance is designed to hold the lateral segments apart with acrylic while the premaxillary area is free to be molded by the lips. Soft heat-pliable acrylic within the cleft itself retains the obturator comfortably in place. The infant readily accepts the appliance and feeding is improved immediately.[14] This prosthesis functions as both a splint and an obturator. In addition to preventing the collapse of the lateral palate segments, the orthopedic appliance facilitates feeding, tongue posture and function, and if used for a prolonged period, the development of speech.[11]

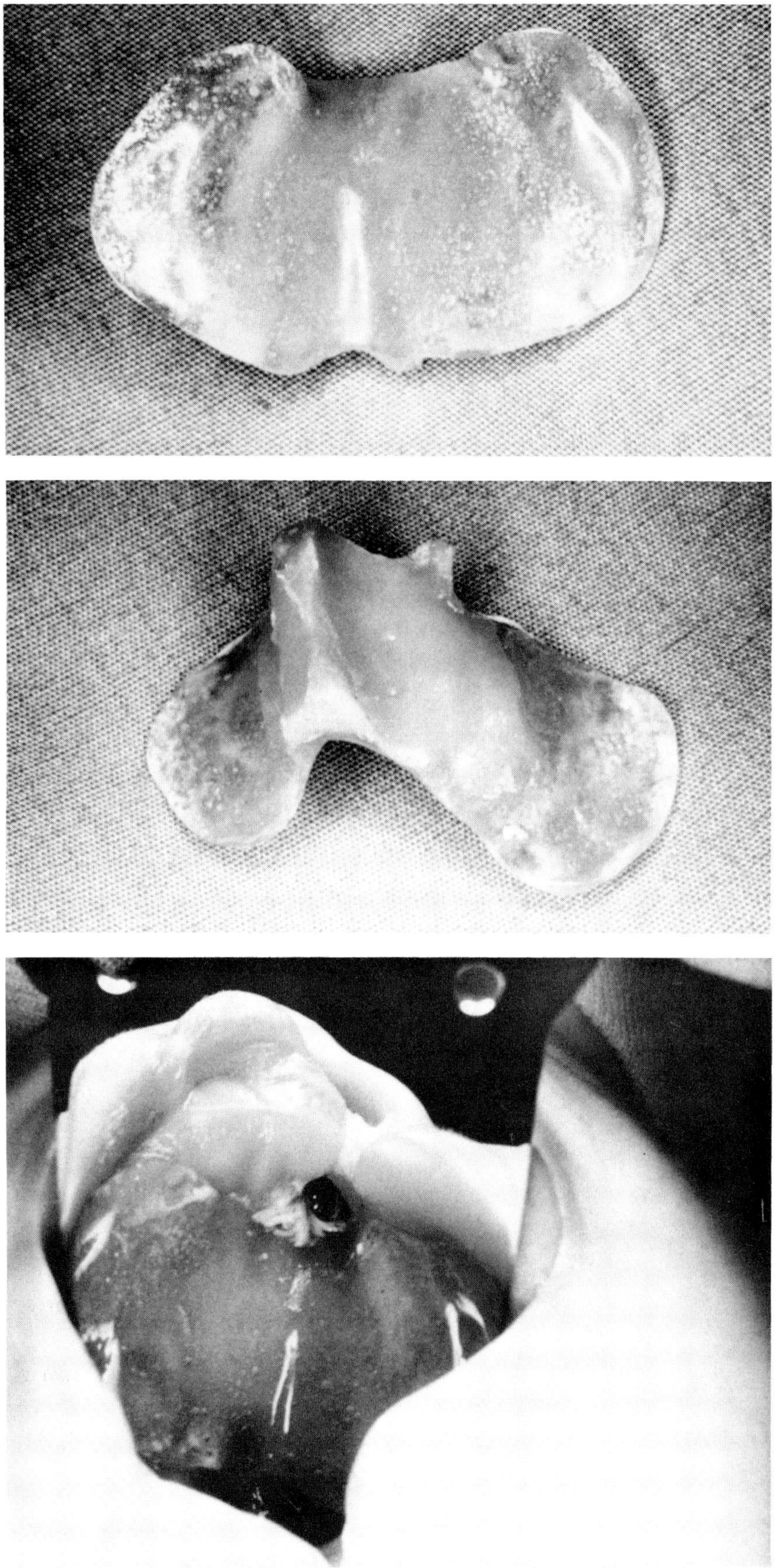

Figure 7-3. (a) Palatal view of the intraoral orthopedic appliance. (b) Cleft view of the obturator. (c) Appliance in place in a cleft lip and cleft palate before lip surgery.

The technique for obtaining an impression of the maxillary arch and cleft in the newborn and the design and construction of the orthopedic appliance have been described and illustrated very adequately by Jacobson and Rosenstein.[11,14] Troutman[13] treated 17 infants with complete unilateral clefts of the lip and palate with the maxillary lateral segments in good arch alignment prior to lip surgery. His study showed that with a passive orthopedic appliance there was no buccal crossbite or medial collapse in the primary dentition in eight (47%) of his cases. Six (35%) showed a partial collapse or crossbite of the primary canines only. Three (17.6%) showed a complete crossbite or medial collapse of the total buccal segment on the cleft side. Troutman recommended that the appliance should maintain the lateral segments in an acceptable position prior to and immediately following lip surgery and that it should be worn until the palate is closed.

In bilateral clefts of the lip and palate where the newborn presents with a protruding "floating" premaxilla, an extraoral "headgear" appliance has been used to facilitate surgical closure of the lips. Jones[15] in a case report, describes how such an appliance retracts the premaxilla. An acrylic cap fits over the premaxilla and a length of 0.036-inch wire connects the cap to elastic straps sewn into a head bonnet worn by the infant.

Early involvement of the pediatric dentist in the treatment of the cleft lip and palate newborn can contribute significantly to the rehabilitation of these children. Prominent in this treatment is the orthopedic management of the developing lateral segments of the palate and premaxilla before and following lip and palatal surgery to assure optimal alignment of the maxillary arch and the emerging dentition.

Dentition

Once the primary teeth in the maxillary arch erupt the pedodontist should be available to evaluate the effect of the cleft lip and palate upon the developing dentition. Supernumerary teeth occur more frequently in these children, possibly because the cleft produces a fold in the embryonic dental lamina and the attached tooth germ. A larger defect in the alveolar process could result in aplasia due to a rupture of the dental epithelium.[16] Of 119 cleft palate patients at Northwestern University Cleft Palate Institute, 21 percent had one or more supernumerary teeth. Fifty-nine patients (49.6%) had congenitally missing teeth.[3] A rupture in the dental epithelium either distal or mesial to the tooth germ could explain why the lateral incisor sometimes develops in the premaxilla and at other times in the lateral palatal segment. A disturbance created by the cleft often affects the permanent central incisor on the cleft side and causes it to be rotated or tipped and to have abnormal form[16] (Fig. 7-4).

Delayed eruption and asymmetrical development in the dentition of cleft children have been blamed on nutritional disturbances and surgical intervention. The most probable cause, however, is a genetic factor which is responsible for the occurrence of the cleft and the associated malformations.[16]

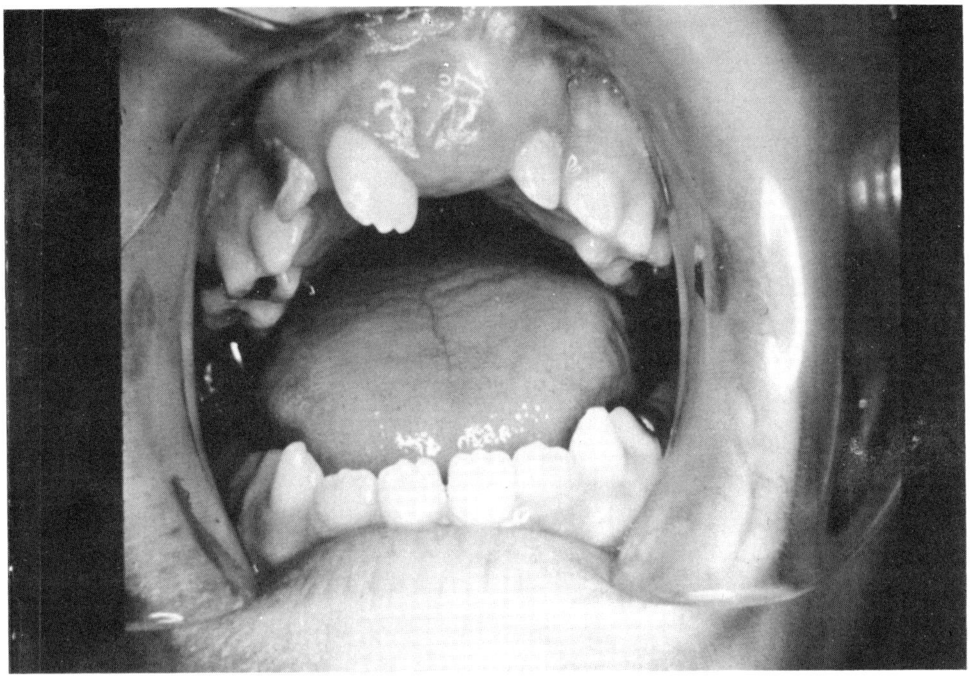

Figure 7-4. Mesially rotated permanent maxillary right central incisor in a surgically repaired complete bilateral cleft lip and palate patient.

Abnormalities and Dental Implications

Jordan[17] reviewed the study models of 105 cleft and 87 noncleft individuals along with tooth buds of 10 human fetuses with cleft lip and/or palate and found a total of 15 separate and distinct dental abnormalities. It is of interest that many specimens in the prenatal and postnatal cleft populations displayed multiple abnormalities of both maxillary and mandibular dentitions, while others showed either single aberations or in some cases none whatsoever.

Missing primary and permanent teeth are the most common dental abnormality in cleft patients. Thirty-five (25.7%) of the cleft models had missing teeth. The tooth most often missing is the lateral incisor at the site of the cleft, but there is also a higher incidence of missing bicuspids in the cleft palate patient.[18] Missing teeth are more common in the permanent dentition (25.7%) than in the primary dentition (8.3%).[17]

When a tooth is lost, the space must be carefully maintained so as not to compound tooth placement problems later.[8] If primary incisors are missing in the cleft area and the child is still rather young, one should consider replacing the missing teeth for aesthetic reasons. The dentist can provide an opportunity for the child with a cleft lip and palate to look the same as other young children his age.[1] Teeth can be attached to a removable acrylic partial denture or a fixed arch and retained in the mouth with relative ease. Many of these young children, in fact, are proud of their "new" teeth and seem genuinely happy to have them.

As the permanent incisors erupt their normal position should be established and maintained orthodontically until a permanent fixed bridge or partial denture can be constructed by the prothodontist.

Abnormalities resulting in malformed anterior teeth found by Jordan[17] were: thick curved central incisors, excess mamelons or "saw tooth" incisal edges, exaggerated mamelons, peg-shaped incisors often with a prominent lingual tubercle, t-shaped maxillary lateral incisors presenting with prominent lingual tubercle connected to the incisal edge by a ridge, irregular mamelons and labial tubercles. These conditions can be treated by selective grinding or restored to normal contour with bonded composite resins. Lingual tubercles may require equilibration to reduce occlusal interferences.[8] With the development of acid-etch bonding techniques the restoration of malformed anterior teeth is a relatively simple dental procedure with often dramatic cosmetic results.

Other abnormalities described by Jordan that would not normally require dental treatment are: malformed mandibular and maxillary first primary molars, missing or reduced distolingual cusps on maxillary second primary molars, fused mesial buccal and lingual cusps and deviant mandibular bicuspids.[8]

Jordan found that supernumerary teeth occur most frequently in the lateral incisor region adjacent to the alveolar cleft.[17] An early radiographic examination will reveal their presence and location. When these teeth erupt into the cleft site they bring in additional alveolar bone. This bony wedge helps hold the cleft segments in position. With conservation of alveolar bone in mind, the practitioner usually should advise keeping the tooth as long as it is not in the path of a proposed surgery, is asymptomatic and can be kept free of disease.[19] Because these embedded teeth often are very difficult to clean they are predisposed to dental caries. Extraction of ectopic supernumerary teeth is recommended when their position prevents adequate restoration[3,8] (Fig. 7-5).

Ectopic eruption of the maxillary permanent molar occurs in one of four cleft lip and/or palate children.[20] When the first permanent molar erupts with a mesial inclination, the roots of the second primary molar may completely resorb, causing it to be prematurely lost. As the first permanent molar drifts and tips mesially, the space for the developing second premolar is reduced. If this condition is allowed to occur, a space regainer must be placed to distalize the first permanent molar. This should be followed with a space maintainer until the second bicuspid erupts into position.[8]

Prevention of the premature loss of the primary second molar can be accomplished with early diagnosis. In addition to a good radiographic survey, ectopic eruption should be suspected when there is a delay in the eruption of the maxillary first permanent molar, supra eruption of the distal of the second primary molar or emergence of the distal before the mesial cusps of the first molar. Every attempt should be made to correct the eruption path of the permanent molar without loss of the second primary molar. This can be accomplished with a brass separating wire or

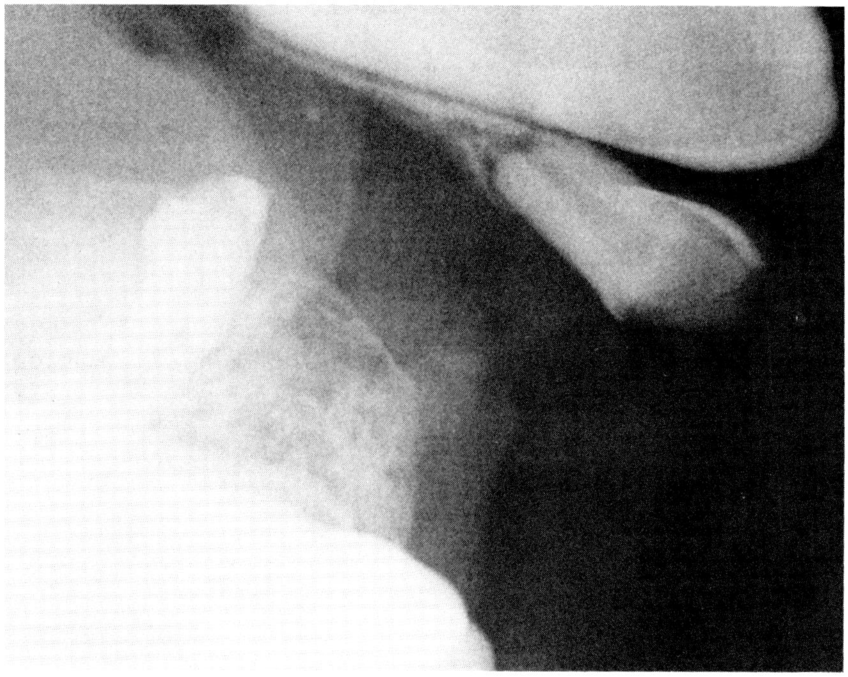

Figure 7-5. Radiograph of an ectopic supernumerary tooth in the alveolar cleft that needs to be extracted.

spring appliance to dislodge the mesial marginal ridge of the first molar from the area of resorption on the distal root of the primary second molar.[21] Once freed the first permanent molar will erupt into its normal position distal to the primary second molar.

Because dental anomalies frequently are encountered in cleft lip and/or palate children, the availability of a pedodontist to diagnose and treat these conditions is important for proper maintenance of the teeth and supporting structures.

Comprehensive Preventive Dentistry Program

An an integral part of the cleft palate team the pedodontist should be available to counsel the parents regarding the dental health of the child and the importance of sound teeth and supporting tissues for successful rehabilitation. Before eruption of the primary teeth the parents must be instructed in a comprehensive preventive dentistry program. This should include a reduction in the ingestion of cariogenic foods, plaque control and increasing the resistance of the teeth with fluorides and sealants. The necessity of periodic recall visits should also be emphasized so the teeth, periodontal tissues and occlusion can be examined carefully and, if necessary, restored to health before time and neglect have taken their toll.

The frequent snacking of cariogenic foods has become incorporated in the lifestyle of many Americans. Starting from birth infants are given nursing bottles filled with sugared fluids such as milk laced with sweeteners, juices and flavored drinks. Often constant companions, these bottles are used as pacifiers during waking hours as well as at nap and bedtimes. When an infant falls asleep with the bottle still in the mouth, the sweetened milk or juice puddles around the erupting incisor teeth creating an ideal environment for plaque growth and tooth decay. It is not unusual for these habits to persist until the child is two or three years old, long after most of the primary teeth erupt into the mouth. This prolonged nursing habit often results in rampant caries. In addition the typical preschool child is a constant snacker. Bombarded by television commercials lauding sugar treats, children are encouraged to seek them out or to ask their parents to buy the promoted sweetened cereals, cookies or candies. To counteract the devastating effect of frequent carbohydrate intake upon the teeth, parents must be counseled early to intercept poor eating habits before they have a hold on the child. This is particularly important for parents of cleft lip and palate children. These patients, because of their handicap, often require prolonged and frequent feedings,[5] which if coupled with cariogenic liquids and solids encourage the development of dental caries.

Because malposed, malformed, maloccluded, missing and supernumerary teeth appear more frequently in cleft palate children than in noncleft children, and because food entrapment and plaque formation is more likely to occur on the surfaces of malposed and malformed teeth and around orthodontic and prosthetic appliances, these children are usually more susceptible to dental caries.[4] Surprisingly, cleft lip and/or palate children have only a slightly higher caries experience than noncleft lip and palate children.[22] But this is not to diminish the importance of good oral hygiene in these children. Future orthodontic and prosthetic appliances will require sound, healthy dentitions for their retention. Unnecessary loss of teeth and teeth compromised with periodontal disease or extensive restorations will make rehabilitation more difficult or impossible.

Like dietary counseling, oral hygiene instruction must be given to the parents early in the child's life so that the primary teeth and surrounding tissue can be flossed and brushed on a regular basis starting in the first year. As soon as children are able to manage a toothbrush they should be instructed and encouraged to clean their own teeth and the cleft area after every meal.

Oral hygiene practices are interrupted occasionally by visits to the hospital for surgical repair of the lips or palate. Because there is fear that brushing will interfere with wound healing or the oral cavity is sore to the touch, cleaning is discontinued. What the parent and patient must be aware of is that plaque and food debris are teaming with bacteria and are capable of producing infection which would compromise healing. As soon after surgery as the child can eat solid foods, cleaning with a soft bristle brush is recommended. While the child is on liquids or eating blended foods, rinsing the mouth with warm salt water is an effective means of removing food particles and promoting healing.

The greatest advancement in the prevention of dental caries is the introduction of fluoride to community drinking water. By adjusting the fluoride content to one part per million, dental caries can be reduced by 60 percent and dental extractions by 80 percent. In addition to the systematic effect of ingested fluorides rendering teeth more resistant to dental caries, topical fluorides in the form of dentrifrice, rinses and professionally applied agents have helped in the remineralization of incipient lesions. The combination of water fluoridation and topical fluorides has reduced greatly smooth surface caries in the United States.[23]

Adhesive sealants for preventing dental caries in occlusal pits and fissures of teeth fill a special need in caries prevention because fluorides prevent decay less effectively in retentive grooves and pits than on smooth surface. Sealants, when fully retained, form a physical barrier to decalcification by acid. This resin coating covering the occlusal surface prevents food and bacteria from getting into the pits and fissures that cannot be reached with a toothbrush. The successful placement of sealants requires fastidious attention to meticulous technique and can be applied by either the dentist or trained auxiliaries with an increased protection of 20 percent in a fluoridated community. Sealants undoubtedly are important in the caries prevention armamentarium of dental practice. When they are combined with fluorides, particularly community fluoridation, dental decay can be prevented entirely in many children.[24]

If parents can be made aware of these preventive procedures their benefits for the cleft lip and palate patient have a chance to be realized. Except for water fluoridation, all the other aspects of a comprehensive preventive program must be discussed with the parent at a time and in a manner which will assure their effective utilization. Parents and children will have to be motivated to brush and floss, eat the right foods and see that the teeth are protected with fluorides and sealants. To assure a healthy dentition the pedodontist or family dentist must do everything possible to be sure that the parent and child are seen on a regular basis. An effective recall system is the key to a good comprehensive preventive program.

Restorative Treatment

The pedodontist has an obligation to the cleft palate team to provide the best restorative dentistry possible. Often he is called upon to determine the restorability of malformed and malpositioned teeth and even to prognosticate as to their expected useful life in the oral cavity.[4] It is essential, then, that the pedodontist be present at all evaluation sessions to appraise the oral structures and to ascertain possible dental problems through clinical examination and radiographic interpretation. The pedodontist then should see that the patient is recommended for treatment when indicated and that the best possible care is made available.

Olsen[3] and Jacobson[8] have described some special problems that would have to be taken into consideraion in rendering dental care to children with cleft lip or palate. For example, the tautness of the upper lip as a result of the primary and revisional surgery may lead the dentist, parent and child to believe that there is inadequate space for performing restorative and oral hygiene procedures. If access to the upper teeth is not as adequate as desired, the operator is encouraged to use smaller-sized instruments: mirror, contra-angle burs, etc.[3] If the condition is severe it can be corrected surgically by deepening the gingivolabial sulcus.[8] The patient should be instructed to use a small-headed toothbrush to clean in the cramped areas created by an insufficient upper lip. With a little ingenuity the dentist and patient can gain access to this restricted area and maintain the teeth and supporting tissues in good health.

Associated with the cleft palate there is often some deviation of the nasal septum with the resultant blockage of one or both of the nasal passages.[8] As with any patient who has difficulty breathing through his nose, working in the mouth, particularly with a rubber dam, may cause him to fear that he cannot breath. This can be alleviated by making sure the patient has an adequate airway. The rubber dam can be positioned to one side or modified with air holes so that the patient can breath through his mouth.[5] Cotton rolls used sparingly or an assistant using an evacuator can be used instead of a rubber dam to maintain a dry field without blocking the airway.

Special consideration should be given to the use of local anesthetic for the cleft palate patient for procedures in the upper arch. Olsen, in discussing the innervation of the maxillary dentition of cleft palate patients, suggests that there may be considerable variation depending upon the location and degree of clefting.[1] For example, in cases of bilateral cleft lip and palate the nasopalatine nerve alone supplies the maxillary incisors. It would be anatomically impossible for the anterior superior alveolar nerve to bridge the alveolar cleft and innervate the premaxillary area in these patients. To be assured of profound anesthesia to the pulps of the incisors it would be necessary to deposit some anesthetic solution high in the incisive canal to block the nasopalatine nerve. Teeth posterior to the cleft can be anesthetized in the normal manner by supraperiosteol injections in the area of the middle superior alveolar nerve and/or a posterior superior alveolar block injection. Palatal anesthesia can be obtained by injecting a few drops in the area of the greater palatine foramen anesthetizing the anterior palatal nerve. The use of painless local anesthesia technique to assure a minimum of discomfort is important in establishing a positive rapport between the cleft palate child and dentist. These precautions should be used to assure that this patient will return regularly for examinations and needed treatment.[8]

The restoration of malaligned incisor teeth often can pose difficulties in cavity preparation.[8] Generally the cavity should be prepared as though the tooth were in proper relation to the adjacent and opposing teeth. Later the orthodontist will be aligning the tooth in its proper position. If "proximal" caries occur on the labial or lingual surface because it is rotated, it should be restored so that when the tooth is later placed in proper relation the margins will be in self-cleaning areas.[8]

As discussed earlier, malformed and hypoplastic teeth are common defects seen in the cleft lip and palate patient. Often the central and lateral incisors immediately adjacent to the cleft site appear pitted, stained or malformed. Fortunately the root development usually is adequate enough so that if the crown can be restored the tooth can be maintained indefinitely. Where there is adequate enamel composite restorations or veneers can be bonded to these incisor teeth with stable, aesthetic results. Newer adhesive agents are being developed so these materals can be bonded to dentin as well as to enamel.[25] Young anterior teeth that once had to be restored with unsightly stainless steel crowns now can be restored to normal color and contour with strong, wear-resistant composite resins.

The dentist may be requested by the prosthodontist or orthodontist to prepare the maxillary dentition to receive a prosthesis, such as a speech appliance, obturator or removable orthodontic appliance. Well-fitted stainless steel crowns with soldered buccal lugs cemented to primary molars or composite prominences bonded to the buccal enamel serve as excellent retention points for these appliances. Removable maxillary partial space maintainers to replace congenitally missing or extracted incisor teeth also can be designed with clasps to engage the buccal surfaces of these modified abutment teeth. If a full denture is placed over the maxillary dentition to restore vertical dimension the teeth should be covered with gold crowns to protect them from dental caries.[1]

All of these restorative procedures are direct ways the pediatric dentist can provide the child with cleft lip and palate with the opportunity to look the same as other young children. It would be justified to state that orthodontic therapy cannot be instituted or carried to a successful conclusion unless the dentition present is in the best possible condition. It also is obvious that a successful prosthesis cannot be constructed or utilized to its fullest advantage without sound supporting structures. Even the effectiveness of speech therapy can be lessened unless the dentition is in good condition. Poor dental aesthetics undoubtedly can contribute to the patient's already complex psychological problems. Good surgical results can be minimized if available dental apparatus is not aesthetically maintained. In all these instances the pedodontist and family dentist play a key role in the total rehabilitation of the cleft palate child.

REFERENCES

1. Olsen NH: Pediatric dentistry, in Grabbe W, Rosenstein S, Bzoch K (eds): *Cleft Lip and Palate.* Boston, Little Brown & Co, 1971.
2. Vincent CJ: The pedodontist in cleft palate rehabilitation. *Cleft Palate Bull,* 10:68, 1960.
3. Olsen NH: Responsibility of the general practitioner to the cleft palate patient. *J Am Dent Assoc,* 60:706, 1960.
4. Vincent CJ: The pedodontist and cleft palate rehabilitation. *J Dent Child,* 29:172, 1962.
5. Hagerty RF: The role of the dentist on cleft palate teams. *Birth Defects,* 16:111, 1980.
6. Kennedy TJ, Miller SH, Tooze FM, et al: The team approach to treatment of the cleft lip and palate. *Am Fam Physician,* 18:74, 1978.
7. Gottlieb MA: Congenital defects, in Nowak AJ (ed): *Dentistry for the Handicapped Patient.* St Louis, C V Mosby Co, 1976.
8. Jacobson BN, Rosenstein SW: The cleft palate patient: Dental help needed. *J Dent Child,* 37:17, 1970.
9. Gorlin RJ, Pindborg JJ, Cohen MM: Facial clefts and associated anomalies, in Gorlin RJ, et al (eds): *Syndromes of the Head and Neck,* ed 2. New York, McGraw-Hill, 1976.
10. McNeil CK: *Oral and Facial Deformity.* London, Sir Isaac Pitman & Sons Ltd, 1954.

11. Jacobson BN, Rosenstein SW: Early maxillary orthopedics: A combination appliance. *Cleft Palate J,* 2:364, 1965.
12. Rosenstein SW, Jacobson BN: Early maxillary orthopedics: A sequence of events. *Cleft Palate J,* 4:197, 1967.
13. Troutman KC: Maxillary arch control in infants with unilateral clefts of the lip and palate. *Am J Orthod,* 66:198, 1974.
14. Rosenstein SW: Cleft lip and palate and other craniofacial anomalies, in Forester DJ, Wagner ML, Fleming J (eds): *Pediatric Dental Medicine.* Philadelphia, Lea & Febiger, 1981.
15. Jones JE: Early management of severe bilateral cleft lip and palate in an infant. *J Dent Child,* 48:50, 1981.
16. Berkowitz S: Section III: Orofacial growth and dentistry. *Cleft Palate J,* 14:288, 1977.
17. Jordan RE, Kraus BS, Neptune CM: Dental abnormalities with cleft lip and/or palate. *Cleft Palate J,* 3:22, 1966.
18. Olni WH: Dental anomalies in cleft lip and palate patients. *Angle Orthod,* 34:119, 1964.
19. Mulick JF: Orthodontics in common craniofacial problems, in Stewart RE, Barber TK, Troutman KC, Wei SHY (eds): *Pediatric Dentistry.* St Louis, C V Mosby Co, 1982.
20. Carr GE, Mink JR: Ectopic eruption of the first permanent maxillary molar in cleft lip and palate children. *J Dent Child,* 32:179, 1965.
21. Bayardo RE, Grandel ER, Milos WE: New concept in treatment of ectopically erupting maxillary first permanent molars. *J Dent Child,* 46:218, 1979.
22. Lauterstein AM, Mendelsohn M: An analysis of the caries experience of 285 cleft palate children. *Cleft Palate J,* 1:314, 1964.
23. *Decayed, Missing, and Filled Teeth Among Persons 1-74 Years.* US National Center for Health Statistics. Vital and Health Statistics, Series 11, No. 223. DHHS Pub No (PHS) 81-1673. Hyattsville, Md, Government Printing Office, 1980.
24. Horowitz HS: The potential of fluorides and sealants to deal with problems of dental decay. *Pediatr Dent,* 4:286, 1982.
25. Bowen RL, Cobb EN: A method of bonding to dentin and enamel. *J Am Dent Assoc,* 107:734, 1983.

CHAPTER 8

ORTHODONTIA

STANLEY G. BIEL and HAROLD T. PERRY

> *. . . A person who has a beautiful soul always has some beautiful things to say, but a person who says beautiful things does not necessarily have a beautiful soul.*
>
> *. . . Confucius*

NUMEROUS dental anomalies are associated with clefting. Usually coincidental with a cleft palate is a maxillary deficiency and a pseudoprognathic mandible.[1,2] Anterior and/or posterior crossbites are generally present.[2] Frequently teeth are congenitally missing in the cleft area[3] (usually lateral incisors[4,5]) and sometimes, in addition, other permanent dental units also are absent. At other times supernumerary teeth will be present.[2,3,6]

Treatment Philosophy

The orthodontist must consider some or all of these problems in various combinations when formulating a treatment plan for the patient.

We ordinarily prefer to delay treatment until eruption of the permanent dentition. If appliances are placed during the deciduous or mixed dentition phases and therapy continues through the eruption of the permanent dentition, the patient will be in treatment from childhood until early adulthood. We feel that this protracted treatment is discouraging to the patient, and that it reduces the patient's enthusiasm about orthodontic therapy. A poor attitude can be the result, and this would affect the cooperation we so vitally need from the patient. The patient's cooperation is essential for many things, such as elastic wear and oral hygiene. Without it, the orthodontic result is doomed from the start. Because of the clefting we are forced into a circumstance where we have to struggle merely to achieve a funtional occlusion, and a lack of cooperation from the patient would only make this difficult situation much worse.

Orthodontic Records and Diagnosis

Orthodontic records are used to diagnose the patient's problem and to determine the treatment plan. They also are used to follow the progress of the case while it is in treatment, and medicolegally, they are a permanent record of when treatment began. Orthodontic records consist of plaster study casts, a cephalometric radiograph, a panoramic radiograph, a hand-wrist radiograph, a complete series of periapical radiographs, intraoral photographs and frontal and lateral facial photographs.

Study models allow visualization of the malocclusion in three dimensions. They also permit various measurements, such as arch length, to be made. The cephalometric radiograph permits the analysis of the relation of the maxillary and mandibular teeth to each other, the relation of the maxilla to the mandible and the relation of the maxilla and mandible to the cranial base. Because the cephalometric radiographic technique standardizes the patient's head position and the target to film distance in relation to the x-ray source, successive yearly radiographs may be traced serially (Fig. 8-1). Serial tracings superimposed on one another allow the clinician to observe the effects of growth and treatment on the teeth and osseous structures of the face. The panoramic radiograph allows the inspection of all the teeth and the contiguous bone of each jaw. In addition, the sinuses, nasal cavity, temporomandibular joints and other areas can be examined for anomalies and pathology which might not be demonstrated on the other radiographs. Periapical radiographs give detailed information about individual teeth, crown-root ratios, bone support, root length, root morphology, carious lesions and so on. The hand-wrist radiograph is used as a predictor of growth.[7] There is a high correlation between skeletal age and the prediction of future growth.[7] The hand-wrist radiograph can tell us where the patient is in relation to pubertal growth spurt, and we can adjust our treatment mechanics accordingly.

After the orthodontist has all the diagnostic records he determines a treatment plan for the patient. He then schedules the parents and the patient for a consultation, at which time the ramifications of treatment are explained.

Elementary Cephalometrics

This will be a very generalized discussion of cephalometrics. It is not meant to substitute for a graduate level cephalometrics course. To obtain sound principles of cephalometric landmark identification, cephalometric interpretation and diagnosis, one is obliged to take a course in cephalometrics. No diagnosis should be attempted without understanding the fundamental principles.

Cephalometrics is a division of anthropomorphics and is the study of the head.[8] Orthodontists use cephalometric radiographs as an adjunct to the other orthodontic diagnostic records to determine if the problem is primarily skeletal in nature, primarily dentoalveolar in nature, or if it is a combination of skeletal and dental problems. It gives the clinician direction in planning the mode of treatment for the patient.

The cephalometric radiograph is a standardized radiograph. By means of ear rods, the patient is positioned in the cephalostat with the midsagittal plane 60 inches from the x-ray source. The central beam of the x-ray is coincidental with the ear rods. In this manner the head position is kept constant in relation to the x-ray source and central beam, so that longitudinal x-ray studies can be performed to analyze growth.

Each clinician has preferred particular landmarks to establish a diagnosis. The landmarks[8,9] we prefer, as shown in Figure 8-1a, are:

Sella (S). The center of the pituitary fossa.
Nasion (Na). The frontonasal suture where it intersects the most posterior point on the curve at the bridge of the nose.
Subspinale (point A). The deepest point on the premaxilla between the anterior nasal spine and prosthion.
Supramentale (point B). The most posterior point in the concavity between infradentale and pogonion.
Gonion (Go). The point which is most posterior, inferior at the junction of the body and ramus of the mandible.
Menton (Me). The lowest point on the symphyseal outline.
Pogonion (Pog). The most anterior point on the contour of the chin.
Porion (Po). The top of the ear rods.
Orbitale (Or). The lowest point on the orbital rim.
Maxillary central incisor (*1*). The long axis of the most anterior maxillary central incisor.
Mandibular central incisor (1). The long axis of the most anterior mandibular central incisor.

With these points, various planes and angles can be constructed on acetate tracing paper. Again, each clinician has favorite planes and angles to use. We prefer the following: SNA, SNB, ANB, FMA, IMPA, SN-MP, *1*-SM, and *1*-1 (Fig 8-1b).

By inspection of the angle ANB (which is the difference between angles SNA and SNB), we can get information about where the maxilla and mandible are in relation to each other and where they are relative to the cranial base (line SN).

The average value of the angle SNA is 82° and that of SNB is 80°. Most often we are interested in the difference between SNA and SNB rather than the absolute values of SNA and SNB themselves. For instance, in a case where SNA might be 77° and SNB 72° with the soft tissue profile of the upper lip not appearing to be deficient, we probably can assume safely that the maxilla is properly positioned relative to the cranial base. The difference of 6° would then tell us that the mandible is posteriorly positioned relative to the maxilla and also relative to the cranial base.

The line formed by the intersection of the line GoMe and line SN is the mandibular plane angle. The more obtuse the angle, the more we can expect our patient's mandible to grow in a vertical direction. A reading near the average of 32° would tell us that the mandible probably will grow in a more favorable direction as far as orthodontics is concerned, which is down and forward. A low plane angle (less than 32°) may indicate that the patient is a horizontal grower and that he may have a tendency to grow into a Class III jaw relation.

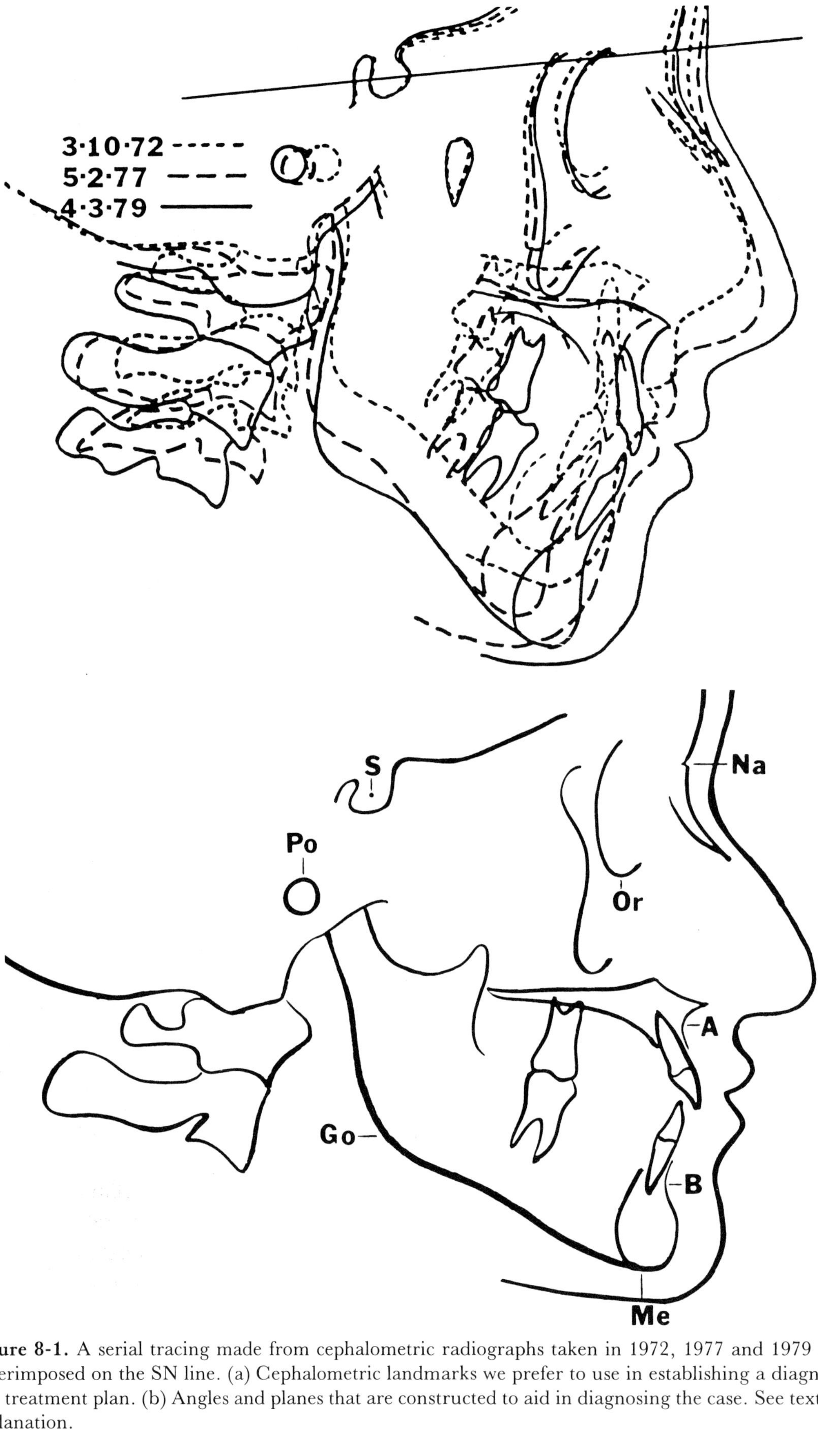

Figure 8-1. A serial tracing made from cephalometric radiographs taken in 1972, 1977 and 1979 and superimposed on the SN line. (a) Cephalometric landmarks we prefer to use in establishing a diagnosis and treatment plan. (b) Angles and planes that are constructed to aid in diagnosing the case. See text for explanation.

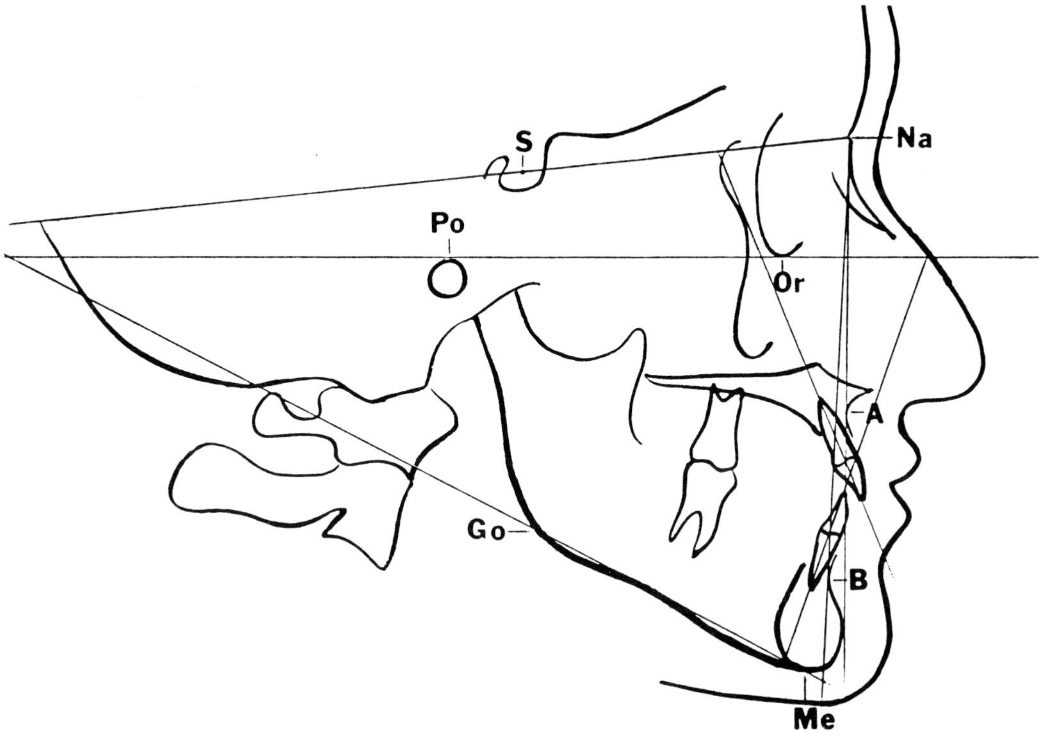

The FMA angle (the Frankfort mandibular angle) is another method by which we inspect the mandibular plane angle. It is formed by the intersection of the Go-Me line with the PoOr line (the Frankfort horizontal plane).[2] The average is 25°. Again, readings greater than the average may indicate vertical growth, while those less than the average may indicate horizontal growth.

The IMPA (incisor mandibular plane angle) is the angle formed by the intersection of the mandibular plane and the long axis of the mandibular incisor. The average is 90°. Sometimes the IMPA helps the orthodontist in determining the fullness of the face and is an aid in the decision to remove permanent teeth to alter the facial profile. The IMPA sometimes tends to become more acute as the mandibular plane angle increases. This is a means by which nature uses dental compensation to improve the soft tissue profile created by a skeletal problem.

The angle formed by the long axis of the maxillary central incisor where it intersects the SN line gives the orthodontist information on how upright or procumbent the incisors are. The average reading is 103°. If the incisors are less than average, they may be too upright and their roots may have to be torqued lingually. If the incisors are procumbent, the crowns may have to be tipped lingually to place them nearer the ideal.

The angle formed by the intersection of the long axes of the maxillary and mandibular incisors gives the orthodontist an idea of how the incisors relate to each other. The average is 132°. Readings less than the average may indicate that the incisors are too procumbent, while readings greater than the average may mean the teeth are too upright.

Theses are the landmarks, angles and planes we use in our diagnostic regimen. There are other analyses available to the clinician such as the Steiner analysis, the

Tweed analysis, the Downs analysis, the Ricketts analysis and so on. Every one of these is a valid analysis and can be used by the orthodontist to diagnose the case. We happen to be comfortable using the set of angles and planes just described. The important thing is to improve the occlusion and the function for the patient. It does not matter which analysis is used as long as the result of treatment is the same.

Facial Growth

Generally speaking, the face grows in a direction that is down and forward in relation to the cranial base. Where the growth is more horizontal, the facial profile would tend to be prognathic. On the other hand, vertical growth would tend to produce a long face or even a mandibular retrusion.

But these are not hard and fast rules. Anything may occur during growth; the direction can change from vertical to horizontal or from horizontal to vertical. It is impossible to predict a pattern.[8]

If we have only a cephalometric radiograph available, we can make a reasonable prediction of the direction of facial growth based on the mandibular plane angle and the overbite and overjet. A low angle will be present in an individual who will tend to grow more horizontally. If the mandibular plane angle is near the average, growth will tend to be downward and forward. In a high angle case, one will probably see growth that is predominantly vertical or even downward and backward.

Where serial tracings can be made from successive yearly cephalometric radiographs, the orthodontist is able to make a more accurate prediction about the direction of facial growth. When superimposed on the SN line, the serial tracings will graphically show the direction of growth (Fig. 8-1).

Approximately 30 percent of the patients with a cleft palate problem exhibit some degree of retrognathism of the maxilla. There is a retardation of maxillary growth leading to pseudoprognathism of the mandible.[10] The facial profile appears to be Class III in nature but in reality is due to a maxillary deficiency.

However in cleft cases, as with any biologic entity, any combination can occur. Both jaws may relate normally to the cranium, the maxilla may be deficient with the mandible normally related, the maxilla will be normally related with a prognathic mandible, and so on. It is the responsibility of the clinician to diagnose the condition and to formulate a treatment plan best suited to the patient's case.

Treatment Planning

In the stage of development in which the deciduous dentition is present, we usually prefer not to initiate treatment. The patient is placed on an observation schedule and is periodically checked to follow the exfoliation of the deciduous teeth.

During the next mixed dentition phase, we are still reluctant to begin orthodontic treatment. However, there are instances when we have not hesitated to institute serial extractions, the placement of a Crozat appliance or some sort of expansion appliance (Fig. 8-2).

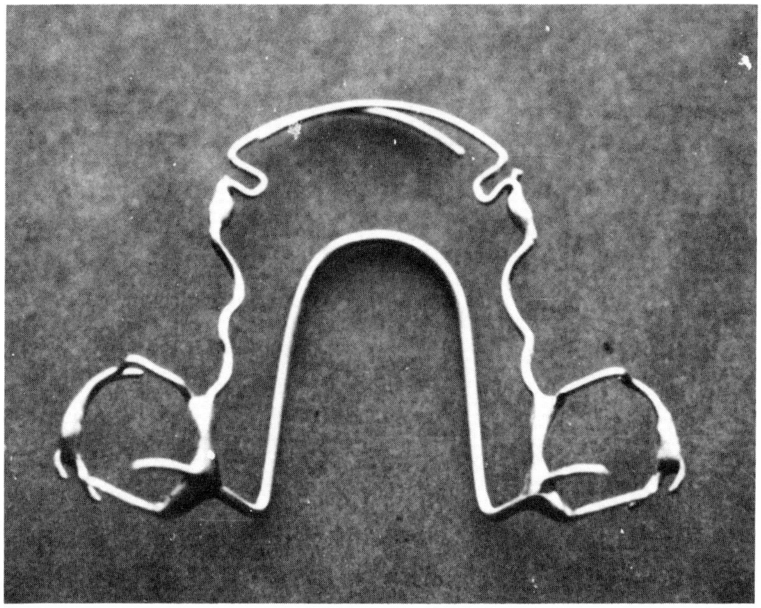

Figure 8-2. A Crozat appliance.

After the permanent dentition has erupted we usually begin full orthodontic treatment. Of course no two treatment plans will be exactly alike because no two malocclusions are exactly alike, but generally speaking, there are similarities in treating malocclusions of most cleft patients.

Most often the maxillary arch segments have collapsed (Figs. 8-3, 8-3a), so the initial task is to expand the maxillary dental arch to obtain a normal width in relation to the mandibular arch.

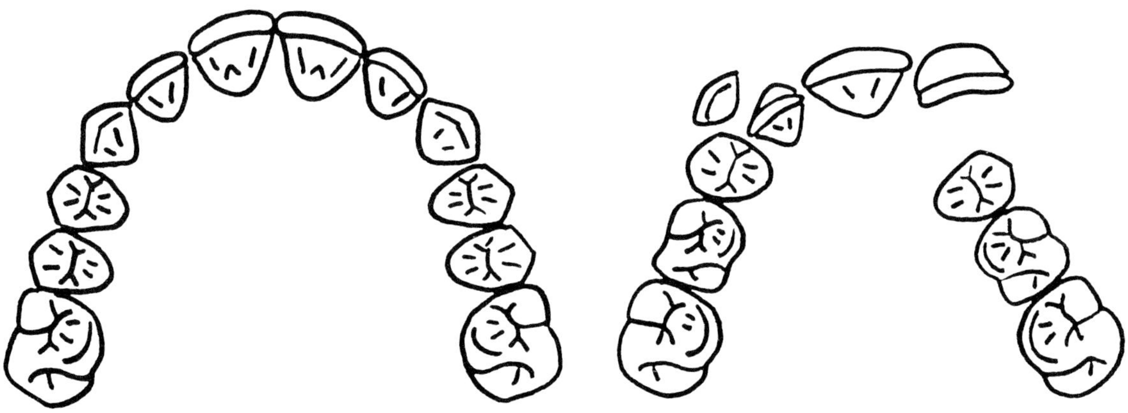

Figure 8-3. Ideally related arch segments. (a) Collapsed arch segments.

We have several means at our disposal to expand the collapsed segments of the maxillary arch. One method is to place bands with lingual extensions (Fig. 8-4) on the first molars. Then an 0.045 inch round gold labial expansion arch is fitted into the buccal tubes on the molar bands (Fig. 8-5). The patient is seen on a monthly basis and the labial arch is expanded at each visit. Another method is to use a removable Crozat appliance (Fig. 8-4) which also is expanded on a monthly basis. Another technique by which to expand is the use of expanded arch wires and crossbite elastics.

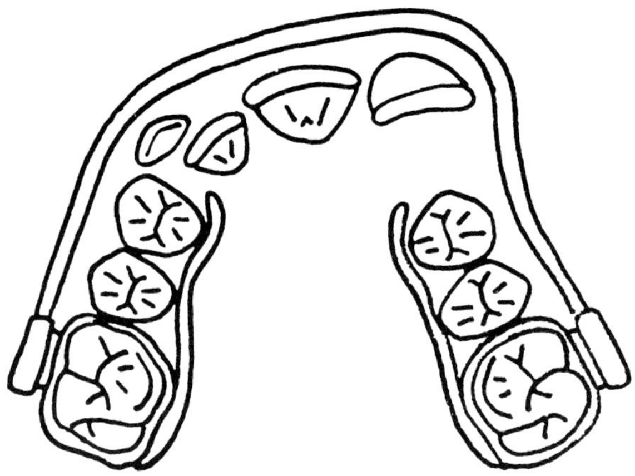

Figure 8-4. 0.045 inch gold expansion wire, occlusal view.

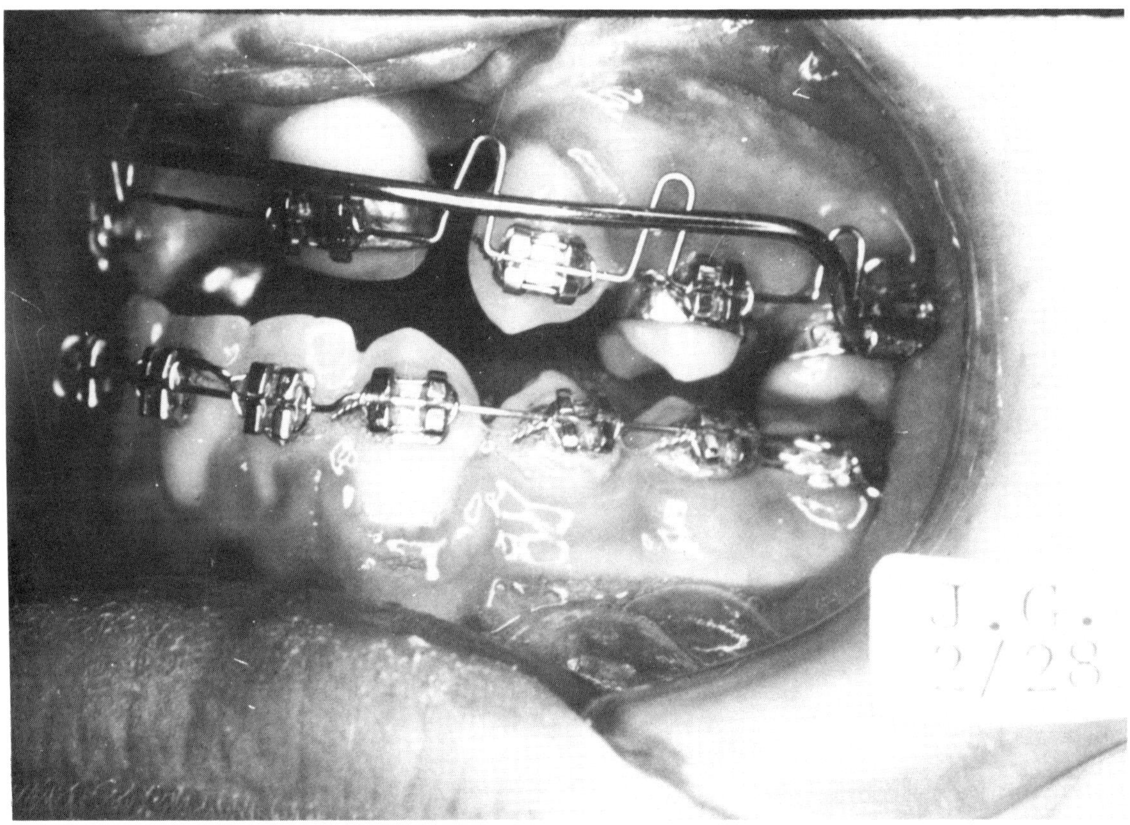

Figure 8-5. 0.045 inch gold wire expansion arch, lateral view.

After we have successfully expanded the maxillary arch and coordinated it to the mandibular arch we place full appliance. At this time we begin to correct rotations, to level the curve of Spee and to advance the maxillary incisors.

Usually the lateral incisor is missing in the area of the cleft. Many times we can use an open coil spring to generate space for the placement of a pontic for the missing tooth (Figs. 8-6, 8-7, 8-8). This way the patient does not have to contend with the unesthetic appearance of the cleft in that area.

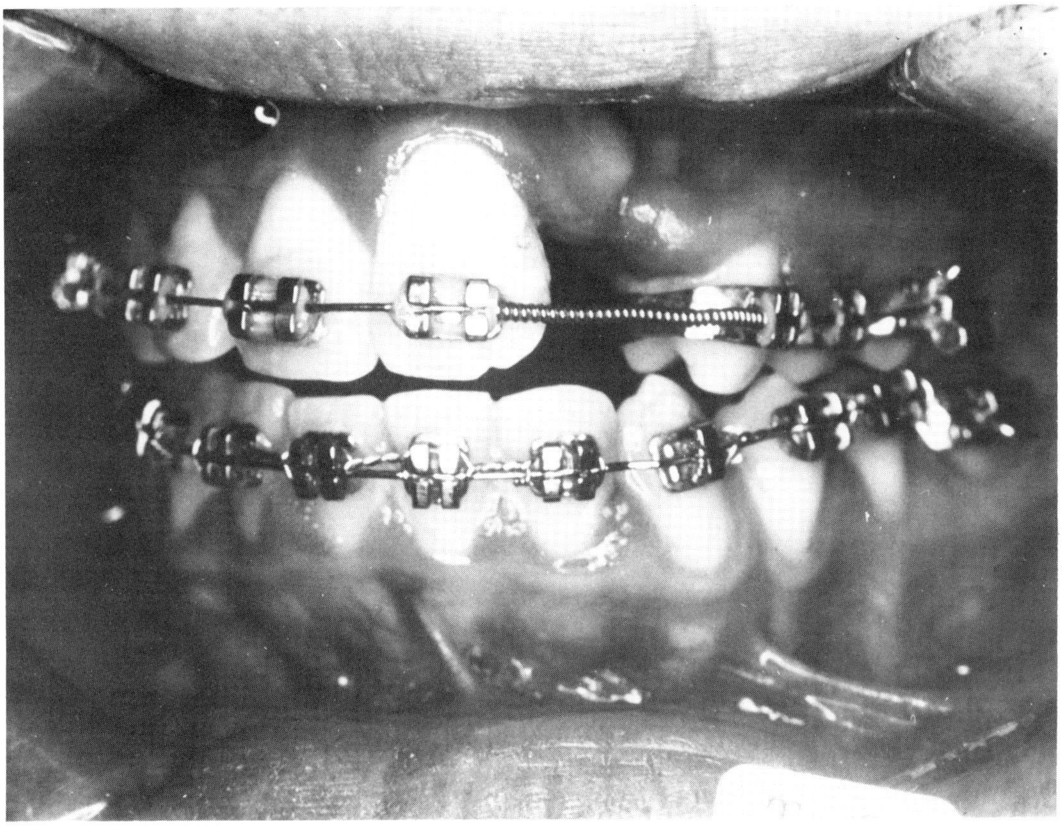

Figure 8-6. Open coil spring creating space in which to place a pontic.

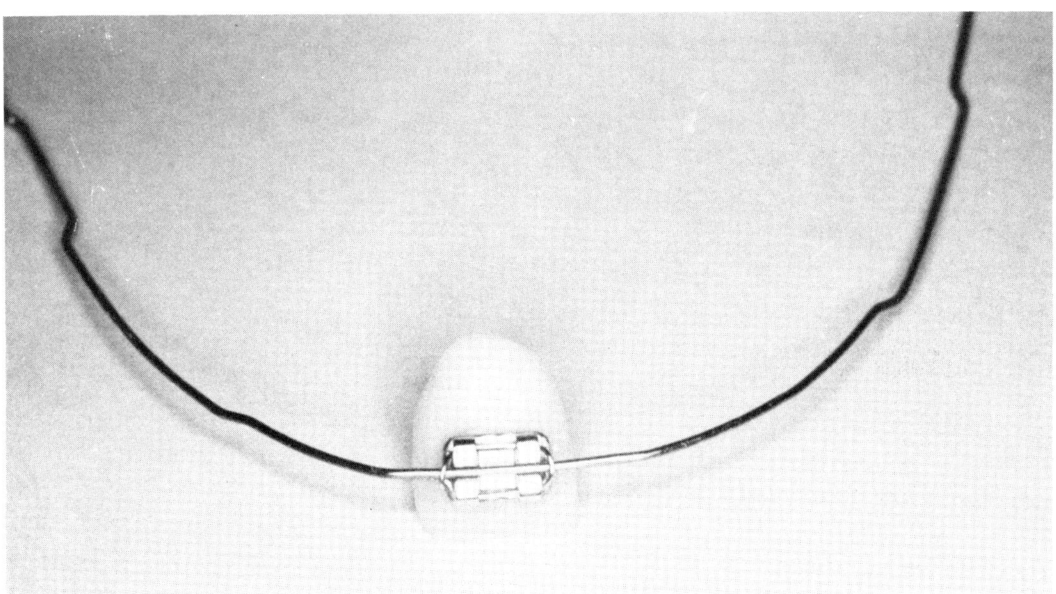

Figure 8-7. A pontic on an arch wire.

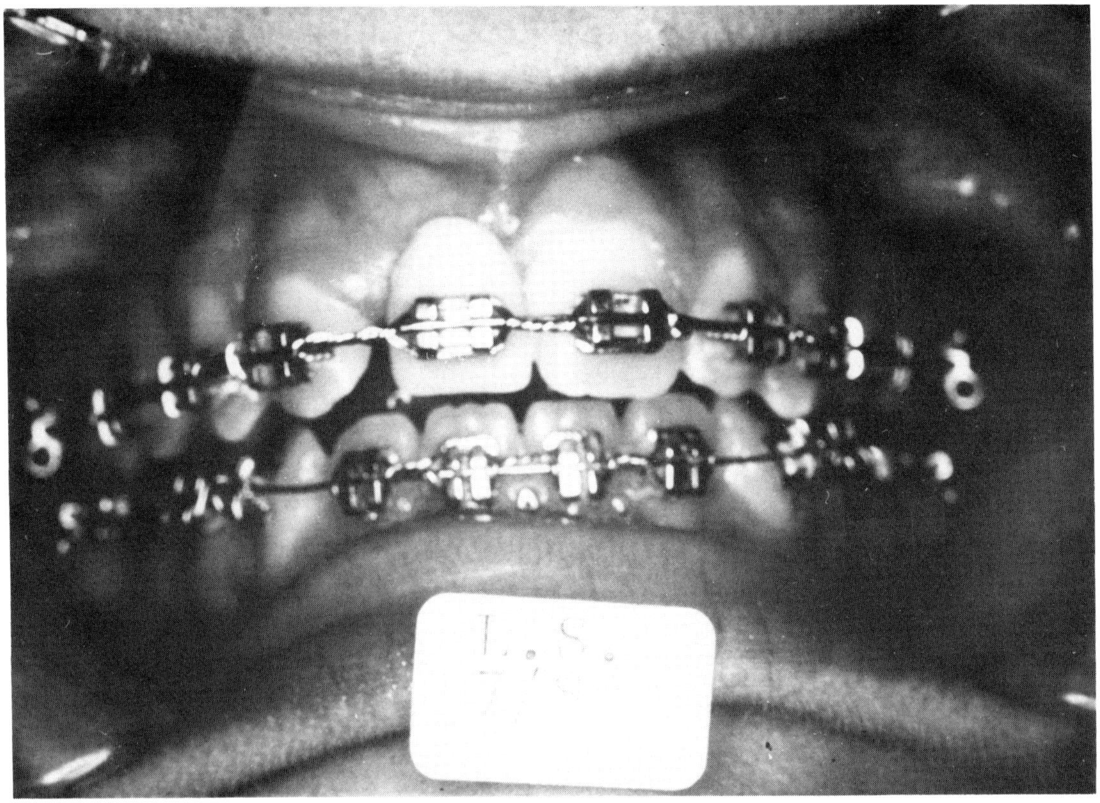

Figure 8-8. A pontic in place in the patient's mouth.

Active orthodontic treatment lasts from two to three years. This is followed by a retention phase during which the patient wears retainers and is checked at intervals of four to six months. At the time of removal of orthodontic appliances we construct a Hawley retainer with pontics attached to it to replace any missing teeth (Figs. 8-9, 8-10, 8-11).

The main purpose of a retainer is to hold the teeth in the position in which the orthodontist has placed them. Ideally the patient wears a retainer for two years, but the retention phase may last until the patient is perhaps 21 years old. Usually, though, at 18 years we advise the patient to see his dentist for restorative dental procedures.

The dentist may elect to place a bridge in the cleft area or even a partial denture, if it is indicated. After the dental restorative procedures are completed, we usually follow the patient's progress at six-month intervals for another year or two.

Although cleft palate cases are more difficult to treat than the average orthodontic case, the majority can be handled successfully by the orthodontist. Through their efforts, orthodontists are doubly rewarded: A challenging case has been restored to a functional occlusion, and a service has been performed which improved the masticatory efficiency and aesthetics for the patient.

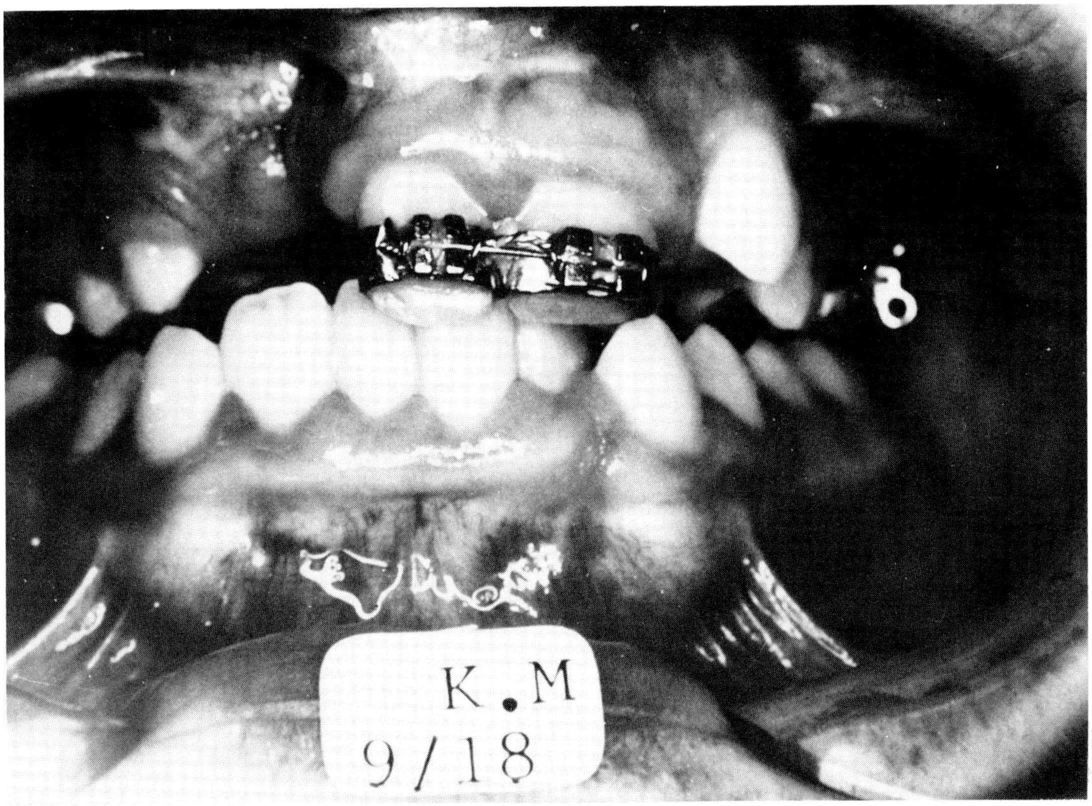

Figure 8-9. Case K.M. after arch expansion, but before full orthodontic treatment.

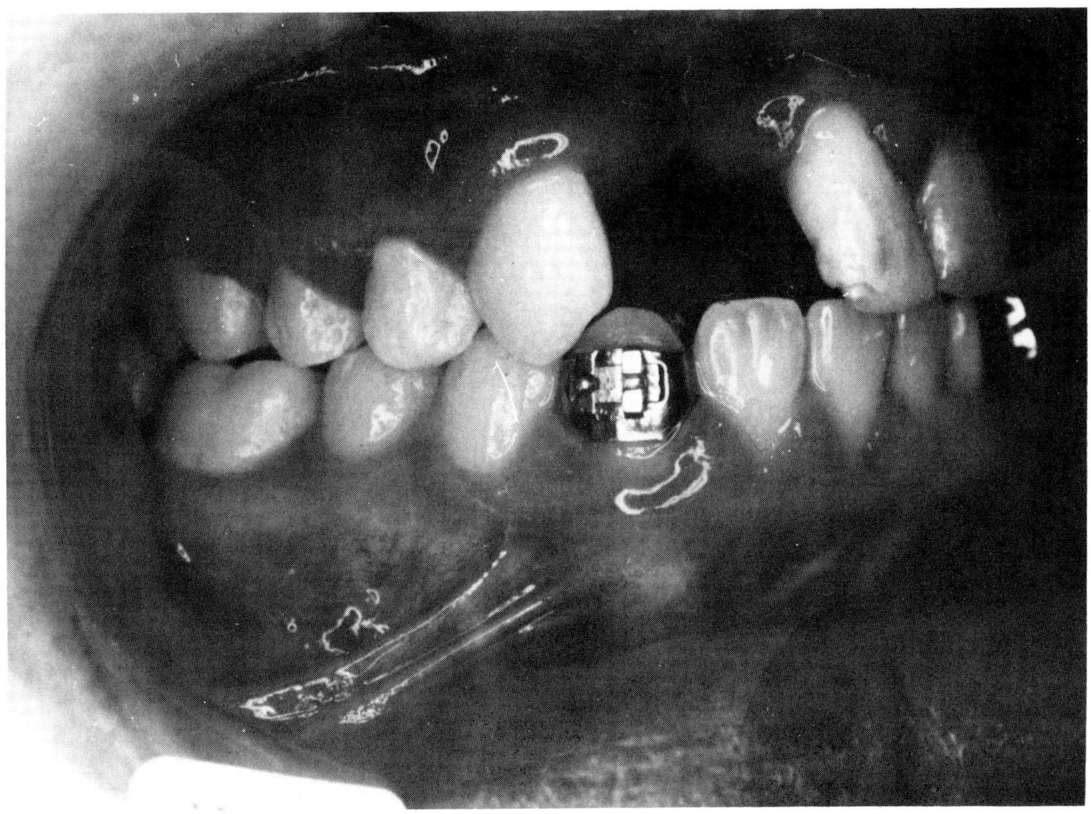

Figure 8-10. Case K.M. at the time of retention before the placement of a maxillary Hawley retainer.

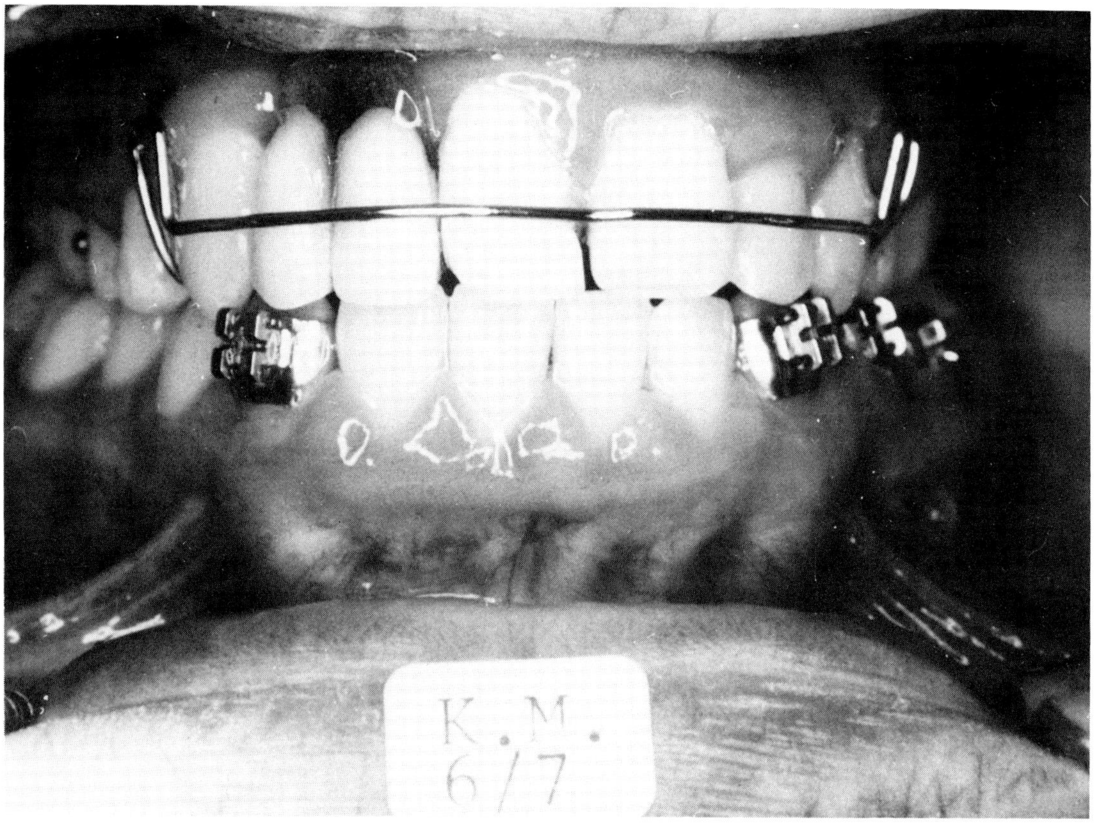

Figure 8-11. Case K.M. with a Hawley retainer with pontics in place.

Surgical Orthodontics

As with many anomalies, clefts vary in their severity. The less severe cases can be treated reasonably successfully with orthodontic appliances alone, but some cases require a surgical correction of the osseous structures in concert with orthodontics.

We strongly recommend in these cases that the orthodontist work in conjunction with a surgeon. This is because a better functioning occlusion can be obtained than would be achieved by either practitioner working independently. If the orthodontist attempted to correct a skeletal problem without a surgeon, the result would be just as compromised as if the surgeon attempted a correction without the orthodontist.

Surgical Orthodontic Records

The surgeon requires the same records that the orthodontist uses. Additionally the study casts are mounted on a dental articulator.

Orthodontic study models allow the surgeon to visualize the dentition in three dimensions, but when mounted on an articulator they show the surgeon how the dentition relates to the cranial complex. The surgeon can perform "surgery" on the models to visualize what can be accomplished. They aid the surgeon in planning surgical cuts and indicate the effects of surgery on the occlusion. The intraoral photographs and facial photographs also are referred to while making a treatment plan. Facial photos enable the surgeon to see the preoperative state and to approximate the postoperative soft tissue changes. Intraoral photos serve as a record of conditions before treatment was initiated. The periapical radiographs give detailed information about individual teeth, crown-root ratios, bone support, carious lesions and so on. The panoramic is a general survey film. It allows the surgeon to observe any gross pathology of the jaws and to picture the size of the ramus and body of the mandible. The cephalometric radiograph permits the surgeon to study the relation of the maxillary and mandibular teeth to each other, the relation of the maxilla to the mandible and the relation of the maxilla and mandible to the cranium. Since the soft tissue of the face can be seen on the cephalometric radiograph, the facial profile can be analyzed. In addition "surgery" can be performed on the cephalometric tracing, so the surgeon can hypothesize, by means of a prediction tracing (Fig. 8-12), what surgery will do to the patient's profile and dentition.[11,12]

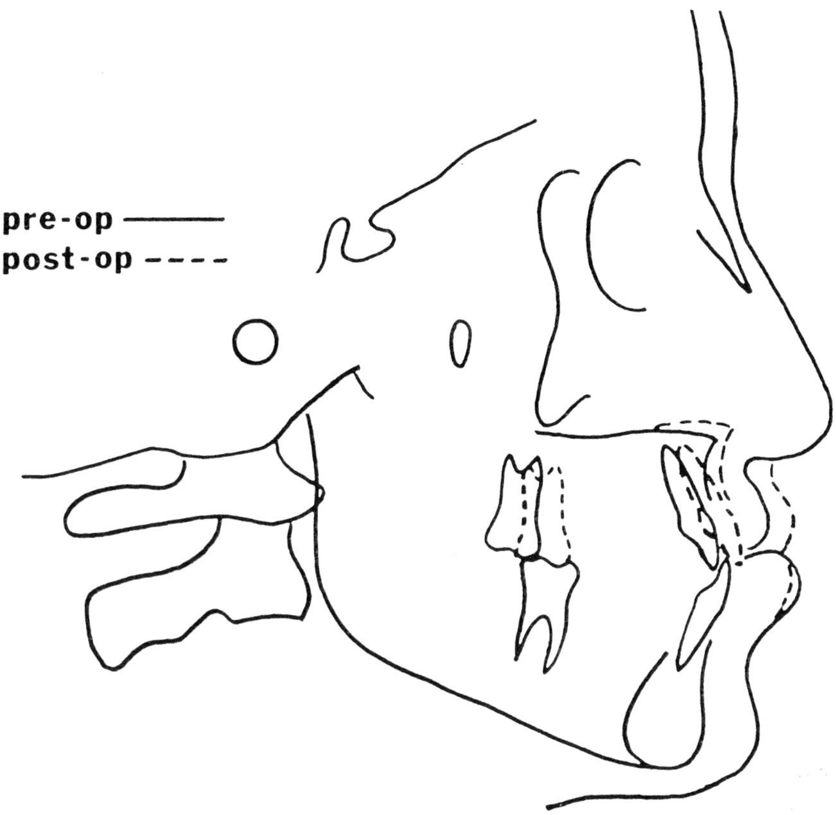

Figure 8-12. A prediction tracing which is used to hypothesize the effect of surgery on the profile and dentition.

The Treatment Plan

Each patient will have a treatment plan suited to the requirements of the individual case. Gans and Kallal[13] stated that a surgical orthodontic treatment plan should be formulated by keeping in mind the following principles:

1. Normal jaw relationships must not be changed to compensate for abnormal tooth relationships.
2. Teeth must not be tipped beyond the limits of their normal position to compensate for abnormal jaw relationships.
3. Malposed teeth first should be properly positioned and aligned on malrelated jaws. The jaws then should be repositioned and final adjustments of teeth made on the newly related jaws.
4. Correction of positional discrepancies of the jaws should be done by moving the malposed jaw into proper relation with the normally positioned jaw.

Generally, a cleft patient will have a maxillary deficiency and pseudoprognathic mandible. Repositioning a normal mandible to fit under a posteriorly positioned maxilla will produce an unacceptable facial profile. The more suitable treatment is to advance the maxilla to improve the middle third of the face, the contour of the lip and, therefore, the entire facial profile.

Not all patients have a maxillary deficiency. Figure 8-13a-d shows a patient with a cleft and a prognathic mandible; the most efficacious treatment was a mandibular setback procedure. The surgery was performed completely intraorally so no external facial scarring would result.

Not every cleft patient will require a surgical orthodontic procedure, but when it is indicated it is usually the responsibility of the orthodontist to recognize that need. The patient should be referred to the surgeon for evaluation, and the surgeon and orthodontist will confer and formulate a treatment plan.

It is imperative that the surgeon and orthodontist work in conjunction on these cases to achieve optimal results. The patient may then acquire an aesthetic facial profile and an aesthetic functional occlusion.

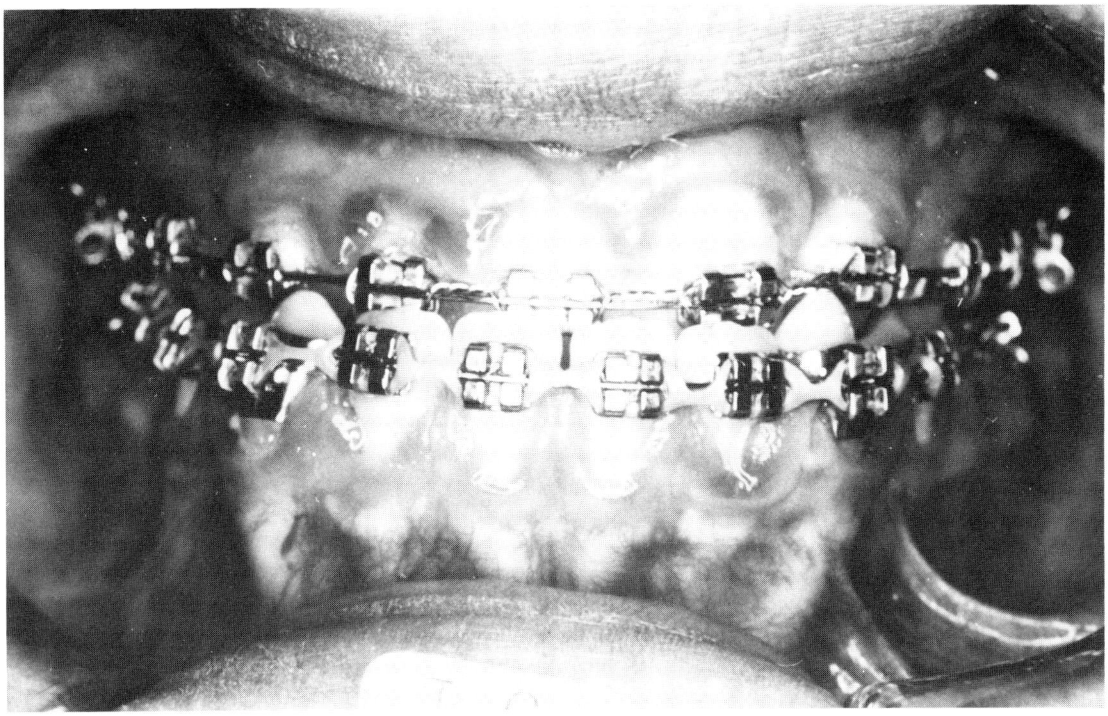

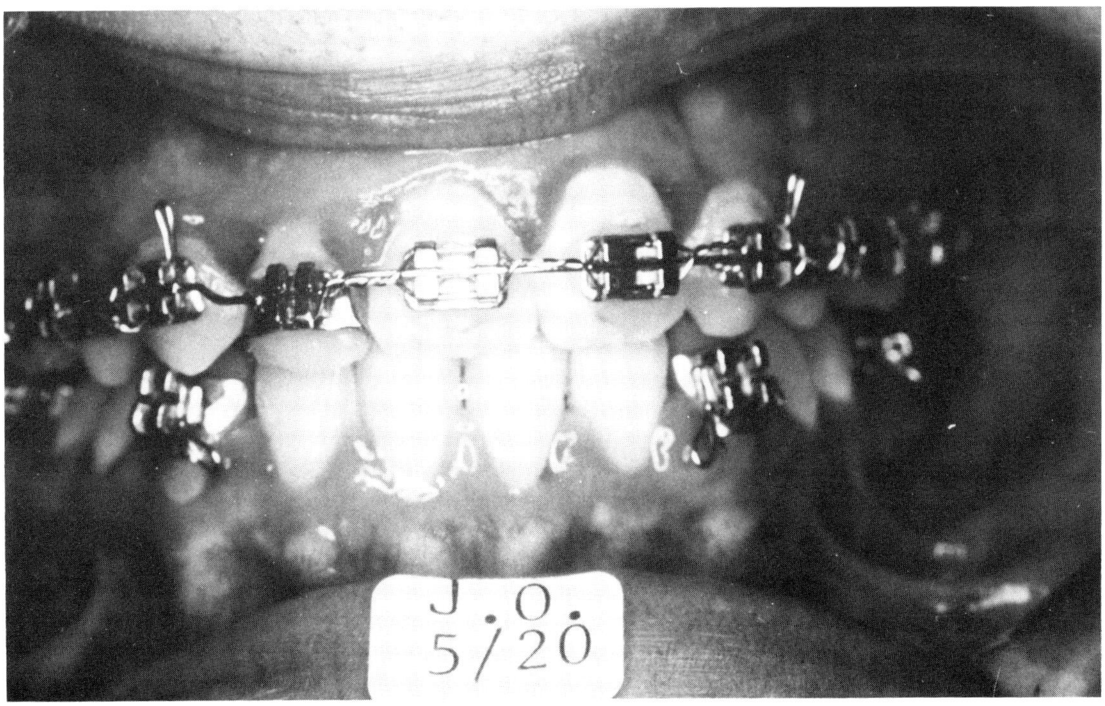

Figure 8-13. (a) Before surgery. Observe that the mandibular teeth are anterior to the maxillary arch due to the prognathism of the mandible. (b) Case 1. After surgery and out of fixation. The maxillary teeth are now properly related anteriorly to the mandibular teeth. (c) Case 1. Tracing the pretreatment cephalometric radiograph. Notice the prognathic mandible. Cephalometric analysis demonstrated that the maxilla was properly related to the cranial base, and that the mandible was positioned too far anteriorly. (d) Case 1. Tracing of the postsurgical cephalometric radiograph. Observe how the profile has improved. If this patient had a pseudoprognathic mandible, as do most cleft palate patients, moving the mandible posteriorly would have devastated the patient's profile.

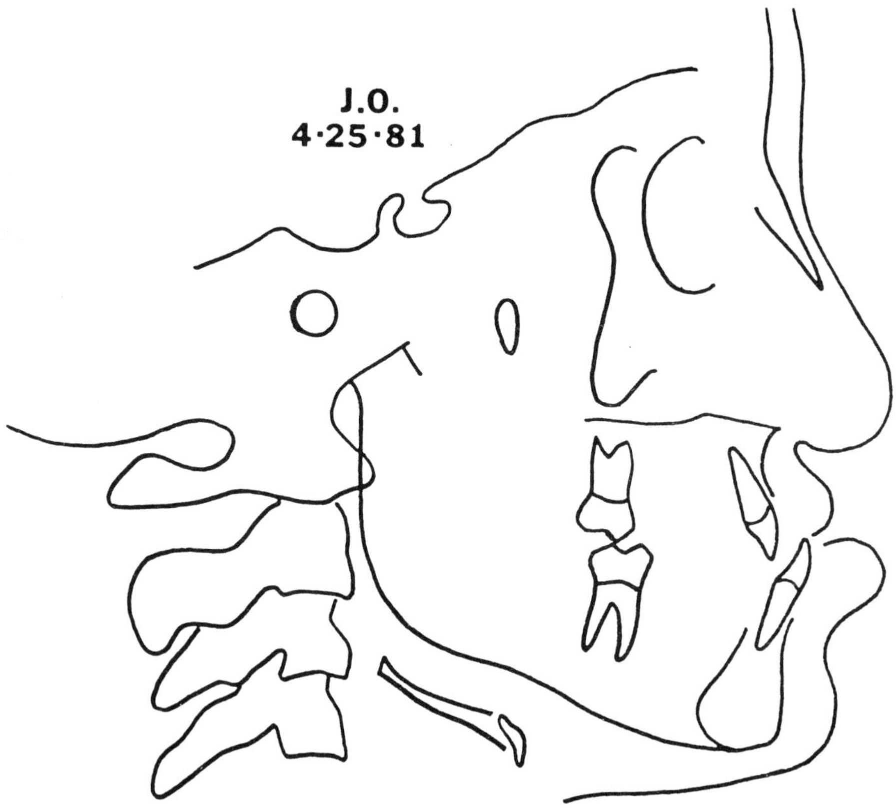
J.O.
4·25·81

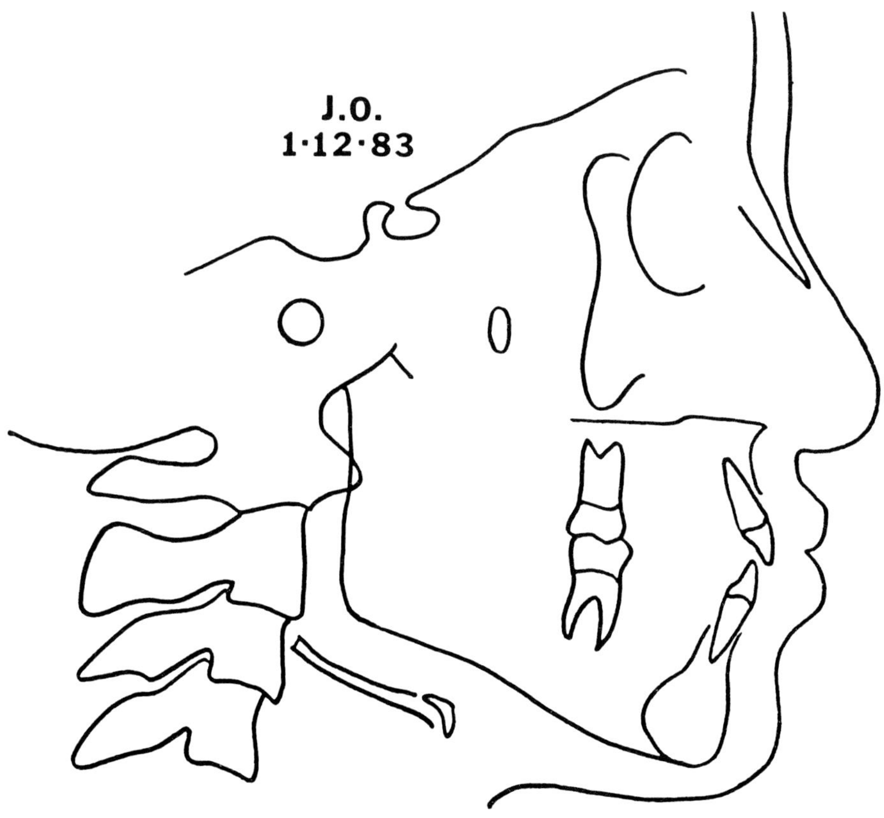
J.O.
1·12·83

REFERENCES

1. Levin HS: A cephalometric analysis of cleft palate deficiencies in the middle third of the face. *Angle Orthod,* 33:186, 1963.
2. Swanson LT, MacCollum DW, Richardson SO: Evaluation of the dental problems in the cleft palate patient. *Am J Orthod,* 42:749, 1956.
3. Jordan RE, Kraus BS, Neptune CM: Dental anomalies associated with cleft lip and/or palate. *Cleft Palate J,* 3:22, 1966.
4. Olin WH: Dental anomalies in cleft lip and palate patients. *Angle Orthod,* 34:119, 1964.
5. Vargervik K: Orthodontic management of the unilateral cleft palate patient. *Cleft Palate J,* 18:256, 1981.
6. Schroeder DC, Green L: Frequency of detail trait anomalies in cleft, sibling, and noncleft groups. *J Dent Child,* 54:802, 1975.
7. Greulich WW, Pyle SL: *Radiographic Atlas of Skeletal Development of the Hand and Wrist.* Stanford, Calif, Stanford University Press, 1959.
8. Graber TM: *Orthodontics Principles and Practice.* Philadelphia, W B Saunders Co, 1972.
9. Hunter WS: Elementary principles of cephalometrics, in Enlow DH (ed): *The Human Face.* New York, Hoeber Med Div, Harper Row Pub, 1968.
10. Olin WH: Orthondontics, in Grabbe WC, Rosenstein SW, Bzoch KR (eds): *Cleft Lip and Palate.* Boston, Little Brown & Co, 1971.
11. Worms FW, Isaacson RJ, Speidel TM: Surgical orthodontic treatment planning: Profile analysis and mandibular surgery. *Angle Orthod,* 46:1, 1976.
12. Fish LC, Epker BN: Surgical-orthodontic cephalometric prediction tracing. *J Clin Orthod,* 14:36, 1980.
13. Gans BJ, Kallal RH: Surgical management of orofacial deformities, in Graber TM, Swain BF (eds): *Current Orthodontic Concepts and Techniques.* Philadelphia, W B Saunders Co, 1975.

CHAPTER 9

PROSTHODONTIA

MORT ROSEN

. . . There may well be those who can do without knowledge, but I for my part am certainly not one of them.

. . . Confucius

Prosthodontic Rehabilitation

A CLEFT PALATE might be defined as a fissure located in the palate and completely surrounded by a human being. This definition could then emphasize a prosthodontic rehabilitative goal—namely, the rehabilitation of the human being born with the cleft palate deformity. Many years of experience in this work have shown that this goal is seldom reached simply by closing the defect through surgery or plugging up the defect through prosthetics. However, the experience of treating over 1,000 persons with cleft lip and/or palate has established beyond any doubt the importance of the prosthodontist's role in the total treatment plan of many patients.

Prosthetic treatment of the cleft lip and palate condition is so wide in scope that one may generalize by saying that it starts at birth and ends with death. This treatise will be concerned with some of the major problem areas subdivided into groups according to anatomical orientation.

Under this category the first problem area that comes to mind is the foreshortened or cleft palate either before surgery or after surgery, and the importance of prosthetic speech appliance in its treatment. Unfortunately much misunderstanding and misinterpretation of the purpose and the limitations of the speech aid still exist, even among medical and dental specialists.

Purpose of a Speech Appliance

The basic purpose of the prosthetic speech appliance is twofold: first, to restore the physical division between the oral and nasal cavities normally accomplished by the intact hard and soft palates; and second, to make possible the recurrent closing and opening of the nasopharynx normally accomplished by the complex velopharyngeal function.

Although the speech aid is designed to be a substitute for the cleft portion of the palate, the modern appliance is not designed to be a substitute palate. No attempt through the use of hinges or movable parts is made to duplicate the velopharyngeal valving of the musculo-fibrous soft palate shown in Figure 9-1, above left and right.

Rather, as indicated in Figure 9-1, below, the rigid extended posterior section of the appliance is positioned high in the region of the nasopharynx, where it is finely adjusted in size and shape to allow it to act as semiobturator of this region.

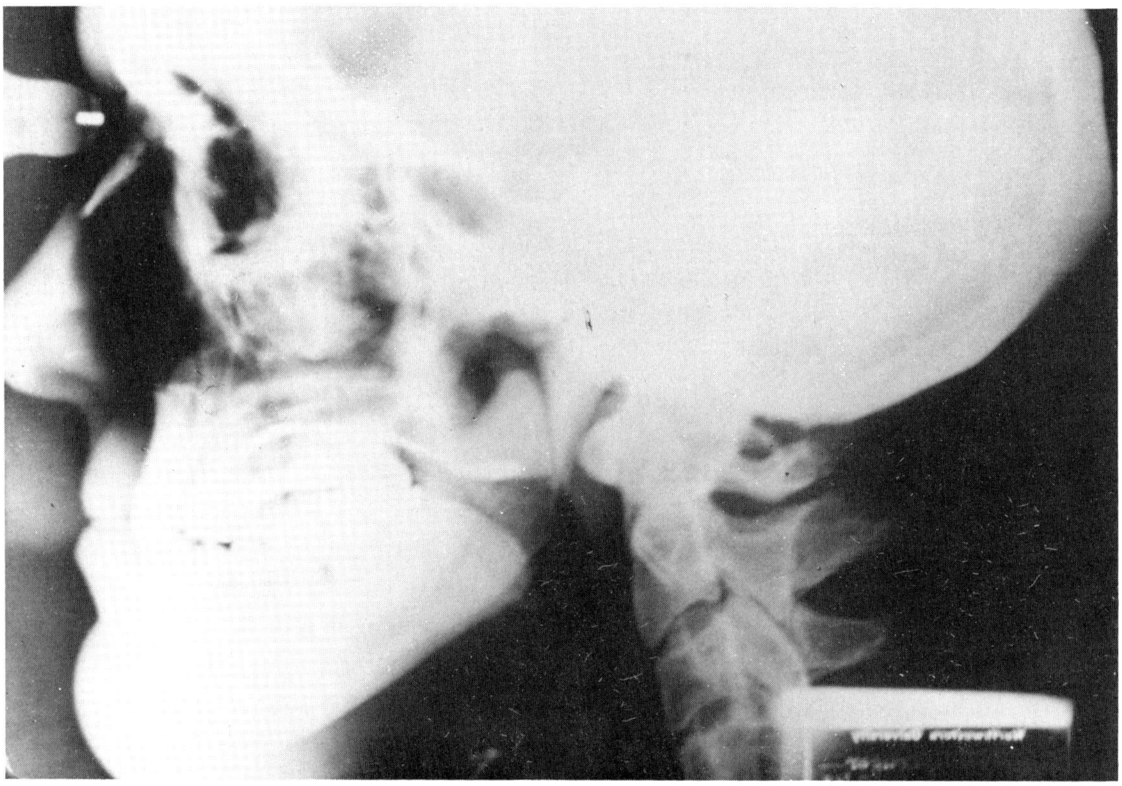

Figure 9-1. Position of prosthetic speech appliance.

The complete speech appliance is shown in Figure 9-2. The body portion attaches to the teeth of the maxillary arch and covers the hard palate on the oral surface. Any remaining cleft of the hard palate or any perforation in this structure is completely obturated by the body section.

The tailpiece section suspends the speech bulb in the nasopharynx. It is a narrowed posterior extension of the body section. The speech bulb is usually positioned high in the nasopharynx by the tailpiece (Fig. 9-1). The size and shape of the speech bulb is adjusted to conform to the anatomy and physiology of each individual in order to allow air to pass freely through the nasopharyngeal port for breathing and yet

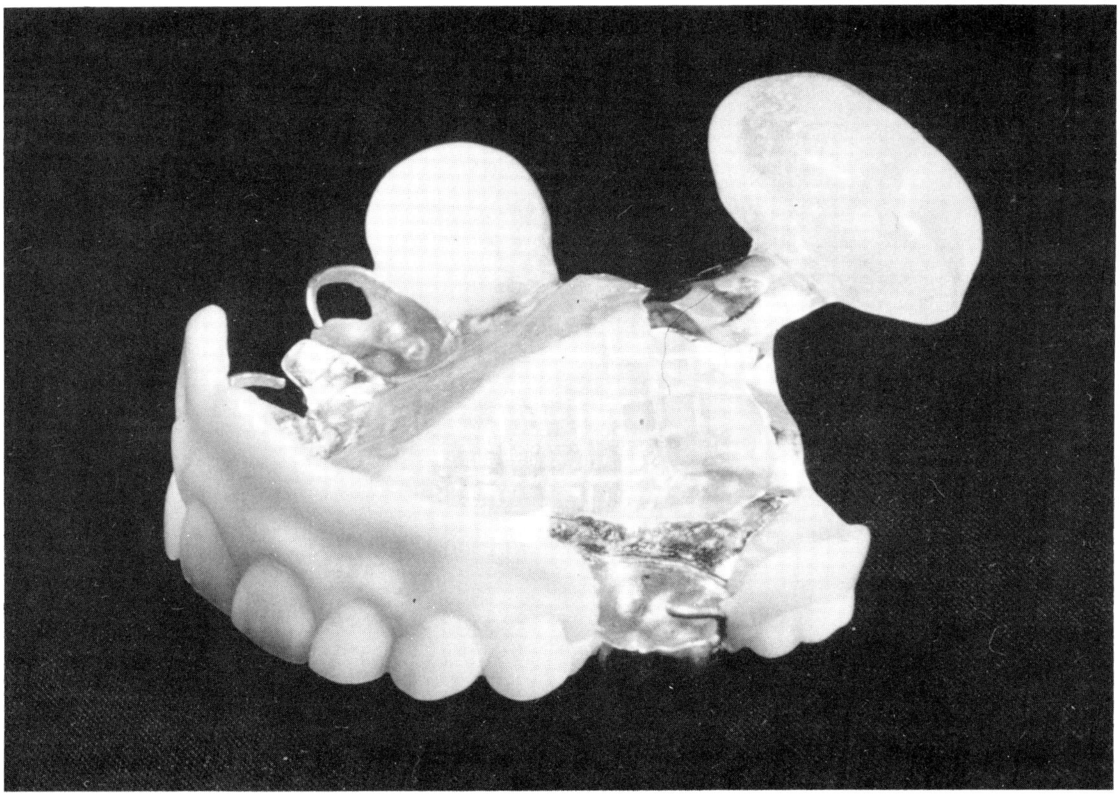

Figure 9-2. The complete speech appliance.

to make possible the closure of this airway space for speech. The greatest portion of the muscular valving against the speech bulb is accounted for by the medial movement of the lateral walls of the nasopharynx. The muscle action of the pharyngeal constrictor, sphinctor-complex, and salpingo-pharyngeus muscles against the stable speech bulb accomplishes this closure for speech.

Uses and Limitations of the Speech Appliance

Hypernasality (or nasal twang) is the subjective impression the speaker's voice makes on a listener when an excessive amount of overtone resonance occurs in the nasal chambers. A speech appliance, of itself, can eliminate hypernasal voice quality and, if carefully adjusted, can eliminate the distortion of consonant sound elements due to audible nasal emission; but it cannot, of itself, correct any habits of misarticulation the patient may possess.

Voice quality can be altered mechanically to the extreme of hyponasality (insufficient overtone resonance in the nasal chambers) by enlarging the size of the speech bulb. A fine adjustment of the size of the speech bulb will make possible a pleasing voice quality. It will also eliminate the distortion of certain pressure sound elements, such as "p," "b," "f," "s," "ch" and "j" sounds, due to audible puffs of air rushing through the nose at the instant of their articulation. If the bulb is adjusted by the prosthodontist to the point where the user can produce a clear "p" and a sustained "f" or "s" sound without emission of air through the nose and also can produce the nasal sound "m," the appliance is adjusted adequately. (The "s" sound gives a finer test of nasal emission than the "f," but should not be used if it is not made in the normal fashion by the patient.)

From this point on the elimination of the remaining speech differences will depend on the motivation and cooperation of the patient in overcoming habits of misarticulation. These habits are learned and reinforced from early childhood. Relearning, therefore, usually can be accomplished best by working with a skilled speech correction teacher. Under favorable conditions, that is, with an intelligent and motivated parent and a well adjusted speech appliance, the prognosis for normal speech is very good, even for adolescent and adult persons with cleft palate.

Certain cautions must be emphasized in regard to the prosthetic speech appliance. If it is not properly managed by the prosthodontist, the appliance could result in: (1) disappointment on the part of the patient over less intelligible speech with the appliance; (2) a possible threat to dental oral health; (3) a causal factor in the development of mouth breathing; (4) a threat to the preservation and stabilization of the maxillary dentition; and (5) disturbance of the normal drainage through the nasal pharynx which could result in otological complications.

To a great extent the speech of patients with cleft palate is deficient on a functional or habitual basis. In a recent detailed analysis of the speech of preschool children Bzoch[1] found that the habit of articulating consonant sounds in the larynx and oral pharynx was typical of children with cleft palate and atypical of similar normal children. Related studies by Starr[2] and Counihan[3] showed that these substitute articulations diminished with age but continued to be a considerable factor in the speech defect.

It is the characteristic functional defect in the speech of patients with cleft palate which the speech appliance per se will not improve. Often these unusual articulation habits are not perceived by the patient or his family because of the gross distortion of speech through hypernasality and nasal emission. When the speech appliance eliminates these two factors of the speech defect, the misarticulations may become perceivable for the first time. The temporary result may be a period of less intelligible speech. The patient and his parents should be prepared for this possibility, and it should be explained that only with the appliance and speech training can these habits be changed.

It is obvious that a patient must have, or be willing to acquire, good oral hygiene habits if he is to wear a speech appliance. The appliance is relatively larger than the more common dental prosthesis and has more irregular surfaces. Also it frequently will be worn by younger patients who need supervision and persuasion from their parents even for routine toothbrushing. If the importance of good oral hygiene is strongly emphasized to both the patient and his parents, no problem need arise. A clear procedure should be outlined by the prosthodontist for care and cleaning of the appliance, and the motivation actually can be utilized to improve or establish good oral hygiene habits.

Sometimes the speech bulb is made too large, or after it has been properly adjusted allergic or infectious conditions cause a swelling of the surrounding membranes. Significant muscular development sometimes takes place after the placement of the appliance (due to the increased activity of the muscles against the resistance of the speech bulb). Any of these conditions could lead to complete obturation of the nasopharynx. This might cause mouth breathing habits to form or otological complications. The condition can be corrected easily by adjusting the speech bulb. Some system of vocabulary or routine reexamination should be instituted, therefore, to guard against such occurrences. Such reexaminations are also important to assess the need for enlargements and adjustments of the bulb after periods of growth.

Finally it should be cautioned that a speech appliance, if not properly adjusted and retained, could act as a reverse orthodontic appliance. The muscle action of the velum and pharynx could transmit intermittent pressure to the teeth, causing them to tilt or shift and thereby affect the occlusion. Proper retention and adjustment eliminates this hazard.

The prosthetic speech appliance can be, and often is for many human beings, the key by which the door to normal life is opened. When the tissue is insufficient for successful surgical closure, prosthetics becomes the rehabilitation method of choice. When surgery is to be postponed through speech readiness and development periods, a temporary speech appliance makes possible the acquisition of acceptable and even normal speech habits. For many adults who have cleft palate and deficient maxillary development, the speech appliance combined with an anterior split and denture plus the skill of the plastic surgeon in adjusting the upper lip and nasal structures, may bring them for the first time in their lives normal speech, normal eating and normal appearance.

Prosthetics Stabilization of the Premaxilla

A second problem area that presents itself, when a defect in the normal configuration of the maxilla is created by the occurrence of a congenital bilateral cleft lip and palate, is the stabilization of the mobile premaxilla, especially when bone grafting either is contraindicated or has failed (Fig. 9-3).

A method to correct this situation and to provide continuity and symmetry of the patient's dental arch, which is so necessary for speech, facial aesthetics and adequate dental function, is to construct a fixed bridge from cuspid to cuspid or even extended to the bicuspids. The maxillary bicuspids and cuspids are not within the premaxillary area and thus become available for abutments.

The replacement of missing teeth and properly shaped and contoured malposed and/or misshaped anterior teeth will give the dental arch continuity and symmetry for proper tongue tip articulation (Fig. 9-4). A good concept of facial aesthetics is of paramount importance when the dental arch form is being restored.

With the advent of new surgical techniques, the prosthodontist is not called upon as frequently as before to aid in the rehabilitation process, but his skills are

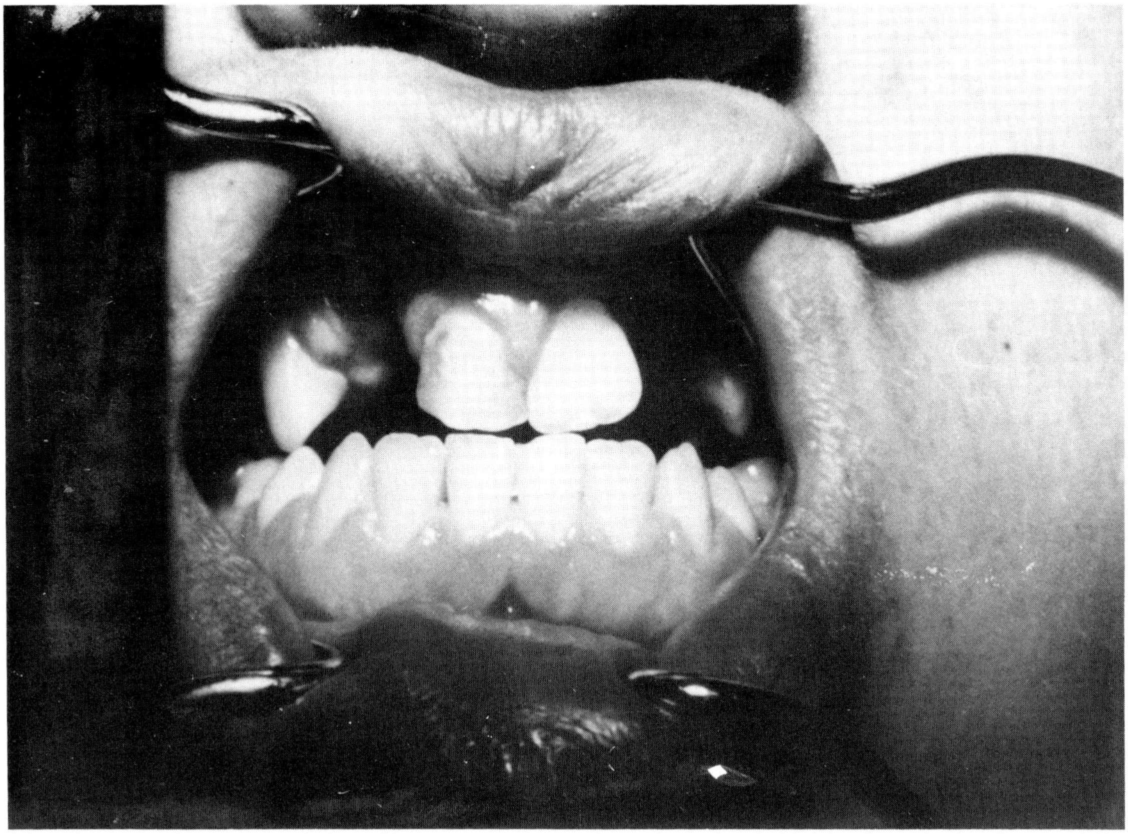

Figure 9-3.

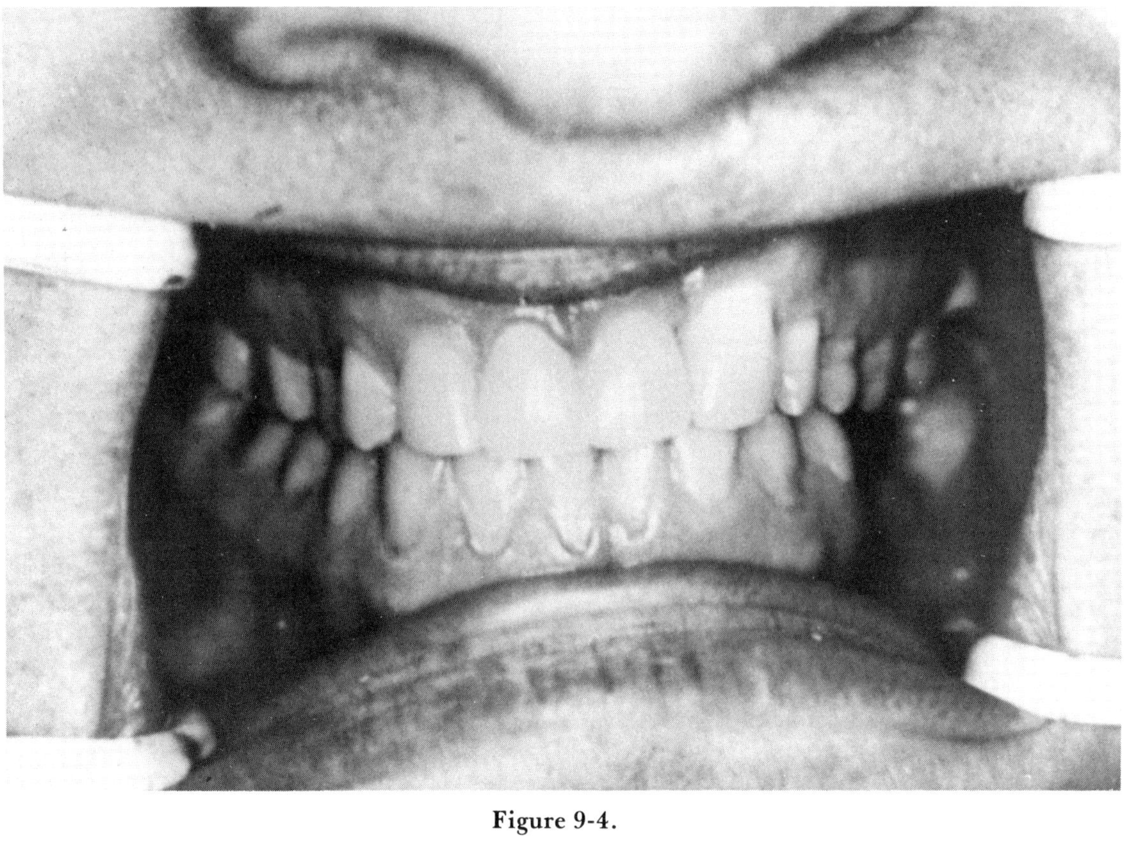

Figure 9-4.

necessary instead of surgery for clefts: (1) when there is insufficient tissue for surgical closure; (2) when surgery has been attempted and failed; (3) in conjunction with surgery when the palate has been redivided; or (4) in combination with surgery with partial surgical and partial prosthetic restoration.

The prosthodontist, by virtue of his ability and training together with inventiveness and perseverance, is the solution to many of the dentofacial problems confronting patients. Prosthodontics can be most gratifying when, in conjunction with other clinical specialities, it gives one the ability to transform a disfigured and disillusioned human being into a normal acting and normal looking person who can take his place in society.

REFERENCES

1. Bzoch KR: *Investigation of the Speech of Pre-School Cleft Palate Children,* thesis. Northwestern University School of Speech, Evanston, Ill, 1956.
2. Starr, C: *Study of Some of the Characteristics of the Speech and Speech Mechanism of a Group of Cleft Palate Children,* thesis. Northwestern University School of Speech, Evanston, Ill, 1956.
3. Counihan DR: *Clinical Study of the Speech Efficiency and Structural Adequacy of Operated Adolescent and Adult Cleft Palate Persons,* thesis. Northwestern University School of Speech, Evanston, Ill, 1956.

CHAPTER 10

PERIODONTAL DISEASE

HARRY STAFFILENO

. . .A gentleman does not mind failing to get recognition; he is too busy doing things that entitle him to recognition.

. . .Confucius

PERIODONTAL disease is the greatest single cause of tooth loss in adults. Children as young as 5 or 6 years of age may show early signs, such as bleeding of the gums after brushing. It is an interesting disease in that it progresses slowly over a long period of time with little or no pain. With time this disease can destroy the gum tissue, bone tissue and other related structures that support the teeth. The main structural unit that is affected by periodontal disease is the dentoperiodontal unit. This unit consists of the tooth, the attachment epithelium, the connective tissue attachment and the ligamentous structure that attaches the tooth to the supporting alveolar process.

Changes that begin to manifest disease in this structure more specifically will reflect clinically at the dentogingival junction because that is primarily where the epithelium attaches itself to the tooth structure. In essence this is a sealing mechanism that seals the outside environment from inside the body. In terms of kinds of periodontal disease in outline form, first would be gingivitis. This is an inflammatory manifestation of the gingival tissues immediately about the neck of the tooth. This condition can be acute, with much pain and discomfort, or chronic, with little pain and discomfort. It can be infective, hyperplastic, desquamative, necrotizing and allergic. A gingivitis problem can be localized to one or two teeth or generalized throughout the mouth.

Periodontitis is simply a progression generally of a preexisting gingivitis to the deeper tissues and, specifically, the bone tissue thereby affected, the supporting apparatus or periodontium. This disease process can be acute or chronic and it can be localized or generalized.

A third category of periodontal disease is dystrophic in nature and referred to as juvenile periodontitis or periodontosis.[1]

Diseases of the dentoperiodontal unit are three in number: caries, pulpal disease and periodontal disease. Any one of these three diseases left untreated results in morbidity of this structure. Specifically, with periodontal disease there are seven signs that are looked for to identify this disease process: (1) bleeding gums when brushing or cleaning the teeth, (2) bad breath, (3) soft, swollen or tender gums, (4) pus from the gumline on compression, (5) loose teeth, (6) gums shrinking away from the teeth and (7) any change in the way the teeth come together.

It is not necessary that all seven of these factors be present. Any one that is present can be indicative of a periodontal disease process. Gingivitis and peridontitis are initiated and sustained in most instances by a sticky bacterial mass called "plaque" on the tooth surface. The portion of the plaque that lies in the vicinity of the gingival sulcus produces gingival lesions. Since plaque also produces caries, its removal is a critical step in the management and control of both periodontal disease and caries. However, once removed the plaque begins to form within 2 hours and is well established in 24 hours. Therefore, frequent removal of plaque is essential to good clinical management of periodontal disease.

If this plaque is not removed, it gradually hardens into a calcified bacterial debris which helps to force the gingival tissue away from the tooth; pockets of infection form between the teeth and the gums. If this is left unchecked, the disease attacks and destroys the supporting bone and then the process is in progress for the loss of teeth.

Anatomically the area of the dentoperiodontal unit referred to as the dentogingival junction is the only one of its kind in the human body.[2] It is the only area in the body in which a tissue structure such as the tooth, which is of epithelial and connective tissue origin, exits the body with an attachment apparatus of epithelium in the form of hemidesmosomes attaching themselves to the surface of the tooth.[3] It is this attachment system that is easily jeopardized by the proliferation of bacteria, as well as their products, in the gingival sulcus so that a destruction of that structure can take place. Ensuing inflammatory response in turn begins to jeopardize the entire integrity of the dentogingival junction. In order to prevent and control periodontal disease, it is essential that this sticky film called "plaque" is removed daily through the use of a brush and floss.

There are other characteristics modifying this gingivitus condition which may be observed at times. There is the infective gingivitis, which is a highly inflamed gum tissue. It is caused by streptococcus organisms resulting in a very red, intensely inflammed, painful gingival tissue. Many times the inflammation is not limited to the gingiva but extends to the mucosa. In addition to the signs, the patient has symptoms of pain, elevation in temperature and general discomfort.

Another form of gingivitis is hyperplastic gingivitus, in which the gingival tissue has increased in size. This may be an exuberant fibrous growth of the gingiva that occurs in certain conditions following the administration of such drugs as phenytoin sodium (Dilantin Sodium) or in certain genetic anomalies. It is referred to as hereditary fibromatos gingivae, for which there is no known cause.

There is also another condition which is characterized by hyperplasia of the gingival tissues. This occurs in people who have difficulty with nose breathing due to preexisting conditions such as adenoids, deviated septum or allergic problems. These people breathe through the mouth, which in turn causes the oral mucous membrane and specifically the gingival tissue to dry. This results in increased size. However, the size increase is not as great as that seen with the administration of phenytoin or in hereditary fibromatous gingivae.[4]

Certain hormonal changes in patients, particularly female patients, can be observed in the integrity of the gingival tissues. This is primarily manifested in puberty when the gingival tissue tends to be enlarged, edematous and bleeds easily.

A very common problem in young people between the ages of 14 and 25 is referred to as "necrotizing ulcerative gingivitis" (NUG). This occurs in those hosts who respond to stress situations and body fatigue with periodontal disease. It seems that these patients have the oral cavity and specifically the periodontal unit as a *target zone.* NUG, also referred to as trench mouth and Vincent's infection, is a noncontagious periodontal disease characterized by many ulcerations of the gingival tissue with pain, halitosis and possibly cervical and submandibular lymphadenopathy and a general malaise of the patient. When a culture is taken there is a high count of the fusiform bacilli as well as the spirochetes. However, these organisms are always present in the mouth; they are simply opportunists which tend to grow profusely at this particular time.[5]

The onset of the acute problem is sudden. Chronic asymptomatic conditions may have existed before. The outstanding symptoms are salivation, a metallic taste, pain, general malaise and elevation in body temperature.

The dentist must make a decision on the immediate management of this patient and identify the clinical signs of the disease. When a patient demonstrates debris on the tooth surfaces, particularly at the dentogingival junction, and widespread or isolated areas of ulceration with a greying, yellowing membrane in the region of the dentogingival junction, it would be valid *tentatively* to diagnose NUG. On some occasions this disease is manifested only in areas of erupting third molars and referred to as ulcerative operculitis or in areas of malaligned teeth such as in alveolar clefts or unerupted teeth.

The significant predisposing factors are poor oral hygiene, inadequate plaque control and tissue stimulation, open contacts, overhanging restorations and erupting teeth. A very important overlying factor is the systemic condition of the patient. Lowered resistance, stress or inadequate care of one's body are also predisposing factors. This disease is sometimes referred to as the "ulcer of the upper alimentary tract."

Management of the NUG Patient

Factors to be evaluated are emotions, antibacterial, nutrition, fatigue, vasomotor mechanism and lifestyle. The management of this acute problem requires examination and interrogation of the patient. Is the patient taking medications for a preexisting medical problem? Has the patient done something that could have precipitated this condition in the oral cavity due to physical contact or drug exposure?

If not, proceed over the next 48 hours with the management of this problem as NUG. The acute phase control program should consist of:

1. Debridement and cleansing. This can be initiated in the office by brushing and, if tolerable, by ultrasonic debridement of the dentogingival junction.
2. If the patient is not allergic to penicillin, it is the drug of choice for acute infections.
3. The patient should be made comfortable and analgesics prescribed along with instruction for plaque control and oral hygiene. In NUG where anaerobic organisms predominate, it is important that the patient be advised to rinse the mouth at least four times a day for at least one minute. An oxygenating mouthwash can be used, such as hydrogen peroxide 3 percent liquid, which can be diluted 1:1 with warm water, or there are packaged materials available such as Amosan, Vince and others.

Advise the patient to use a sulcus-type or soft brush with a minimal number of bristles, if the patient can tolerate brushing the teeth and soft tissue. Rest, proper diet and vitamins are advised.

In summary, the acute phase control program for this patient includes: (1) debridement and cleansing of the oral cavity, (2) antibiotic regimen, (3) analgesics as necessary, (4) plaque control, oral environment control utilizing a special mouthwash that releases oxygen and personal brushing and (5) supportive care consisting of diet, rest and vitamin-mineral supplements.

Although one initiates a program of management for the acute stage, one must be aware that, from a diagnostic point of view, there are other problems that mimic the acute ulcerative gingivitis problem.[1] Some of these are:

1. *Acute herpetic stomatitis,* which involves many areas of the oral cavity other than the gingiva;
2. *Erythema multiformae;*
3. *Streptoccal stomatitis,* which includes generalized malaise, elevated body temperature and general involvement of tissues other than the immediate gingival tissues;
4. *Agranulocytosis;*
5. *Leukemia.*

Within the first 48 hours NUG generally responds dramatically to the regimen just described. At the initial appointment there also should be a hematological examination consisting of a complete blood count with a differential review. A culture of the mouth is not significant. It would be appropriate to contact this patient by phone within 24 hours and mandatory to clinically examine the patient in 48 hours. At that time the cellular blood count should be available. In most instances one will find no particular abnormality in the blood cell count. Leukemia and agranulocytosis consequently can be ruled out. There will be dramatic response by the patient in terms of feeling better, reduced regional lymphadenopathy, less pain and less odor within the oral cavity. The patient is advised to continue the regimen. One should see the patient again in two to three days. At that time, five days post initial examination, the patient will have made a complete reversal with very little evidence of preexisting acute NUG.

In the second phase of management of NUG patient, long-term control, many dentists fail to continue treatment and management. It is mandatory to help the patient find, so to speak, *shock absorbers* within the psychophysiological system in order to prevent further acute flareups. Included as part of this regimen are:

1. A daily routine with an oxygenating mouthwash is strongly advised.
2. Dietary habits should be reviewed to assure good, balanced nutritional support.
3. Adequate rest must be advised to prevent physical fatigue.

In essence a program for local management as well as general supportive management is advised to develop a *resiliency* within the patient. He develops an ability to "roll with the punch" when undergoing additional stress. He becomes aware of when stress is occurring and, with the dentist's advice, will slow down and be particularly careful with plaque control and his general physical behavior.

Generally the experience is that patients with acute NUG as described do not repeat the acute phase if given secondary long-term management as discussed and provided they follow their instructions and their regimen carefully.

Allergic Gingivitis

Another gingivitis problem that is identified from time to time is referred to as allergic gingivitis.[5] Histologically, on a microscopic specimen there will be dense aggregates of plasma cells. They are confined to the marginal gingival tissue. After much study and review of the patient, it can be determined that this patient has responded in an allergic manner to some toothpaste, chewing gum or could even be reactive to animal dander. The gingiva becomes red, swollen, sometimes granular and has a burning sensation. The discomfort is far less than the clinical appearance would indicate. In all of these gingivitis problems that have been mentioned management should consist of cleansing of the oral cavity and the establishment of a plaque control regimen. If there is infection and submandibular lymphadenopathy with elevation in temperature, antibiotics are indicated, primarily those for gram-positive organisms, such as penicillin and/or erythromycin. If there is evidence of calcified debris about the teeth and subgingivally, professional attention should be instituted. If there is a problem that is in response to drug administration, then there should be research as to whether this patient can be transferred to a medication that will not cause this response by the gingival tissue. Any desquamative problem that is free of infection can be treated by surface or topical application of steroids.

If there is a condition that has much discomfort as well as inflammatory response and lymphadenopathy, then antibiotics should be utilized. Generally, in any of these problems response is significant within 48 to 72 hours, bringing the problem down to a low-grade, chronic state. Then further dental management and periodontal management are necessary either to arrest the disease process or to keep it under control. It is advisable in those conditions such as NUG and infective gingivitis to have hematologic studies. They will assure that this is not a manifestation of a systemic disease such as leukemia, agranulocytosis or some other problem.

As mentioned earlier, periodontitis is generally an extension of a gingivitis problem characterized significantly by bone involvement. This change is a resorption of the coronal aspect of the alveolar process. Clinically, without probing, the dentogingival junction may resemble a gingivitis when in reality, upon probing and studying dental x-rays, it is a very definite periodontitis. Pockets can be measured beyond the 2 mm range into 4, 5, 6 and up to 9 or 10 mm. This means that there is a breakdown or detachment of the tissue apparatus that formerly was intact. Besides bleeding there may be a purulent exudate and tooth mobility present. This does not necessarily mean that a tooth will be lost, but it certainly indicates that some bone support has been affected. The two most important characteristics of periodontitis are bone destruction, as demonstrated by x-rays, and pocket formation that is demonstrated by periodontal probing.

In addition to dental plaque as a causative agent for periodontitis, there are other local irritants such as faulty restorations, loose dental contacts and malocclusion, or irregularities within the bite. Again, as with gingivitis, there are changes in color and tissue character showing edema, hyperplasia or recession, formation of clefts or little grooves on the root surface and, as mentioned before, tooth mobility. Those people who do not eat balanced diets consequently have inadquate nutrition. They may have a heavy carbohydrate intake, which makes sugar available and from that dextran is formed. Dextran is a sticky substance that attaches plaque to the teeth. Since bacteria require sugar to form dextran, if the amount of sugar eaten is limited, the amount of plaque formed is reduced.

There is another very important clinical behavior of patients—clenching, or in some instances grinding of the teeth. This puts undue pressure upon the dentoperiodontal unit and, depending upon the host, will precipitate a breakdown of the supporting apparatus and will help precipitate periodontitis.

Another form of periodontal disease is found in 4-8 percent of the population. It is referred to as "dystrophic periodontal disease" and more specifically in adults as "periodontosis." In adults, and particularly in people from the Middle East, Near East and Far East, it occurs in women of childbearing age. It seems that the anterior teeth, particularly the incisors, are generally involved. The clinical features include migration of the teeth, diastemas, extrusion and malocclusion. There is also a similar condition that is observed in a small percentage of teenagers and is referred to as juvenile periodontitis. It seems that rapid destruction of the bone occurs in these patients, causing a lossening of teeth and eventually, within a short period of time (just a few years), loss of significant numbers of teeth. It has been found in these juvenile periodontitis patients that there had been a particular characteristic of the polymorphonuclear leukocytes which is significant in the peripheral blood studies. There is also a periodontitis-like lesion that is observed in patients who have Papillon-LeFevre syndrome, which includes hyperkeratosis of the palms and soles. This again manifests early in life and is seen as a juvenile periodontitis.

In more recent studies there have been identified in the pockets of teeth with periodontitis of these different types, certain organisms which are not identified with gingivitis or very early grade periodontitis problems. Overall treatment of periodontal disease begins with the removal of the causes. Depending on the severity of the disease, this may be done by the general dentist or by a periodontist. In the earliest stages simple removal of the calcified bacterial debris on the tooth crown by scaling and root planing suffices to restore health.

There are times when a further step in treatment is indicated, consisting of curettage of the gum tissue in order to permit the gingival tissue to adapt tighter to the tooth surface. With the more advanced disease conditions surgical removal of the diseased tissue may be necessary. A combination procedure of soft tissue flap reflection with underlying management of the bony tissue, through either osteoplasty or osseous grafting procedures, is done at times to reestablish the integrity of the dentogingival junction. These surgical measures are performed in order to give access to areas about the teeth that are inaccessible to personal cleansing or professional management, and to leave a healthier anatomical form that can sustain itself in the future.[6]

There are other procedures performed in periodontal disease management, such as bite adjustment and prosthetic appliances to replace teeth and give support that was lost through the resorption of bone in the disease process.

Periodontal disease can always recur; however, it is extremely important that once the disease process has been identified and treated, the patient practice a daily regimen to prevent its recurrence. Periodontal professional review and therapy may be necessary to arrest early recurring disease conditions.

Other forms of therapy in the management of periodontal disease are directed to the intraoral plastic surgical reconstruction of the dentogingival junction unit. This kind of measure is indicated when:

1. Disease causes loss of soft tissue about a tooth:
2. Disease causes loss of soft and hard tissue supporting structure about a tooth;
3. Growth and developmental abnormalities precipitate a dystrophy of tissue structure resulting in the denudation of a tooth or inadequate masticatory mucosa at the dentogingival junction area of the tooth.

Therapeutic philosophies have undergone complete reorientation in the plastic surgical repair of the disease dentoperiodontal unit as their reconstructive procedures have become increasingly predictable.

Full Thickness Versus Split Thickness Flaps

Currently measures in periodontal therapy have progressed so that treatment of the patient is very predictable except in extreme situations. This has been made possible because of advancement in the technology of clinical therapy and because of the information that has been learned through experimental research in the laboratory and clinic. With the progress of periodontal disease there is a disruption of the immediate soft tissue morphology in the dentogingival junction region. The progression of peridontal disease is quantitative in nature—more tissue structure becomes involved with its movement in an apical direction. The deeper connective tissue and the coronal area of the alveolar process are affected by the destructive nature of this disease. Consequently the gingival attachment appartus moves apically along with a loss of bone at the crestal area of alveolar process and possibly the eventual lossening of teeth. Correlating with this process is pocket formation, and with the existence of a pocket there is further bone loss and tooth mobility. This process eventually may lead to the loss of the tooth or teeth involved. The objective in periodontics is the maintenance of a functional morphology of the dentoperiodontal unit and then, once disease has initiated, to treat it and to restore the integrity of the periodontal tissues. Primary in periodontal therapy is the elimination, if possible, of the etiology of the periodontal disease and removal of pockets that have formed resultant to the pathology. In the past two decades periodontal therapy has progressed so that today therapy consists of many methods, depending upon the nature and advancement of the disease. This contrasts to some years ago when simple gingivectomy was the universal treatment of choice, and this resulted in the removal of marginal, gingival tissue that formed the disease wall of the pocket. However, where osseous pathology has taken place and a deformity in the osseous architecture existed, a correction to this tissue through gingival resection was not achieved.

The concept of pocket elimination today is a fundamental objective of periodontal therapy. It also has been demonstrated in recent years that in order to eliminate the periodontal pocket successfully there must be a correction of the underlying osseous lesion. This has moved periodontics through a period of strictly gingival resection into an era where several methods of therapy have been made available on the basis of the nature of the periodontal lesion. The more advanced methods of therapy consist of mucogingival surgery for those pockets transversing the mucogingival junction and when deep or moderate osseous lesions prevail. These methods of therapy have made possible the reestablishmnt of the integrity of the dentogingival junction so that there is a proper working relationship of the clinical crown of the tooth, masticatory mucosa and lining alveolar mucosa apical to the mucogingival junction. This also has permitted more predictable periodontics with results in which the patient could better maintain oral health and prevent further periodontal disease. This led to surgical endeavors in the area of mucogingival surgery and subsequently motivated astute clinical observers to broaden the horizon in the development of many refinements for correcting deformities of the dentogingival junction. Clinicians realized that the objective was to establish a functioning dentogingival junction enveloped by masticatory mucosa that had no direct conflict with the mucogingival junction. Approaches in this direction in some instances provided disappointing results, however sophisticated they were. It was only after laboratory research by Wilderman,[7] Staffileno and associates,[8-12] Cohen and Ross,[13] Chacker,[14] Hellburn,[15] Pfeifer,[16] and Friedman and Levin,[17] that the findings revealed certain procedures could be done with predictability, though others were extremely traumatic and destructive to the existing supporting structures.

The primary surgical procedure in mucogingival surgery is the flap. Because of recent laboratory studies the flap most desirable to utilize is the partial thickness or split thickness flap. This permits the periosteal connective tissues to remain intact on the bone and a flap with epithelium and its underlying connective tissue to manipulate in whichever way desired. This flap, which has been referred to as the split thickness or partial thickness flap, is probably used in the majority of mucogingival procedures. The full thickness or mucoperiosteal flap, as it is sometimes called, is used less frequently in mucogingival surgery. It is significant at this point to outline the indications of one type of flap over the other, and in order to do this one must consider not only that clinical problem at hand but also a review of the histological response of the immediate tissues involved when there is either the split thickness or full thickness flap developed in a surgical procedure.

The basic difference in the preparation of the flaps is that for the full thickness or mucoperiosteal flap, an incision generally is made in or near the gingival sulcus region and carried apically toward the crest of the bone, from which point there is total reflection of all soft tissue from the surface of the alveolar process. This may leave a small stump of connective tissue attached to the tooth and a denuded bony surface from which the mucoperiosteal flap was reflected. In contrast the split thickness or mucosal flap is prepared by initiating an incision on or near the gingival sulcus region and proceeding apically through the connective tissue *past the crest of the alveolar bone* so as to leave a layer of periosteal connective tissue intact, covering the vestibular surface of the alveolar process. The flaps themselves are basically the same in tissue components except varied as to their thickness because of the connective tissue variation due to, in one, some of the connective tissue being left on the bone, and in the other, all of it being reflected from the bone.

Histological studies carried out with these two flap procedures reveal that when there is no existing periodontal disease we are able to evaluate the differences in the tissue response to this surgical intervention and gain better insight as to what degree of destruction or change results because of that specific surgical technique. When two flaps are prepared just as has been described, reapposed to their original position and maintained by sutures, there is a definite variation in response of the immediate tissues in the healing process. The findings are: The epithelial tissue repairs itself similarly in both procedures. This is no surprise because whether there is full thickness or split thickness it has no effect on the epithelium, and there is still an interface of epithelium to epithelium. Subjacent to the epithelial attachment region there is the connective tissue and again in both flap procedures there is no significant variation as to the repair of the connective tissue.

However, the difference in repair between the two flaps becomes manifest in the region of the alveolar process because on the one hand we have an interface of bone and connective tissue with the mucoperiosteal flap, and on the other we have an interface of periosteal connective tissue and connective tissue of the flap. This establishes a distinct difference in the stage of repair. In the full thickness preparation this is direct physical as well as biological trauma to the vestibular surface of bone. This results in necrosis, and the associated resorption takes place. In order to remove this necrotic tissue there is intensive activity in this flap connective tissue in order to debride that vestibular surface as well as to prepare the stage for repair between a soft connective tissue and the dense, hard connective tissue of the bone. In contrast, in the split thickness flap procedure the periosteal connective tissue suffers some biological embarrassment which is characterized by increased cellular activity immediately adjacent to the vestibular surface of bone. However, at the same time at the interface between the flap connective tissue and the periosteal connective tissue there are positive efforts taking place to reestablish the integrity of the connective tissue in wound repair. The main difference at this point, which will continue to follow through as far as the alveolar process which has been subjected to one flap technique or the other is concerned, is in degrees of tissue activity and quantity of tissue affected.

It is a quantitative difference in that there is more resorption of the vestibular aspect as well as the crest of the alveolar process with the full thickness flap than there is with the split thickness flap. There is also a distinct difference in the rate of healing histologically. The full thickness flap is a few days behind the split thickness flap in the repair rate. The question arises as to why the variation in the amount of bone tissue resorbed in the two studies and the altered repair of one compared to a complete restitution in the other. The answer is the difference in the surgery performed. In the one study there was total exposure of bone, resulting in direct tissue damage and some surface infection; while in the other there was not this direct physical and infectious embarrassment of the bone. Also the interface was between two soft connective tissues in the split flap, in contrast to a hard connective tissue and a soft connective tissue in the full thickness flap. The degree of activity in the repair response varies; however, the initiation of specific cellular activity occurred at approximately the same time. The main difference is the increased number of cells working in the osteoclastic and osteoblastic phases after the mucogingival surgery. There are many more osteoclasts and osteoblasts in action during their respective times of activity with the full thickness flap. This is related to the degree of damage or trauma by surgery. From a comparison one may conclude that certain periodontal surgical procedures should be performed employing split thickness flap surgery.

Considerations from a histological point of view have been presented on the differences of the healing in the split thickness and full thickness flaps. It is paramount that the clinician consider the problem at hand and what he hopes to achieve with the pathological lesion in resolving the existing periodontal deformity. The objectives of mucogingival surgery are:

1. Eliminate pockets with their base transversing the mucogingival junction.
2. Create an adequate zone of attached gingiva.
3. Eliminate gingival clefts.

4. Relieve the pull of frena and muscle attachments on a gingival margin.
5. Perform mucogingival surgery in conjunction with procedures for the correction of osseous deformities.

Therefore with these objectives in mind the clinician, in reviewing the existing clinical anatomy, may find it necessary to use a mucosal or full thickness flap in spite of the histological disadvantage from a wound healing standpoint.

Primary in consideration of reflecting any flap for periodontal surgical procedure is the maintenance of the integrity of the flap itself, not risking any perforation or deterioration of that biological covering. There are anatomical regions that present themselves with varying physical dimensions of thinness of the soft tissue. Where it is not advisable to raise a partial or split thickness flap because of the increased possibility of traumatizing and perforating the soft tissue of the flap, the full thickness flap should be considered in preference to the split thickness flap. It would be most undesirable clinically to reflect a split thickness flap with soft tissue dimension being very thick and in the immediate postoperative period encounter a situation manifesting perforation and necrosis of the flap. The result would be extensive osseous resorption and an extended period of repair. It should be noted that the full thickness flap causes osseous resorption, but not to the degree that it could not be considered in certain clinical procedures. It is most important to strive to maintain biologic and physical integrity of the flap so that it can be reapposed or repositioned, whichever is desired, and serve that function without further occurrence or a pathological situation. Conversely, with the reflection of the full thickness flap the clinician has no choice but to reappose it at a point near or even with the crest of the alveolar process. An attempt at reapposition of a full thickness flap apical to the crest of the bone is not desirable because of the osseous exposure and the extensive osseous resorption that will follow. This is very strongly supported by the studies of Wilderman.[7] The use of full thickness flaps is not advisable in autogenous or contiguous soft tissue grafts because of the degree of osseous resorption that would follow in the donor site and the decreased rate of repair to the osseous base at the recipient site.

Therefore the full thickness mucoperiosteal flap has restricted application in periodontal mucogingival surgery when we consider those procedures that are to be performed in the facial aspect of a maxilla or mandible. In contrast the split thickness or mucosal flap has many applications in periodontal mucogingival surgery. This flap, once it is raised, can be positioned apically where it was reflected. Also it can be part of a procedure to position it laterally rotate it in order to improve integrity of the adjacent area from the standpoint of masticatory mucosa, and like the mucoperiosteal flap it can be reapposed to its original position with the crest of the alveolar process, causing less osseous resorption than with the mucoperiosteal flap.

It is common in mucogingival surgery to employ a suturing technique in which a flap is attached to the periosteum, stabilizing it in certain positions. This is not possible when there is a full thickness mucoperiosteal flap reflection, but with the split thickness there is always that periosteal connective tissue base into which sutures can be made to hold down the flap.

Any osseous surgery that has to be performed from the facial aspect makes up but a small percentage of the total flap area that is reflected. It is highly traumatic to expose an excessive area of bone simply to use that exposure to visualize the bone for osseous surgery. There is no difficulty in performing osseous surgery utilizing the split flap reflection technique.

When one considers mucogingival surgery as the plastic surgical procedure in periodontics, it is imperative to utilize procedures which enhance an end result that is commensurate with the requirements of a healthy dentogingival junction. Reflecting a split thickness flap achieves thinness with body and permits its reapposition at the gingival margin region with it being better contoured and much more adaptable than the heavy-bodied full thickness mucoperiosteal flap.

This aspect of flap preparation becomes readily observable when the clinician works on the palatal aspect of the maxilla. The preparation of the partial thickness flap in the palate is similar to the preparation of a facial flap. However, there are certain significant aspects that should be considered. The anterior palatal segment is generally thinner in dimension than the posterior palatal segment. It is imperative, in making the initial incision, that adequate flap tissue remains to reappose following the completion of the corrective measures and also to maintain that thinness to the margin of the flap that adapts the root surfaces of the teeth.

There are also times in the facial or lingual aspect when it is necessary, in repositioning technique, to gain in the mesiodistal dimension of the flap and this is accomplished through short vertical incisions. This is facilitated with the split thickness flap.

The dentoperiodontal unit with its diseased structure is easily accessible for corrective surgery with the split thickness flap. The clinician will find very little need postoperatively in the second, third or fourth week to make any corrections to the palatal marginal gingival tissue because of bulkiness or heaviness following the use of a split thickness flap.

Perhaps the lingual aspect of the mandibular arch varies slightly from the approach in the maxillary arch as far as utilization of the split thickness flap is concerned. The lingual anterior of the mandibular arch most generally permits reflecting a split thickness flap, and this would be followed in the same procedure as described for the facial or palatal flap. However, from the second premolar posteriorly in the lingual aspect of the mandibular arch the tissue generally becomes very thin, and it is not advisable to attempt partial thickness dissection. Preferably a full thickness mucoperiosteal flap should be reflected so that the integrity of the soft tissue of the flap is maintained. It is infrequent that the tissue of the thickness necessary to do split thickness dissection is available in the posterior aspect of the lingual arch. In mucogingival surgery it is important to plan the mode of treatment properly so that flap preparation is made that will enhance and make possible a satisfactory end result.

The clinician must decide which flap techniques he will utilize in his mucogingival surgical procedure, keeping in mind the histological response of the two flap techniques, the anatomical morphology that presently exists clinically as a result of the disease process and considering the morphological end result that he hopes to attain in the region of the dentogingival junction. The split thickness mucosal flap affords greater flexibility to the flap as well as the greatest protection and preservation of the existing support structure. However, on the basis of the tissue dimension that may exist at the time of surgery, the clinician may decide to utilize full thickness flap reflection in order not to jeopardize the integrity of flap tissue, and in order not to lose further osseous structure through perforation and the ensuing necrosis, in contrast to the attempt to save bony tissue.

The split thickness mucosal flap is the least traumatic flap technique available in mucogingival procedures today; however, it is not always applicable clinically because of certain existing anatomical configurations and dimensions.

Grafts

Early reports by Nabers[18] recognized the value of mucosal grafts as adjuncts to vestibular extension procedures as well as to techniques directed toward increasing the width of attached gingiva and correcting frenum problems. Becker[19] employed gingival graft in restoring adequacy to a narrow dentogingival junction. Clinically the graft healed with zero sulcus depth and achieved an apparent attachment to tooth surface. Sullivan and Atkins[20] concentrated the use of gingival grafts in predictably treating areas of gingival recession, providing the cases were carefully selected and good surgical principles were followed.

Sullivan and Atkins[20] also presented an excellent paper outlining the rationale and surgical principles involved in the gingival grafting. Paramount among those set forth are a vascular and immobile recipient bed and adequate immobilization of the graft during healing. Gordon et al.[21] presented a histologic survey of healing gingival grafts which primarily described the nature of matured epithelium and underlying connective tissue. In addition they determined the mobility of a healed graft was associated with discrepancies between the connective tissue density of the graft and subjacent tissues. Gargiulo and Arrocha[22] were among the first to describe the early healing phases in healing of gingival grafts. This human study on healing mucosal grafts employed with vestibular deepening procedures pointed out the importance of a primitive "plasmotic" circulation which maintained the vitality of the graft prior to its actual vascularization.

Oliver et al.[23] and Staffileno[24] have presented healing studies of gingival grafts in dogs. Each deals with restoring the dentogingival junction with an adequate zone of functional masticatory mucosa. Both authors echo the work of Gargiulo and Arrocha[22] by stressing the importance of the initial primitive "plasmotic" circulation in the success of each graft. Staffileno[8] refers to the phenomenon as "fluid fusion." Oliver[23] and Staffileno[8] separately stress the sensitivity of epithelium to the reduced vascularity of the graft during initial healing stages. The result is a necrosis and slough of all epithelium except a few basal cells within epithelial ridges projecting deeper into underlying connective tissue. Oliver et al.[23] go on to discuss in detail the revascularization of the graft. Staffileno[8] indicates that the final healing of a gingival graft placed at the dentogingival junction results in the restoration of normal characteristics of the area without deformity.

It is extremely difficult to group mucoperiosteal problems into strict categories of involvements with inadequate vestibular depth and high frenum attachments or narrow zones of attached masticatory mucosa. More frequently the mucogingival problem is quite complex and might be labeled more accuraely as a gingivo-muco-myo-skeletal involvement. To expand this point, one rarely encounters a defect requiring surgical repair of a narrow zone of attached gingiva without an additional superimposed shallow fornix and/or a high frenum attachment. In addition it must be remembered that the mobility of oral lining mucosa is inherently related to underlying orofacial musculature and osseous structure of the maxilla and mandible.

The goal of periodontics is to establish a healthy and properly functioning dento-gingival unit in a previously diseased periodontium. Gingival grafting has been shown to be one effective method in accomplishing this goal, particularly where narrow or inadequate zones of attached gingiva prevail. When a zone of attached gingiva is complicated by a shallow vestibule or a high muscle attachment it is imperative that the situation be recognized for its complexity as a gingivo-muco-myo-skeletal problem. Accordingly, the basic surgical approach to mucosal graft will of necessity have to be altered to circumvent otherwise inevitable failure. At the same time the skilled therapist should be aware that gingival grafts have their limitations. For example, because of the strict requirement of an ample vascular bed, gingival grafts cannot be expected to correct extensive areas of gingival recession. Where the defect of gingival recession is narrow and there is an abundant vascular bed, collateral circulation through the phenomenon of bridging,[20] may permit correction by grafting techniques. Perhaps the horizontal sliding flap as modified by Staffileno[12] or the double repositioned flap of Cohen and Ross[13] are procedures that will manage gingival defects more predictably since the vascularity of these flaps is not normally embarrassed.

Bowers,[24] in an extensive human study, indicated convincingly that mandibular premolars tended to be associated with the narrowest zones of attached gingiva. Of diagnostic importance also are the shallow vestibular depth in the area and the high frenum attachment just mesial to the involved tooth. In order to establish stable wound margins and to minimize the influence of orofacial masculature, preparation of the recipient bed required vestibular deepening accomplished by horizontal relaxing incisions placed at the mucogingival junction. The apically displaced mucosal margin was stabilized by suturing the underlying periosteum. Subsequently the graft was transferred to the prepared bed and fixed with suture.

Of possible related importance to gingival grafts in periodontal therapy is more universal utilization of grafts in periosteal retention areas. According to Oliver et al.[23] gingival grafts tend to minimize untoward reactions in the surgical wound, including edema, degeneration, necrosis and osteoclastic activity. There may be an additional indication for use of gingival grafts—that of protecting exposed periosteal connective tissue and creating an environment conducive to more rapid and uneventful healing.

1. Gingival grafts can be successfully utilized in the surgical repair of a diseased dentogingival unit.
2. Gingival grafts need not be abandoned as a therapeutic modality where a shallow vestibule or high frenum may complicate a surgical approach.
3. Gingival grafts are not the treatment of choice in the surgical management of extensive areas of gingival recession.

The use of osseous grafts to reestablish the periodontium coronally on the tooth has been given considerable attention during the past decade. It was hoped that the new graft material would stimulate the surrounding cells to lay down new bone and eventually recontour the existing bone to its original form and consistency. There are four types of graft material: (1) autoplastic—if bone of the same patient or experimental animal is transplanted into the defect; (2) homoplastic—if the bone of the same species is grafted from one individual member to another; (3) heteroplastic—if the bone is from a different species and (4) alloplastic—if a bone substitute is employed.

The most favorable results can be expected if autoplastic grafting material is used, particularly if the transplant can be kept viable and if it contains marrow type bone rather than cortical bone. When a piece of bone is transplanted the osteocytes, severed from their blood supply, die. However, the osteogenic cells of the periosteal and endosteal tissues, being on the surface, are likely to be sufficiently bathed in tissue fluid to survive. These cells will contribute toward osteogenesis which comes mostly from the bone into which the graft is inserted.

Schallhorn[25] reported the successful use of autogenous implants of hemopoietic bone marrow obtained from the posterior iliac crest. The cancellous cores used are obtained with a Westerman-Jensen bone marrow biopsy needle. Following removal the cores are placed in a sterile glycerol solution. They are frozen using alcohol and dry ice and stored in a freezer. Twenty-five minutes before periodontal surgery the cores are thawed in warm water and then placed in one-half volume of a 50 percent sterile glucose in physiologic saline solution for about 10 minutes. An equal volume of physiologic saline solution is added and allowed to reach equilibrium for one minute. This is necessary to reestablish a compatible osmotic gradient of the cells to tissue fluids. If the marrow implant is to be used within three days, it is stored in minimum essential media. This avoids the need to reestablish the osmotic gradient of the cells.

The bony defect is then prepared thoroughly. All periodontic and endodontic procedures must have been completed, occlusal traumatism eliminated and food impactions corrected before performing transplant surgery. The surgical area must be clean, the root surface thoroughly debrided and all necrotic tissue and excess granulation tissue removed. It is advisable to have some bleeding in the area of the implant, for an implant placed alongside dry bone will certainly fail. The cores are removed from the broth and the bony defect is slightly overfilled. The tissues are repositioned over the osseous transplant, making sure that the sutures are not over the area of the transplanted bone. Care should be taken not to probe the area for several weeks.

Teeth with deep periodontal pockets associated with bony defects adjacent to an edentulous space are good candidates for the osseous repositioning procedure. The maintenance of vital tissue in contact with the periosteum and the periosteum in turn in contact with the transplant will improve the prognosis of any transplant or repositioning procedure. After the recipient site is prepared periodonally, the osseous transplant is freed from the surrounding bone and tipped into the defect so that it completely fills the preexisting void. A narrow intrabony defect is created, and a new attachment can be anticipated if the blood supply is maintained in this way. The donor site heals like the alveolus after an extraction.

Bone swaging collapses as a plate of bone from the buccal surface into an interproximal crater. This technique offers the opportunity to carry periosteum into the defect and, consequently, can be successful if the bony architecture is not too extreme. However, if the periosteum does not remain vital the transposed bone becomes a large sequestrum wedged between the tooth and vital bone.

The use of grafting material to increase the height of the alveolar process should be based on biologic principles. Osseous implants placed coronal to the alveolar crests will fail because this position does not provide a frame for callous formation. Implants are therefore limited to wide-mouth, three-walled, intrabony defects and two-walled craters. It is hoped that with autogenous bone or marrow grafts defects that now have a hopeless prognosis will change to a favorable prognosis. Frequently reentry surgery is necessary following a grafting procedure to reestablish a physiologic alveolar architecture.

It also has been shown that the stimulus for osteogenesis can be enhanced by the use of cancellous bone with its high proportion of periosteal and endosteal cells.

Due to the difficulty in obtaining bone marrow, some use a combination of bone dust and blood, which is called osseous coagulum. Osseous coagulum is prepared by removing fine shavings of bone with a #6 or #8 carbide bur. The bur speed is slow, between 20,000 and 30,000 revolutions per minute. Blood is used as a lubricant with care being taken not to cause excessive heat. As the coagulum is prepared it is stored under any flap of transplant tissue. The coagulum then can be removed from under the flap of tissue and used at the operator's convenience. The source of bone is varied: osseous areas needing recontouring, exostosis, endentulous ridges, tuberosity areas and so forth.

The use of osseous coagulum is identical to the technique used in other bone grafting procedures. Furthermore, more recently freeze-dried cadaver bone has been used with encouraging results.

Most important with bone graft surgery is the establishment of an environment of suppressed bacterial population in the bone graft region. This is accomplished by administering preoperatively and continuing postoperatively for five days penicillin or erythromycin in therapeutic dosages to suppress gram-positive organisms. Then at seven days, when osteogenesis begins to occur, the therapeutic regime of tetracycline is given for seven days and followed by a reduced level of tetracycline for 21 to 35 days to suppress gram-negative bacteria. Use of this regime has been most encouraging and effective because the serum levels of tetracycline in the gingival sulcus is four to seven times that in the bloodstream.

In this chapter the emphasis has been on the recognition of periodontal disease and the possible variations in etiology of the disease process. The causative factors are not always clear and at times leave the clinician frustrated when a successful treatment plan is to be put into effect. Nevertheless, different regimens of therapy were discussed which cover nonsurgical and surgical management as well as some of the rationale for selecting certain modalities of therapy. This includes clinical experience as well as laboratory studies in wound healing.

The patient with alveolar and palatal clefts experiences periodontic disease and in some instances more so because of severe anatomical environmental distortions. This makes it doubly important to implement management to prevent periodontal disease and conserve dental and periodontal tissue structure as well as to optimize the result in treatment of active disease.

REFERENCES

1. Bhaskar SN: *Synopsis of Oral Pathology.* St. Louis, C V Mosby Co, 1977.
2. Friedman N: Anatomy of the periodontium as related to therapy: Alveolar architecture. Read before the Rocky Mountain Dental Seminar in Periodontics, Glenwood Springs, Colorado, December, 1959.
3. Gargiulo AW, Wentz FM, Orban B: Dimensions and relations of the dentogingival junction in humans. *J Periodont,* 32:261, 1961.
4. Grant DA, Stern IB, Everett FG: *Orban's Periodontics.* St. Louis, C V Mosby Co, 1968.
5. Glickman I (ed): *Clinical Periodontology,* ed 3. Philadelphia, WB Saunders Co, 1964, pp 218-224.
6. Caffese RF, Ramfjord S, Nasjileti CI: Reverse periodontal flaps in monkeys. *J Periodont,* 39:219, 1968.
7. Wilderman M, Wentz F, Orban B: Histogenesis of repair after mucogingival surgery. *J Periodont,* 31:283, 1960.
8. Staffileno H, Levy S: Histologic and clinical study of mucosal (gingival) transplants in dogs. *J Periodont,* 40:311, 1969.
9. Staffileno H, Levy S, Gargiulo A: Histologic study of cellular mobilization and repair following a periosteal retention operation via split thickness mucogingival flap surgery. *J Periodont,* 37:117, 1966.
10. Staffileno H, Wentz F, Orban B: Histologic study of healing of split thickness flap surgery in dogs. *J Periodont,* 33:56, 1962.
11. Staffileno H: Histologic study of healing of split thickness and mucoperiosteal flaps in dogs. Read before the Rocky Mountain Seminar in Periodontics, Glenwood Springs, Colorado, December, 1959.
12. Staffileno H: Management of gingival recession and root exposure problems associated with periodontal disease. *Dent Clin North Am,* 1964.

13. Cohen DW, Ross S: The double papillae repositioned flap in periodontal therapy. *J Periodont,* 39:65, 1966.
14. Chacker FM, Cohen DW: Regeneration of gingiva tissue in non-human primates, abstracted. *J Dent Res,* 39:743, 1960.
15. Helburn RL, Cohen DW, Chacker FM: Healing of repositioned mucogingival flaps in monkeys, abstracted. IADR Abstract #324, 1963.
16. Pfeifer J: The reaction of alveolar bone to flap procedures in man. *Periodontics,* 3:135, 1965.
17. Friedman N, Levine L: Mucogingival surgery. *Dent Clin North Am,* 63, 1964.
18. Nabers JM: Free gingival grafts. *J Am Soc Periodont,* 4:5, 1966.
19. Becker NG: A free gingival graft utilizing a pre-suturing technique. *J Am Soc Periodont,* 5:4, 1967.
20. Sullivan H, Atkins JH: Free autogenous gingival grafts. I. Principles of successful grafting. *Periodontics,* 6:121, 1968.
21. Gordon HD, Sullivan HC, Atkins JH: Free autogenous gingival grafts. II. Supplemental findings—histology of the graft site. *Periodontics,* 6:130, 1968.
22. Gargiulo AW, Arrocha R: Histoclinical evaluation of free gingival grafts. *Periodontics,* 5:285, 1967.
23. Oliver RC, Loe H, Karring T: Microscopic evaluation of the healing and revascularization of free gingival grafts. *J Periodont Res,* 3:84, 1968.
24. Bowers GM: Study of the worth of attached gingiva. *J Periodont,* 34:201, 1963.
25. Schallhorn RG: The use of autogenous hip marrow biopsy implants for bony craters defects. *J Periodont,* 39:145, 1968.

CHAPTER 11

CLINICAL EVALUATION AND MANAGEMENT OF PROBLEMS OF SPEECH, LANGUAGE AND HEARING

KENNETH BZOCH

> *. . . He that is really good can never be unhappy. He that is really wise can never be perplexed. He that is really brave is never afraid.*
>
> *. . . Confucius*

THIS CHAPTER will focus directly on three related topics. The first identifies some criteria and guidelines for the role of the Speech Pathologist on a Cleft Palate Team. The second details a specific battery of clinical tests and procedures that have proved most useful for fulfilling that role within the constraints of the usual short time frame available at cleft palate team clinics. The screening tests to be described also have proved useful for conducting clinical research on the comparative efficacy of different management strategies as currently followed at different cleft palate team centers. The third topic discusses the idealistic goal of prevention of communicative disorders for all children born with cleft palate through the team approach. The University of Florida craniofacial team's most recent findings bearing on this possibility or goal will be reported here. The data for this study were drawn mainly from grouped speech and language test data obtained over a recent five-year period from the clinical tests described later in this chapter.

The early individualized intervention and/or treatment of developing communicative disorders through the current "state of the art" team approach holds promise of the more routine prevention, rather than the later rehabilitation, of these disorders found in the cleft lip and palate population.

Guidelines and Criteria for the Role of the Speech Pathologist

It is recommended that routine screening speech and language evaluations be a part of each cleft palate team clinic for each patient. This periodic assessment should begin shortly after birth for each newborn cleft palate patient and his family and should allow time for face-to-face discussions of findings and recommendations with team colleagues.

In most cases an objective screening evaluation focusing on language development and speech articulation error patterns can be accomplished in about a 20-minute period with a young patient and knowledgeable informants from the family. The basic purpose is to identify through case history, observation and objective screening tests the presence or absence of several possible organic and/or functional types of problems causing developmental communicative disorders. These include, but are not limited to: (1) velopharyngeal insufficiency to support normal speech and language development, (2) dental or occlusal hazards which are directly affecting speech articulation or communication behavior, (3) the presence or absence of hearing loss affecting speech and language development and/or needing otologic or audiologic rehabilitation followup or (4) other functional or learning problems such as delay in the normative development of language skills or developing compensatory habits of misarticulation of speech sound elements.

Basically the team role of the speech pathologist should be to help plan for the earliest possible physical management of all organic problems needing treatment through surgery, medical or dental care (such as orthodontics and prosthodontics) with the other team members during each team staffing. The speech pathologist also should plan for the management of functional learning problems of delayed speech and language development or articulation or voice disorders of speech often characteristic of cleft palate individuals. These developing functional habits of speech production can result in the same stigma of "cleft palate speech" for an individual's lifetime as might continued velopharyngeal incompetency. The apparent need to refer patients for early speech or language therapy, as indicated by screening tests and case history, often should be defended with team colleagues and third party providers of the cost of such treatment. The cost effectiveness of preventive treatment over later long-term correction of habituated speech and language disorders can be demonstrated.

It should be possible with a routine test battery (taking only 5 to 15 minutes to administer) to identify the presence or absence of any of the 11 categorical aspects of frequently occurring communicative disorders as previously described by Bzoch.[1] *Yes* or *No* judgments should be made for each and recorded, particularly for the apparent presence or absence of (1) *nasal emission distortions of pressure consonant sounds* during speech utterances, (2) *hypernasal distortion of syllabic elements* during speech or (3) observed *nasal or facial grimacing.* These three findings all are indicative of possible velopharyngeal incompetency to support normal speech production and development. Also, the presence or absence of (4) *hyponasal resonance distortions* is important to assess since this may be an adverse result from overcorrecting pharyngeal flap operations or speech prostheses which may lead to mouth breathing and affect facial growth through the development of the "adenoid faces." Such problems also increase the possibility of sleep apnea complications. (5) *Gross sound substitutions* in speech particularly need to be identified if present, since these suggest the need for early referral for direct speech therapy. (6) Dysphonia through *aspirate (breathy)* voice production, (7) *hoarse voice* characteristics, (8) *articulation distortions related to dental or occlusal abnormalities* or (9) *communication disorders related to hearing loss* all need to be identified, if present. Finally, (10) identification of any *significant delays in either receptive or expressive language development* or (11) the development of the more common types of *misarticulation disorders,* severe enough to affect intelligibility of speech, need to be identified, if present. This is a tall order for the speech pathologist in the usual noisy environment of a cleft palate team clinic.

The best criterion for effective assessments by the speech pathologist on a cleft palate team is his ability to make and defend the kinds of clinical judgments represented by the recording form in Figure 11-1. With experience using this short battery of screening tests it should be possible for a speech pathologist to discuss or actually record on this form all the indicated *yes* or *no* judgments required—e.g., the presence or absence of (1) velopharyngeal insufficiency for speech (probably requiring consideration of an early secondary operation to correct this disability), (2) functional problems requiring speech therapy, (3) dental-related articulation disorders (lateral lisping requiring consideration by the dental consultants for a temporary prosthesis of a missing lateral incisor tooth) or (4) the need for direct speech therapy with a 2-3-year old infant (the usual criteria being the presence of a gross substitution error pattern on the screening articulation test).

Hearing Assessments

Ideally a cleft palate team also should have as an integral part of the clinic an audiologist and an otologist to monitor, measure and refer for treatment any hearing problems occurring over time.

A routine complete audiometric assessment should be conducted for each patient at or just before each team visit. Air/bone pure-tone measures, speech reception tests for older children and tympanometric tests for infants should be an integral part of the evaluation data obtained and discussed for management decisions at each clinic. Objective audiometric tests should be supplemented with otoscopic examinations by either pediatric or ENT experts (preferably by pneumatic otoscope). Recommendations by the team audiologist and/or pediatrician for referral for treatment of suspected or confirmed hearing loss problems should follow routinely each clinic visit for each cleft palate patient.

Frequency of Reexaminations

It is recommended that all cleft patients be seen by the entire team at least once a year through the period of their followup, from birth to young adult life. It also is recommended that all infants (i.e., newborn cleft palate and craniofacial patients) and young children be reevaluated from birth to five years of age at least twice each year, if possible.

I.	ORGANIC PROBLEMS NEEDING PHYSICAL MANAGEMENT:	YES ☐	NO ☐
	1. Velopharyngeal insufficiency	YES ☐	NO ☐
	2. Dental - occlusal hazard	YES ☐	NO ☐
	3. Hearing loss: conductive _______ Sensori Neural _______	YES ☐	NO ☐
	4. Other ________________________________		
II.	FUNCTIONAL PROBLEMS NEEDING THERAPY	YES ☐	NO ☐
	Rx ________________________________		
	________________________________		
	________________________________		
	________________________________		
III.	CATEGORICAL ASPECTS CHECK:		
	1. Nasal emission distortion, ratio: : ______/10	YES ☐	NO ☐
	2. Hypernasal, resonance distorton, ratio : ______/10	YES ☐	NO ☐
	3. Nasal and or facial grimace	YES ☐	NO ☐
	4. Hyponasal distortion, ratio: : ______/10	YES ☐	NO ☐
	5. Gross substitution error pattern, ratio: : ______/30	YES ☐	NO ☐
	6. Dysphonia; aspirate voice:	YES ☐	NO ☐
	7. Dysphonia; hoarse voice:	YES ☐	NO ☐
	8. Dental related artic errors:	YES ☐	No ☐
	9. Artic errors related to hearing loss:	YES ☐	NO ☐
	10. Developmental dyslalia (functional artic):	YES ☐	NO ☐
	11. Delayed speech and language: Reel Scale RLA _____ ELA _____	YES ☐	NO ☐
	(Language Test scores ________________________________		
	________________________________		
IV.	FOLLOW-UP RECOMMENDATIONS:		
	________________________________		
	________________________________		
	________________________________		
	________________________________		
	________________________________		
	________________________________		
	________________________________		

Figure 11-1. The Oral Facial Communicative Disorders Clinical Evaluation Form. 1980-A. K. R. Bzoch, Ph.D.

Speech and Language Therapy Referrals

These can add to the early cost, but also do save third-party providers or parents a great deal of money. Therefore the appropriateness of all speech program referrals for therapy should be recommended and defended by the speech pathology consultant and agreed to by the team members at each team staff review following each clinic. The effectiveness of any direct speech or language therapy program needs to be reevaluated at the time of each succeeding clinic and changed or modified as the measures of progress indicate.

The need for direct speech therapy for this population varies and often should include very young children (i.e., from two to three years of age) when they speak primarily with glottal stops and/or evidence probable inadequacy of velopharyngeal function to support normal speech following primary surgical closure. Clinics should include a pragmatic home language stimulation program caried out by counseling with parents. This is always appropriate during the first and second years of life, either separately or during team clinics as time and circumstance allows.

Recommendations for speech therapy also might include adult patients being reviewed who need articulation retraining following dental, prosthodontic or surgical treatment which has modified their speech mechanism. A direct early language therapy program also might need to be instituted for a preschool or early school age patient with a marked delay in expressive language skills and much higher level of receptive language competency, when stimulation at home is not possible or is ineffective.

Each case is individual and cannot be definitively listed in guideline recommendations. However, most judgments and the defense of recommendations for the need for functional speech and/or language therapy can and should be justified on the basis of objective findings, such as the short battery of clinical tests described below.

Specific Objective Tests and Procedures Useful for Team Evaluations

A short battery of objective tests screening speech, normative language development scale measurements and hearing tests has proven most useful for the routine evaluation for communicative disorders of infants and children in the cleft palate team clinic setting. It is equally useful for adult patients. Such routine tests also provide data for more objective clinical research of the comparative efficacy of differing treatment procedures.

Speech Evaluation Tests

The following is a brief discussion of the rationale and procedures to be followed for conducting and recording the test battery illustrated in Figure 11-2.

TEST 1. The Nasal Emission Test. The nasal emission test has proved to be the single most valuable speech evaluation procedure for drawing an inference of the adequacy or inadequacy of velopharyngeal function to support normal voice and articulation development following primary surgical reconstruction of a cleft palate. It is particularly useful for testing 2- to 4-year-old cleft palate subjects.

Name ______________________________ Birth __________ Age ___ Sex ___ No. __________

Examiner ______________________________ Date __________ Stimulus Oral/Reading/Pix

I. Nasal Emission Test:

Circle words or syllables uttered that evidenced nasal air flow (i.e., indicated Velopharyngeal insufficiency); air flow checked by FLA II ☐, Paddle ☐, Bubble ☐, other ____________ .

a. people paper puppy pepper piper

baby Bobby bubble B.B. bye-bye

b. For infants test (pi) syllable ten times:

P P P P P P P P P P

Nasal Emission Score _____/_____

II. Hypernasality Test:

Circle words or vowels on which a shift in tone quality occurred when nares were closed (i.e., indicated Velpharyngeal insufficiency); ask patient first to repeat word loudly then to say again while nares are pinched.

a. Beet bit bait bet bat

bought boat boot but Bert

For infants or speechless try simpler test of alternately pinching and opening nares as patient utters prolonged vowels /i/ as in **see** and /u/ as in **new**; circle those that shift.

b. /i/ /u/ /i/ /u/ /i/ /u/ /i/ /u/ /i/ /u/

Hypernasality Score _____/_____

III. Hyponasality Test:

Circle words or nasal sounds which sound the same (i.e., indicated block nasal passages) when nares are pinched closed as when open; otherwise proceed as above.

a. meat mit mate met mat

moat moot mut Mert might

For infants or speechless, have patient hum (i.e., prolong /m/ then /n/ as tested).

/m/ /n/ /m/ /n/ /m/ /n/ /m/ /n/ /m/ /n/

Hyponasality Score _____/_____

IV. Phonation Test

	Duration	Aspirate	Hoarse
/i/	Sec. _____	Yes/No	Yes/No
/a/	Sec. _____	Yes/No	Yes/No
/u/	Sec. _____	Yes/No	Yes/No

V. Error Pattern Screening Articulation Test

C = Correct Ĩ = indistinct from nasal emission alone
D = distortion (.5 error) SS = simple substitution (1.0 error)
GS = gross substitution (1.5 error) O = (2.0 error)

	PLOSIVES	C	Ĩ	D	SS	GS	O
/p/	aPPle						
/b/	baBy						
/t/	mounTain						
/d/	canDy						
/k/	chiCKen						
/g/	waGon						
	FRICATIVES						
/f/	elePHant						
/v/	shoVel						
/θ/	tooTHbrush						
/ð/	feaTHer						
/s/	bicyCLe						
/z/	sciSSors						
/ʃ/	diSHes						
/ʒ/	televiSion						
	AFFRICATES						
/tʃ/	maTCHes						
/dʒ/	briDGes						
	GLIDES						
/w/	sandWich						
/l/	baLLons						
/y/	onIOns						
/r/	aRRow						
	NASALS						
/m/	haMMer						
/n/	baNana						
/ŋ/	haNGer						
	BLENDS						
/sp/	SPider						
/str/	STRawberries						
/st/	STar						
/SK/	SKirt						
/sm/	SMoke						
/bl/	BLock						
/kl/	Clown						
/br/	BRoom						

ARTICULTATION SCORE C̄ + Ĩ = ______________

.5x__ 1x__ 1.5x__ 2x__

ERROR SCORE = ______________

Figure 11-2. Craniofacial Center Communicative Disorders Clinical Tests—1982-A, currently in use at the University of Florida. K. R. Bzoch, Ph.D.

The role of the speech-language pathologist on a cleft palate team is, in part, to make a decision as to the adequacy or inadequacy of the palate and velopharyngeal mechanism to support normal voice and articulation during the rapid speech development period of time shortly after primary reconstructive surgery is completed. At that usually early, critical age, when objective studies (such as speech cinefluorographic recordings, nasopharyngoscopy, PERCI, or more sophisticated forms of oral-nasal air flow studies, inferences from accelerometer tests, spectrographic analysis of speech or other instrumental measures) are difficult because of age and inability to cooperate of most subjects, this simple, short diagnostic procedure can be completed easily by an experienced speech-language pathologist, even in a 2-5 minute period of direct testing. The test can and does reveal important diagnostic information related directly to velopharyngeal function for speech.

The validity of the nasal emission test procedure for the clinical evaluation of velopharyngeal function during speech seems evident from principles of speech physiology and speech science. That is, if there is any leak in a pneumatic system, air under pressure should flow (be released) through that leak. If the palate is intact and the velopharyngeal mechanism is able to seal completely, air should not flow through the nose under the conditions of this test procedure.

Our own validity study of the specific procedure for Test 1, the nasal emission test in Figure 11-2, was conducted on a rural pediatric screening clinic population of 100 children, 50 males and 50 females, ages 2 years, 6 months to 5 years, 7 months. All tests (100%) yielded an index of 0/10 (no clinical evidence of nasal emission) through this specific test procedure. Finally, a recent study of the agreement between judgments from speech cinefluoroscopic analysis and this test, as to judgment of the adequacy or inadequacy of the velopharyngeal function in the act of speech of 40 patients revealed a 96 percent agreement.

The nasal emission test procedure was standardized on a set of 10 two-syllable words, each containing two unvoiced or two voiced bilabial plosives, /p/ or /b/. The words are to be repeated by the subject while the examiner observes and records a judgment concerning the presence or absence of abnormal nasal air flow by circling those words on which such abnormal air flow occurs. A simple air flow paddle, as described by Bzoch,[2] is sufficient for conducting this clinical test to obtain a base 10 index of nasal emission. Experience indicates that most 2- or 3-year-old cleft palate subjects can be tested in this manner. The nasal emission test always should yield an index of 0/10 if cooperating subjects have an adequate velopharyngeal mechanism to support speech development.

However, subjects can pass this test, which requires only simple two-syllable utterances, and they still may be unable to obtain adequate velopharyngeal closure in running speech or in longer utterances with fricative consonants. Therefore, if nasal escape is detected accompanying the bilabial contact on these simpler words, it is indicative of a more severe level of organic or functional velopharyngeal incompetency.

The test is invalid if glottal stop coarticulation occurs with the habituated bilabial articulations. This possibility can be determined by first holding the paddle, mirror or hard plastic (stethoscope) listening device to the lips, to assure the presence of impounded air pressure for the explosive phase of the plosive productions on /p/ and /b/ syllables.

TEST 2. The Hypernasality Test. The hypernasality test was standardized on a set of 10 one-syllable words, each beginning with /b/ and ending with /t/ and sampling vowels from high front to low back to high back tongue positions. The specific test and the clinical procedure for its completion have been described previously by Bzoch.[2] Its purpose is to yield a count of 10 clinical judgments as to the presence or absence of atypical hypernasal resonance on the vowels in these words by having the patient repeat each word two times. On the second utterance of each word, the test procedure simply requires the nares to be pinched closed. A comparison by ear is made of the two utterances of the same word. Words that shift in quality under the "cul-de-sac" resonance test condition are circled. The number of words so circled provides the base 10 index for hypernasality.

The validity of this "cul-de-sac" clinical resonance test was demonstrated recently in an unpublished master's thesis[3] by a 91+ percent agreement of data from this procedure and that obtained from vocalic peak amplitude measures of oral or nasal syllables obtained from a piesoelectric microphone transducer attached to the bridge of the nose of 10 subjects. The variable of gender of the subjects was found to have no significant effect on the ability of either the instrumental or the clinical test procedures to detect the presence or absence of hypernasal resonance.

TEST 3. The Hyponasality Test. The hyponasality test is similar to the hypernasality test but changes the set of one-syllable words from oral to nasal by standardizing on words initiated by /m/. The alternate open and closed cul-de-sac resonance test procedure also is followed. Under normal velopharyngeal function conditions, therefore, a shift in resonance quality is expected when the nares are alternately closed. When a change in resonance quality of the words is *not* heard as it should be, that test word is circled on the form in Figure 11-2. An index of hyponasality is obtained by counting the number of words so circled during the procedure.

TEST 4. The Phonation Test. A short sustained vowel phonation test, as previously described by Bzoch,[2] may be used to determine the presence or absence of hoarse or aspirate phonatory voice characteristics. Since vowels rarely are defective in early speech, and since phonatory quality judgments are influenced most by the consonantal environment,[4,5,6] this test of aspirate or of hoarse voice quality characteristics is limited to judgments of isolated prolonged vowels only. The duration of vowel phonation on one inhalation on the vowels /i/, /a/, /u/, on three attempts each, was used as an added indication of habituated aspirate phonation for subjects unable to sustain phonation for 10 seconds.

TEST 5. The Error Pattern Screening Articulation Test. The error pattern screening articulation test has been described previously and briefly discussed by Bzoch,[2] along with its rationale (based on findings from a longer 100-element, initial, medial and final word position test). Experience has indicated that the 31 words selected for this screening test, including medial position plosives, fricatives, affricatives, glides, nasals and a sample of common two- and three-consonant blends, yield findings most typical of the articulation errors in connected speech and of the frequency and type of habituated error patterns for each subject. As can be seen from Figure 11-2, attempts at articulation of the target sound or blend simply are checked in the C (correct) column if correctly articulated. Errors that essentially are articulated correctly but sound distorted due to nasal emission alone are checked in the Ĩ (indistinct due to nasal emission alone) column. The nasal air flow paddle or mirror should be used throughout testing to confirm such judgments. Errors that are allophones of the target sound but sound distorted due to imprecise or incorrect movement patterns of the articulators are checked in the D (distortion) column. The air flow paddle held to the middle and lateral portions of the lips can and should be used to confirm suspicions of lateral lisping distortions related to dental and/or occlusal abnormalities. These also should be recorded in this D column with a note of probable *dental*-related etiology. Whenever an error on a target sound is perceived more like an allophone of another standard phoneme, that error should be recorded in the SS (simple substitution) column and recorded as such (e.g., p/f, w/r) even if slightly distorted. Gross substitution errors should be distinguished from SS errors and recorded in the GS (gross substitution) error column with the appropriate symbol, if possible (i.e., ?/p). The reliability of clinical judgments of omission errors for medial word position sounds is simplified since the word has to be uttered as a single syllable for such errors to occur. Errors of omission of the target sound simply are checked in the O column.

The error pattern screening articulation test is best conducted by having the examiner say the word first, which is then repeated by the test subject. This eliminates self-correcting errors in children during a normal developmental period of articulation skill maturation, saves much time during testing and results in recording only strongly habituated error patterns for each subject.

Language Assessment Tests

Use of the REEL Scale. The REEL scale can be used routinely to assess quickly language skill development in all subjects under 3 years of age. This scale assesses both receptive and expressive language skills in children from birth to 3 years. The development of this scale was based on the biolinguistic concept that there is an inherent and predictable pattern of emergent language development for all children, particularly in the first 36 months of life.

The REEL scale uses a short parent interview format applicable to the time limits available during most cleft palate clinics. The greatest number of language behavior changes occur in the first year of life, due to rapid maturation at this time. There are six items on this scale, three receptive and three expressive, for each month of age for the first 12 months of language development. The second year is assessed in 2-month intervals, with six items in each interval. The third year is assessed in 3-month intervals, with six items in each interval. Technical vocabulary is avoided, and a glossary of terms is provided in the manual *Assessing Language Skills in Infancy,*[7] which gives directions for the current use of this language test scale.

Normative data for this test were taken from a sample of environmentally language-advantaged Caucasian infants likely to be functioning at their best linguistic potential. No infants with any organic or sensory disabilities were included in these norms, so that the comparison of any cleft palate child on this scale is a comparison with advantaged normal subjects.

The REEL scale can have a twofold purpose in cleft palate clinics. It may be used for the assessment of the levels of each child's language development and also as a counseling tool for parents. During each clinic visit a general discussion of the child's progress gives parents an opportunity to verbalize their feelings about their child's progress with language skills since their last team evaluation. Any concerns they have can be discussed and noted to assure that all questions are answered fully.

It also is important during the language screening evaluation that the clinician directly observes parent-child interactions during the parent interview and while eliciting the child's responses. The clinician can gain some insight into the type and amount of language stimulation provided by each parent. Frequently, parents do not know what to expect from their child in terms of early language development. They often respond to the child's requests when the child uses only gestures and do not expect the child to attempt verbal communication. This can set a pattern that can be detrimental to any child's development of expressive language skills.

Because there are critical time limits during cleft palate team clinics, it is difficult to assess language by any of the more recent direct test-response tests or methods which might be used more standardly in speech clinic settings for more complete evaluations of this parameter of development. The **Preschool Language Scale**[8] or the **Birth to Three Scale**[9] have proved most similar and useful when time and/or level of development of language skills allow or dictate. Other more recent procedures, particularly the **Early Language Milestone Scale**[10] now might be used similarly for this purpose. Whatever language screening procedure is followed, assessment and management of early receptive and expressive levels of language skills is considered a most critical part of the evaluation role of the speech pathologist on a cleft palate team.

Audiological Test

In our most recent cleft palate team experience report[11] all children with cleft palate were seen for complete and audiological examinations by a certified audiologist as soon as possible, regardless of their age. The tests that were attempted with each child included free field, pure tone, air-bone conduction, speech and impedance audiometry, followed by an otological examination, if indicated.

Included in the audiological assessment were basic questions to the parents with regard to each child's speech and language ability at home. In addition information was obtained from the family concerning the child's response to sound in his home environment and any recent history of ear problems. The case history information obtained from the parents was recorded and considered a valuable part of the audiological diagnostic evaluation.

Each of the possible audiological tests was attempted regardless of the age or cooperative state of the child at the time of testing. Much information was obtained, even from a crying, screaming child. Based on this experience it was found that the audiologist needs to be very flexible and first should utilize test procedures that allow for maximum responses from each child.

It has been the experience of Bzoch et al.[11] with very young children that the first auditory response attempted should be a speech awareness threshold in sound field. This provides information about the child's potential for hearing and speech and also provides an estimate of hearing sensitivity. For this test the infant or young child generally was seated in the mother's lap between two speakers in a sound-treated room. An observer also was in the room to note changes in behavior and to increase the reliability of the observations. Conditioned behavioral audimetric thresholds may be impossible to establish for young infants or for some very young children. However, the audiologist should be able to detemine if a sensorineural hearing loss exists.

Next, pure tone, sound-field measures were made, beginning at 4,000 Hz (if a sensorineural hearing loss exists, the loss most often will be in the high frequencies). If audimetric responses cannot be obtained beyond these two measures (speech awareness and 4,000 Hz) there is at least a sufficient baseline to assist the audiologist in counseling the parents with regard to language development and future management. Next, additional responses at 2,000, 1,000, 500 and 250 Hz were obtained whenever possible.

If the responses to either speech or pure tone sound-field stimuli were greater than 70dB for children 0-3 months, an immediate followup examination was scheduled. There are many references[12,13] in the literature concerning responses of infants and young children, beginning with the reflexive responses at less than 1 month, to pointing at familiar pictures and possible conditioned play audiometry at age 2-3 years.

Dr. F. Joseph Kemker[11] commented on the use of (1) bone-conduction audiometry, (2) impedance audiometry and (3) tympanometry during cleft palate clinics as follows:

> Bone-conduction audiometry was next attempted to determine the integrity of the sensorineural system. Many different types of congenital abnormalities are seen in the craniofacial clinic, and children with atresia are frequently evaluated. In addition, a finding of some sensorineural loss in the cleft palate population has been reported. Sensorineural reserve, therefore, should be obtained, if possible, for proper management of each child's language and educational growth. An air-bone gap was considered significant when it was either equal to or greater than 10dB.
>
> As stated previously, many children can show 0 – dB hearing level by air conduction alone and yet have substantial middle-ear problems. Therefore, the next test attempted was a measure of middle-ear function. Every child seen by the team, regardless of the level of hearing sensitivity obtained, was administered impedance audiometry. Impedance audiometry, as used in our clinic, consists of the tympanogram, acoustic stapedial reflex measures, and Eustachion tube functions tests. Whenever possible, Eustachion tube function should also be assessed. The Eustachion tube function test provides infor-

mation with regard to tubal opening, presence of tympanic membrance perforation, and/or function or lack of function of ventilating tubes. The positive finding is a change in compliance or pressure when the child swallows or performs the Valsalva maneuver.

Impedance audiometry is considered an extremely valuable tool to use with this population since bone-condition audiometry is frequently unsuccessful with the young child. However bone-conduction audiometry should be attempted on each child, even if unmasked, to determine the level of sensorineural hearing. A child with a sensorineural hearing loss can have a normal middle-ear system or a pathological middle-ear system. If either the pure tone and/or impedance results suggested aural pathology, a referral should be made for a complete otologic evaluation. Following medical management of the aural pathology, the cleft palate infant or child should be seen for regular audiometric screening to determine the effect of either medication or the function of ventilating tubes. These follow-up visits should be at 3- to 6-month intervals for the young child.

The importance of maintaining good auditory sensitivity during the critical period of language development when aural pathology is common in this population cannot be overemphasized. Although the conductive hearing loss found with the majority of the cleft population seems to be reversible, it should not be allowed to exist! Systematic audiological and otological care for the young cleft palate child is difficult, but it is a necessary part of all routine cleft palate team evaluations.

Based on this and more recent clinical research, it is recommended that cleft palate teams regularly provide early, and as complete as possible, objective data on each child's hearing level function. Routinely these objective data are needed to provide the information necessary for individualized management of each child's development toward achievement of the goal of essentially normal speech and language development and language communication skills, particularly during the most critical preschool years of development.

Goal of Prevention of All Communicative Disorders of Cleft Palate Children

A review of the literature on the subject of communicative disorders of children born with cleft palate clearly indicates that three different kinds of communication disorder handicaps have been found frequently for the 1 of 600-700 infants born with this congenital defect in each community each year. The three most common problems are (1) the frequent development of severe and often complex forms of habituated voice and articulation disorders of speech production, (2) a measurable delay in expressive language development norms in infancy and early childhood and (3) a mild to moderate hearing loss, particularly from chronic or more frequent than average recurrent bouts of otitis media. The following is a selected review of the literature bearing on the nature and usual prevalence of each of these types of communicative disorders from recent clinical research on the subject.

Articulation and/or Voice Quality Disorders. In the past the early occurrence of severe forms of articulation or voice disorders appeared to be a usual problem following the birth of a child with cleft palate. Based on the literature as well as past clinical experience, the frequency of such problems may be estimated to occur for up to 75 percent of this population.[1,14-18] Although cleft palate is an obvious congenital organic disorder, past studies of cleft palate speech indicate that the majority of such long-persisting disorders become mainly functional in nature (i.e., only secondarily related to the later effective management of velopharyngeal insufficiency, dental or occlusal abnormalities, or hearing loss). The specific disorders most often encountered may include any of 11 categorical aspects of cleft palate speech as operationally redefined by Bzoch[2] and listed above. The following is a brief discussion of our current clinical rationale for the prevention and/or early management of each of the past major types of speech disorders found.

The articulation disorders of patients with cleft palate may be classified into four types, each requiring different management decisions for intervention and correction. Each type of frequent communicative disorder can be defined by the pattern of errors found mainly on standardized screening articulation tests of speech. A short 31-word screening test that has been developed for use in the limited time available during cleft palate clinics has been found to be generally adequate for this differential diagnostic purpose. However, close attention to the error patterns that occur, when five different possible error types are defined and recorded, leads best to an early diagnosis and a management plan for each specified type of error pattern.

Two of the articulation error patterns definable by screening test data are primarily functional in nature. They may be treated best by early referral for direct speech therapy. The other two error patterns suggest a rather probable direct, organic etiology. These may be managed best by referral to dental or medical specialists for correction of the underlying dental or velopharyngeal organic disorders.

Gross Sound Substitutions and Developmental Dyslalia. Early functional articulation disorders of 2-, 3-, 4-, and 5-year-old children with cleft palate may be of two kinds. The articulation error pattern that seems almost exclusively related to learned compensations of children with velopharyngeal incompetency is the pattern of substitution of glottal stops and/or velar and pharyngeal fricatives for normally oral and more anteriorly articulated speech sound elements by most infants during the preschool years. This error pattern has been termed "gross sound substitutions." More recently, Trost[17] has specified additional gross substitutions. She would add the pharyngeal stop, middorsum palatal stop and posterior nasal fricative as a part of this error pattern.

Empirically, it appears that most functional articulation differences of this nature in early speech develop inconsistently and almost only occur when velopharyngeal incompetency is prolonged through the second, third and/or later years of life for any reason. More normal articulation skills may develop and sometimes do, even in the face of uncorrected congenital velopharyngeal incompetency. However, such gross errors seldom are found without this specific underlying etiology.

When gross sound substitutions do develop in the speech behavior of a child with cleft palate, speech is characterized by the frequent use of glottal, pharyngeal or middorsum stops and/or velar, pharyngeal or posterior nasal fricatives for particular pressure consonant sound elements in early speech efforts. When habituated, this type of articulation disorder resists change to more normal articulation patterns with maturation alone, even after later correction of velopharyngeal incompetency or closure of a poorly obturated hard palate left open to enhance maxillary growth. This speech problem most often is caused first by the too-late accomplishment of complete palatal closure and functional velopharyngeal adequacy for speech. Although it is thought to be primarily a functional articulation disorder, it is a speech pattern of articulation compensations learned for producing more oral sounding and intelligible word approximations with velopharyngeal incompetency during infancy. These habits may, and often do, persist even after primary surgical reconstruction (postponed for any reason past 12 months of age).

The elimination of this disorder most often requires early direct articulation therapy and an attempt to verify the possible need for secondary reconstructive surgery to achieve adequacy of the existing speech mechanism. Therapy to correct a gross substitution error pattern is most effective after establishment of velopharyngeal competency to support normal speech production. Diagnostic therapy may be used to determine the adequacy or inadequacy of postsurgically reconstructed palates. If nasal emission distortions of correctly articulated pressure consonants like /p/ or /s/ persist with training, then a secondary palatal reconstruction probably is needed. Bzoch[2] reported this type of disorder to be the most frequently occurring communicative disorder in a sample of 1,000 cleft palate cases studied. This specified type of articulation problem occurred for 56.9 percent of that sample population.

The prevention of such handicapping occurrences in a cleft palate population sample may be achieved best by working closely with plastic surgeons willing to complete total hard and soft palate reconstructions as early as possible in the life of each child treated. Effective total reconstruction between 7 and 12, or even up to 18 months of age for specific reasons, usually averts the development of this compensatory speech disorder. In addition in most cases the early secondary surgical management is needed in those patients who present with repeated clinical evidence of continued velopharyngeal insufficiency after complete primary palatal reconstruction, to prevent their developing gross substitution error patterns in early speech from becoming habitual. An early secondary reconstruction of the velopharyngeal mechanism followed by direct articulation centered speech therapy most often is required in this clinical situation.

Developmental Dyslalia. The second primarily functional articulation disorder frequently found in children with cleft palate may be termed "developmental dyslalia." This problem is characterized by frequent articulation errors with speech sound substitutions such as t/k, p/f, t/s, w/r and omissions of final consonants, in an error pattern more typical of younger individuals, but not typical generally of a child's peers. Such error patterns most frequently are related clinically to early delayed speech and expressive language development in infancy.

When such error patterns are severe enough to affect intelligibility of speech attempts and are judged severe enough in the latter preschool years to interfere with personal adjustment and further speech and language development, a referral for early direct speech therapy also is indicated. Bzoch[2] reported finding such articulation error patterns in the speech of 340 of 1,000 cleft palate cases studied.

Any of these two primarily functional early error patterns of articulation disorders may be accompanied by one or more categorical types of articulation disorders thought to be more directly related to an organic etiology. These need more direct physical management of underlying problems from the other members of the team as follows.

Articulation Disorders Related to Dental and/or Occlusal Abnormalities. This is one of the "organic related" speech error patterns that most generally takes the form of lateral lisping, usually resulting in lateral oral distortions of the /s/, /z/, /ʃ/, /ʒ/, /tʃ/ and /dʒ/ sound elements. These can be observed clinically to be related to an asymmetrical maxillary dental arch, to missing teeth or to maloccluded teeth by lateral air flow related to preceived articulation distortion error observation. Management often involves first consideration of early orthodontic, pedodontic or prosthetic correction or dental replacement of the malpositioned and/or missing teeth. Such articulation errors previously have been found to occur in 12.8 percent of 1,000 case studies.[2]

Management through referral for dental treatment before or instead of speech therapy often may be advisable. This may postpone early important speech therapy efforts to correct such emerging abnormal articulation habits. However, usually such therapy should be initiated before school age, if possible, to be most efficacious. Compensatory speech articulation without distorted speech usually is possible before total dental or orthodontic correction is completed. Speech therapy can be effective even under these conditions and should not be postponed indefinitely, particularly when a dental correction requires a long-term, planned orthodontic program to be initiated between 7 and 9 years of age.

Articulation Distortions of Pressure Consonant Sounds from Nasal Emission Alone. This is a speech problem almost always thought to be caused directly by velopharyngeal incompetency or related directly to continued functional velopharyngeal insufficiency. Such distortions usually are detected by a nasal air flow paddle test or other similar clinical test methods as previously described by Westlake and Rutherford[19] and Bzoch.[2] The distortion or pressure consonant sounds from nasal emission alone should be considered as valid clinical evidence of probable velopharyngeal incompetency for speech. However, nasal emission also can persist on a functional basis for a period of time following primary palate cleft closure or even secondary reconstructive surgery. Diagnostic speech therapy can test this possibility.

Management of such problems usually calls for a period of diagnostic speech therapy training and/or maturation before further palatal reconstruction is recommended. This is especially true when nasal emission distortions are inconsistent (i.e., 2/10 to 7/10 indices are found on the nasal emission test). Management of inconsistent distortions from nasal emission alone should be first through attempts at speech training for the possible total elimination of such abnormal speech distortions. Secondary palatal reconstruction for the adequate correction of an underlying velopharyngeal inadequacy problem is indicated as early as possible after a reasonable period of effort (i.e., only 3 months up to a 1-year period of diagnostic therapy and maturation). If such therapy attempts fail and other objective evidence of velopharyngeal incompetency can be obtained, secondary palatal reconstruction probably is needed. This form of cleft palate speech disorder previously was found to occur in 42.3 percent of 1,000 case studies.[2]

The further communicative disorder of distraction to the listener because of nasal and/or facial grimacing by the speaker occasionally accompanies distortion of pressure consonant sounds from nasal emission. This problem is thought to occur mainly as an effort by the speaker to stop or diminish nasal emission due to velopharyngeal incompetency by using the more peripheral muscles controlling the nares and surrounding facial structures. This relative disorder was reported to have been observed in 4.2 percent of 1,000 cleft palate cases in earlier studies.[2]

Voice quality differences detected during clinical testing also may be of two types. One type has to do mainly with the efficacy of reconstructed palate (velopharyngeal mechanism). Such problems may result in either (1) significant differences in measurable and/or reported hypernasality or in (2) hyponasality distortions of speech utterances. The other two voice deviations relate more to compensatory laryngeal voice generation functions which can develop and present as an impression of either (3) hoarse voice or (4) aspirate voice, or both.

Hypernasality and/or Hyponasality. These are two types of resonance disorders of voice quality that frequently also are associated with speech disorders from congenital cleft palate. They are considered to be the main clinical findings leading to the inference of inadequate reconstruction or of overcorrection of velopharyngeal function from surgical or prosthetic procedures.

Hypernasality is the voice quality symptom that, when diagnosed clinically, along with distortions of pressure consonants from nasal emission, indicates the presence of velopharyngeal incompetency for speech. This problem usually requires some form of physical management through surgical or prosthetic reconstruction of the palate and velopharyngeal mechanism or nasal passages. Hypernasality, as operationally defined by Bzoch,[2] was reported present in the speech disorders of 43.1 percent of a large sample population of 1,000 cleft palate patients treated in the 1960's at cleft palate team centers.

The management of prolonged hyponasal distortion of voice quality sometimes may require further surgery to unblock an obstruction diagnosed radiographically or visually through nasopharyngoscopy. More often and more simply, postsurgical hyponasality is corrected through maturation alone (i.e., by waiting for the anticipated diminution of the bulk of a pharyngeal flap or an adenoid mass, or by medical treatment for chronic allergies or infections). However, the possible adverse effects of such obstructions on speech intelligibility and facial development are real. Nasal passage obstructions may cause mouth breathing and altered tongue carriage, which adversely affect facial growth and appearance during the early years of head and neck growth. The possibility of obstructive sleep apnea must be considered. Chronic obstruction over long periods of time demands correction on a somatic, if not a speech intelligibility basis.

Hoarse and/or Aspirate Voice. These are phonatory voice disorders cited as also frequently occurring in the cleft palate population. A review of the literature implies that hoarseness is a prevalent abnormal voice characteristic of this population.[16,19-23]

Bzoch,[1] Moore[24] and Wilson[18] all cited compensatory glottal stop articulation error patterns as the most probable cause for the frequently found hoarseness of voices in cleft palate populations. Such compensatory laryngeal articulation functions create additional strain and tension on the larynx and, when continued over time, may result in vocal abuse. Such persistent mistreatment of the vocal cords can lead to organic changes causing vocal nodules. Wilson[18] reported that such vocally abusive habits most commonly caused vocal nodules in children with cleft palate. In 1969 McWilliams et al.[16] found that 84 percent of 32 hoarse children with cleft palate at a mean age of 8.5 years had such vocal problems. Twenty-three of these children (71.9%) had bilateral vocal nodules. McWilliams et al.[16] and Bluestone[20] found a high frequency of vocal cord abnormalities in children with prolonged velopharyngeal valving problems. Hoarse voice abnormalities also were found in high frequency in individuals with cleft palate as reported by Morley.[23] Bzoch[2] reported that 15 percent of 1,000 cases studied presented with clinical evidence of hoarse voice abnormalities.

Aspirate voice abnormalities also have been cited as related to cleft palate speech characteristics. Brackett[25] discussed the basis of aspirate phonation in contrast to clear phonation as due to: (1) the vocal folds vibrating without a closed phase, (2) the closed phase involving only the anterior portion of the vocal folds, or (3) the closed phase being considerably shorter in duration than the opening or closing phases. Aspirate phonation is perceived clinically as a weak and breathy quality of voice with the perception of air turbulence.[26]

McDonald and Baker[22] also mentioned aspirate voice as an abnormal quality constituting one of several differences frequently found in cleft palate speech. They stated:

> We believe that an important part of the quality of cleft palate speech is the result of faulty phonation. Subjectively, this seems to vary a great deal from patient to patient, however, it can best be described as an ineffective use of air which adds to the overall quality a feature similar to breathiness, and which prevents the speaker from producing sounds with a wide acoustic spectrum.

Bzoch[7] specified that such a weak and aspirate phonatory voice quality was found in 31.3 percent of 1,000 cleft palate case studies. He stated:

> An aspirate phonatory voice quality appears to be often developed by the children with cleft palate in order to improve the intelligibility of their speech when they must communicate while they have velopharyngeal insufficiency. The distortion from velopharyngeal insufficiency due to both nasal emission and hypernasal resonance characteristics is greatly increased perceptually when the patient speaks with clear phonation as contrasted to weak aspirate phonation.

It appears from Bzoch's findings that aspirate phonation may become habitual for many children with cleft palate who attempt to lessen the perception of distortion of voice from speaking with prolonged velopharyngeal incompetency during early development. The occurrence of aspirate voice in a sample cleft palate population probably could be prevented best by an early team management plan that confirms velopharyngeal adequacy and/or corrects inadequacies when present after primary closure so that normal velopharyngeal function is able to support normal phonatory voice development.

Delayed Language Development. Research on the early language development of children with cleft palate has been sparse in the literature. However, most of the discussion by experts and reports of language research investigators indicate that there has been a frequent occurrence of delayed speech and language development, especially for expressive language skills in the cleft palate population.

Westlake and Rutherford,[19] in discussing the data from the doctoral research of Olson,[27] considered that even the preverbal vocalization differences found for infants with cleft palate, namely more back vowels and glottal consonants in place of labial and lingual fricatives and plosives, partly explained the frequent delay in using words and sentences. They stated:

> The mothers of the operated cleft-palate children reported almost half to have been slow in starting to walk. . .the mean age was about 16 months, four months behind normal. The mean age for combining words was 29 months.

Westlake and Rutherford suggested that because children with cleft palate could not articulate many sounds clearly at this early age, they probably retreated to simpler language, their vocabularies expanded more slowly and their early language was not as elaborate as that of normal children. Faircloth and Faircloth[14] analyzed in some detail the natural language skills of 10 children with cleft palate 6-11 years of age and agreed with this hypothesis. There appeared to be a clear relationship between articulatory proficiency and linguistic competence, including syntactic integrity, in this cleft palate sample. They generalized: "The child who strives for articulophonetic accuracy reduces sentence length, word length, and sentence complexity."

That approximately 50 percent of the cleft palate population evidenced delayed speech and language development is supported by Bzoch's report.[2] He stated that 502 of 1,000 consecutive cleft palate case studies evidenced this significant form of communication disorder based on a comparison of such factors as the first use of true words, sentence utterances, expressive vocabulary, mean length of response and the level of syntactic development. However, the frequency of this problem in the cleft palate population has been estimated to be even higher. Phillips and Harrison[28] used the Language Abilities Test on 137 children with cleft palate aged 18-72 months and compared the results with the use of this test on a control group of 165 children without clefts. The results of this comparative study revealed that the group with cleft palates generally was delayed in both receptive and expressive language skills, with a tendency toward poorer performance with increased age.

Bzoch et al.[29] reported a study using the REEL scale on a somewhat younger population sample of 25 cleft lip and palate subjects with a mean age of 18 months. They found 23 of the 25 subjects evidenced delays, primarily in expressive language skills. Swanson[30] studied the language achievement of a larger group of 37 infants with cleft lip and palate from four cleft palate centers using the REEL scale. She also included analysis of age, sex, type of cleft and order of birth in the family. Her results also showed a consistent receptive-expressive language difference. Females showed higher receptive and expressive skills but had a greater receptive-expressive difference. When cleft types were compared, no significant differences were noted. Her findings showed that children with cleft lips (primary palate only) had as much or more expressive delay in language development as those children with cleft palates only. The finding suggests that facial appearance alone may have an important impact on language acquisition.

In addition, a multiple regression analysis revealed other factors related to expressive language delay, including: (1) postsurgical behavior change (possibly due to a child's hospitalization and/or trauma from surgery), (2) mother's education level, (3) mother's verbal and social interaction with the child and (4) presence or absence of hearing examinations.

Fox et al.[15] compared preschool children with cleft palate to matched controls on three developmental scales, including the Denver Developmental Screening scale (DDS),[16] the REEL scale[9] and the experimental version of the Birth-3 scale.[1] Their results showed that the performance of the cleft palate subjects paralleled but fell below that of their peer group on all 11 behaviors measured by the three screening tests administered. They found that the expressive language subtests of the REEL scale were the most effective measure for predicting subject grouping into cleft and noncleft categories. This study also indicated that the early measures of language skills of children from birth to 3 years of age with cleft palate can predict their later language skill achievement. There is an implied inference from the literature as well that delayed use of expressive language (early speech) probably adversely affects the later receptive language development for this population.

Smit[31] demonstrated the high value of language quotients obtained from the REEL scale in the first three years of life for predicting later language performance. Nine females and 11 males who had been measured on the REEL scale at least three years previous to her investigation were given a battery of language measures, including the Preschool Language scale,[8] the Peabody Picture Vocabulary test,[32] the Boehm Test of Basic Concepts[33] and the Developmental Sentence Scoring test[34] for evaluation of a corpus of spontaneous speech. The results of regression analysis of the data showed that the REEL scale scores, as used in this study, were significant predictors of later receptive and/or expressive language abilities. The REEL scale scores obtained in years 1, 2 or 3 were all valid predictors of later language achievement, and predictability was as high for male as it was for female subjects.

Rationale for the Prevention of Communicative Disorders in the Cleft Palate Population. Our current rationale for the prevention of the usual communication disorders found in past studies of the cleft palate population is to involve the parents and families of each newborn infant with cleft palate in frequent counseling and discussions of their child's hearing, speech and language development based on frequent standardized clinical tests and measures, particularly during the first three years of life. The experienced group of plastic surgeons working with our team generally were able to reconstruct totally clefts of the primary and secondary palatal areas well before 18 months of age, and usually in the first year of life, without evidence of increased problems of restricted growth of the maxillae. With cooperative families and infants with cleft palates who generally had been involved in a home speech and language stimulation program, we were able to evaluate the adequacy or inadequacy of the velopharyngeal mechanism from a clinical speech test battery. As soon as a specific surgical, dental or medical problem affecting hearing, speech or language development could be identified, referral for appropriate treatment was arranged as part of the craniofacial center team report. Whenever functional speech or language learning problems were found or suggested by the test battery (e.g., for inconsistent evidence of velopharyngeal incompetency following surgery), referral for a short period of diagnostic therapy or specific therapy (e.g., training) was made as soon as possible.

The implementation of this rationale required the development of a standard set of short clinical tests that were adequate for the routine differential diagnosis of any or all of the specific communicative disorder problems discussed previously. The team coordinator had to develop an effective method of total team evaluation, referral and followup for the early management of identified problems. The test battery and management procedures are described above. A recent five-year clinical study drawing on data from this test battery and evaluating achievement of the goal of prevention following this rationale is reported below.

Report of a Recent Clinical Study on Preventing the Development of Communicative Disorders in Children with Cleft Palate. Recently it has been demonstrated objectively that it is possible in the early preschool years almost regularly to prevent (rather than later try to correct) the usual speech and language disorders which often occurred in cleft palate population samples studied in the past. Such disorders essentially can be eliminated before school age. However such an effective team management approach requires, among other things, the acceptance of the surgical and dental team colleagues of the priority of this early consideration.

This is a management decision to be made by each team over the possible longer-term priority of perhaps effecting better dental occlusion and/or mid-face growth development through later staged surgical reconstruction procedures. After two decades of research at large cleft palate treatment centers, there appears to be no definitive study, to date, to demonstrate that the early surgical reconstruction of cleft palates measurably exacerbates the mid-face growth development problems or the frequency of dental malocclusions and facial growth problems also of importance in the evaluation of any cleft management of this population. The most recent controlled animal research testing the factor of age at surgery[35] found no effect on maxillary growth related to early as compared to later surgery.

Table 11-1

Comparison of the frequency of occurrence of specific types of cleft palate speech disorders following past and present management procedures.

Categorical speech defects	Past studies (N = 1000) (%)	Present study (N = 50) (%)
1. Gross sound-substitution error pattern	56.4	6.0
2. Hypernasal distortion of voice	43.1	4.0
3. Distortion of articulation from nasal emission	42.3	8.0
4. Developmental dyslalia	34.0	10.0
5. Aspirate voice	31.3	10.0
6. Hoarse voice	15.0	0.0
7. Dental-related articulation disorders	12.8	8.0
8. Hyponasal voice	12.0	2.0
9. Distraction from nasal grimacing	4.2	0.0

Table 11-1 illustrates the possibility of the regular efficiency of a cleft palate team's effort to prevent, rather than later to attempt to correct the frequent communicative disorders of individuals with cleft palate. It seems apparent from inspection of the data in the table that this goal of such early prevention is attainable.

The details of the clinical demonstration study of a population of 50 consecutive case studies of infants born with clefts of the palate were previously reported.[11] The highlights of that report are considered below.

First, the population sample will be described in terms of sex, type of cleft, criteria for selection and age at time of primary complete surgical reconstruction, followed by a statistical analysis of the data from the speech, language and hearing measures.

Table 11-2

Description of the population sample by sex and age.

	I Unilateral	II Oblique	III Overt	IV Submucous	V Congenital VPI	VI Unilateral	VII Bilateral	Total
Males	2	1	3	2	0	15	8	31
Females	2	0	11	0	1	4	1	19
Total	4	1	14	2	1	19	9	50

Population Sample. Table 11-2 presents a description of the population sample in terms of sex distribution and type of congenital malformation. It can be seen that

50 subjects (31 males and 19 females) meeting basic criteria for selection were included. Only patients who had been evaluated a minimum of two times by the entire craniofacial team were included. All 50 subjects were born between December 6, 1975, and October 15, 1980. All presented with one of seven types of congenital disorders, but with no other known medical or developmental disorder that might of itself affect speech, language or hearing development (i.e., neurologic impairment, syndrome with usual severe retardation or deafness or multiple congenital abnormalities). Five case studies of infants with clefts of the primary palate only (including one with combined oblique facial cleft) were included since the language research reported in the literature indicated that such conditions also frequently result in delayed language development. Table 11-2 reveals that 17 cases presented with clefts or deficiencies of the secondary palate only (5 males and 12 females).

As might be expected in most cleft palate population samples, the most frequent type of congenital cleft malformation was a combined unilateral cleft of both primary and secondary palates, and this occurred most frequently in males, but included some females, for a total 15:4 ratio (n=19). The remaining category was combined complete clefts of both primary and secondary palate structures, which occurred for 8 males and 1 female.

Empirically this sample appears to be fairly typical of the cleft palate population in general. Clefts involving the primary palate with or without clefts of the secondary palate, occurred more often in males (n=26) than in females (n=7), for a ratio of over 3:1. Conversely, clefts or malformations involving the secondary palate only occurred more frequently in females (n=12) than in males (n=25). The most common presenting type of cleft was a unilateral combined cleft of the primary and secondary palates, and this occurred mainly in males. It was considered, therefore, that generalizations might be drawn from this clinical sample regarding the efficacy of early complete surgical reconstructions and procedures for prevention of communication disorders in the general cleft palate population.

An empirical basic tenet of this center's program for the effective management and prevention of hearing, speech and language disorders in children with cleft palate is that early, complete palatal reconstructive surgery has a direct and very positive influence on the achievement of this goal. Table 11-3 presents recent experience with regard to the timing of primary surgery for the 50 subjects.

It can be seen that the majority of patients (31 of 50) had their primary surgery completed by 12 months of age, and all but 7 had their primary surgery completed by 18 months of age (5 of those with later dates were treated elsewhere before moving into the district for team management). One child with obvious submucous cleft palate and an initial clinical diagnosis of borderline (inconsistent) velopharyngeal insufficiency to support clear speech, responded well to speech therapy alone and maintained adequate velopharyngeal function for normal voice and speech over the period of the report, so that the total set of dates of completed surgery is 49 rather than 50.

Seventy-four percent of the subjects reported were eligible for the State of Florida's Children's Medical Service program. They were, therefore, drawn from the

Table 11-3

Age at completion of primary reconstructive surgery by type of cleft

Type	I	II	III	IV	V	VI	VII	Total
0-6 months	4	1	1	0	0	0	0	6
7-9 months	0	0	2	0	0	1	0	4
10-12 months	0	0	5	0	0	10	6	21
13-18 months	0	0	4	0	0	6	1	11
19-24 months	0	0	2	0	0	2	0	4
25 + months	0	0	0	1	1	0	1	3
Total	4	1	14	1	1	19	9	49

lower socioeconomic group of the general population. All subjects were from predominantly rural areas, causing difficulty in arranging transportation for frequent team or specialty clinics, child care, preschool placement or weekly speech therapy.

Findings from Speech Test Data. Table 11-1 presented the findings from the speech test data related to the effectiveness of the total management program for the prevention of each of the categorical aspects of cleft palate speech previously defined and discussed. Recent experience is compared to past studies using similar clinical indices. Whereas in the past cleft palate speech disorders were present in an estimated 75 percent of the population, only 20 percent of this group were found to have any form of speech disorder. Most of these were mild forms of developmental dyslalia or dental-related articulation distortions common at this age in the general population.

The data in Table 11-1 reveal the speech problem most uniquely related to cleft palate, gross sound substitution error patterns, was found in only 6 percent (3 cases) of this sample of 50 case studies, as compared to 56.4 percent of a previous sample diagnosed in a similar manner. Two of these case studies showed evidence of continued velopharyngeal incompetency for speech following primary and/or secondary reconstructive surgery. They were scheduled already for further palatal reconstruction. The third already had had a successful secondary palatal reconstruction and was making rapid progress in breaking the gross substitution error pattern through speech therapy.

The problem of hypernasal distortion of syllabic elements in speech was found in only two of the subjects. These same two also presented with a glottal stop error pattern (the other subject with a glottal stop error pattern showed no evidence of hypernasality by the base 10 cul-de-sac resonance test). Under the limits of this clinical investigation, therefore, it appears that operationally defined hypernasality was reduced from 43.1 percent under previous team management to 4.0 percent under the present system.

Distortions of pressure consonant sounds from nasal emission were found in only 8.0 percent (4 cases) in the present study as compared to 42.5 percent in previous studies. Two of these four cases were the same two as presented with hypernasality, gross sound substitution error pattern and velopharyngeal incompetency confirmed by speech cinefluorographic studies and diagnostic therapy. One of the remaining cases presented with a mild nasal emission problem in the range of 2/10-5/10 indices on the base 10 nasal emission test. The cause was determined to be a fistula in the anterior hard palate. This was confirmed both by temporary obturation of the fistula, which then yielded a 0/10 index, and by the fact that no nasal emission occurred on the syllable /ki/ as compared to /pi/ on repeated clinical testing. A dental obturator was planned until such time as surgical closure or spontaneous closure over time could eliminate the problem. The remainder of the cases with nasal emission findings were only mild, with 2/10-0/10 indices on repeated testing without evidence of hypernasality on the cul-de-sac test or perceived hypernasality in running speech by listener judgment. These were thought to be cases of borderline adequate velopharyngeal valving, to be managed by further speech therapy and frequent diagnostic testing.

Developmental dyslalia (functional articulation disorder) is a problem reported in approximately 10 percent of the beginning school age population. Table 11-1 indicates developmental dyslalia also was found for 10 percent (5 cases) of the study group, as compared to 34.0 percent in previous studies. The limitation of functional articulation disorders was thought to be accomplished mainly through routine counseling of parents during cleft palate clinics or through home speech and language stimulation techniques and the prevention of functional delayed speech and language development.

The frequency of findings of aspirate voice characteristics was limited to 10 percent of the study population (5 cases), as compared to 31.3 percent in the past studies. The determination was made from the phonation test of our clinical test battery, and was limited to subjects who were unable to sustain phonation for 10 sec on three trials for each vowel, who sounded aspirate in running speech to the speech pathologist and whose parents confirmed that this phonatory quality was generally typical of speech at home. It is not known what percentage of a normal population sample of similar preschool age children would be judged to have aspirate voice.

Hoarse voice (as operationally defined for this and previously reported studies) generally is of more serious concern because of the frequent finding of vocal nodules with this type of voice disorder. None of the 50 subjects presented with hoarse voice abnormalities. The problem of developing a hoarse voice quality did not occur in this population sample whereas it occurred in 15-25 percent of other previously reported cleft palate population samples.[1,36]

Table 11-1 also reveals that dental related articulation disorders remained at a fairly similar level (8% compared to 12.8%) to that found in a previous, larger population sample. This type of speech disorder may be similar in difficulty of management to the problem of otitis media from poor eustachion tube function. In order to totally prevent this problem, a very aggressive early pedodontic and orthodontic program in the first four years of life probably would be necessary to replace lateral incisor teeth and alveolar cleft areas and to move collapsed buccal segments before mixed dentition.

In the past hyponasal voice distortions were found in 12 percent of a larger, and generally older, cleft palate population sample. This voice abnormality was generally a temporary sequela to the frequent use of the broad obturating pharyngeal flap surgical procedures most frequently used in that era to correct persistent velopharyngeal insufficiency following unsuccessful primary cleft palate surgery. This finding was present for only 1 of the 50 more recent case studies reported here. This subject was one of three presenting with a previously developed gross sound substitution error pattern and was now making good progress with therapy following a recent secondary pharyngeal flap operation. As the hyponasality index was in the range of 2/10-5/10 and the 5-year-old patient was less than one year post secondary surgery, this finding of mild hyponasality was judged to be a tolerable problem.

The final problem of distraction from nasal and/or facial grimacing was not found in the present sample. It occurred in 4.2 percent of past studies and appears to develop only when prolonged development of speech with velopharyngeal insufficiency occurs.

Findings from the Language Development Data. The REEL scale norms used and specific items of achievement of both receptive and expressive language skills are based on the actual achievement of healthy "normal" infants from linguistically enriched environments. The original validity studies[7] showed that 90 percent of well baby infant population samples scored within ± one age interval on this scale, and that sample normal well baby populations should have average language quotients of 105.

The data from 116 REEL scale evaluations of the language development status of 43 of the 50 subjects is presented in Table 11-4. Five of the seven subjects not tested on the REEL were over 3 years of age when first seen, and two were not tested because of time limitations and lack of a knowledgeable informant. The data reveal that the average combined language age quotients were as high or higher than those of the well baby samples reported in the validity studies for this scale.

Table 11-4

REEL scale combined language quotients by mean and standard deviation for the first three years of life.

	N	Number of tests	X	SD
Year 1	32	46	111.67	23.02
Year 2	32	50	107.32	13.49
Year 3	16	20	105.00	12.42

Table 11-4 also shows that 46 REEL scale evaluations were given to 32 different subjects in the year 1 sample, and that calculation of the mean combined Language Age Score yielded a quotient of 111.67 with a standard deviation of 23.02. Twenty of these 32 subjects (78%) had a combined language quotient of 90 or above, and 19 of these (76%) scored above 100. Only 5 (15%) scored between 80 and 90 in the first year of life and 2 subjects (6%) had combined language quotients below 80.

In the second year of life a mean combined language quotient of 107.32 with a standard deviation of 13.49 was obtained from 50 REEL scale evaluations on 32 subjects. In year 2, 30 of the 32 subjects (93%) had quotients of 90 or above, with 21 (70%) of these scoring above 100. One subject (3%) scored between 80 and 90 and one had a quotient below 80.

Test results also were evaluated according to receptive, expressive and combined language skills by sex, cleft type, age at primary closure and socioeconomic status. Changes in language skills during the first three years of life were evaluated using the mean receptive, expressive and combined language quotients.

Table 11-5

Mean combined quotients by sex for the first three years of life.

	N	Number of tests	X
First year			
Male	19	29	113.86
Female	13	17	108.64
Second year			
Male	19	29	101.72
Female	13	21	110.76
Third year			
Male	10	10	107.40
Female	6	10	102.60

The data in Table 11-5 compare the mean combined language quotients for male and female subjects for each of the first three years of life. They reveal that both groups had essentially normal language achievement levels for each of those years. Although there were no substantial differences between the means, males scored slightly higher in the first and third years and females in the second year.

Table 11-6 presents the findings of the mean average Receptive Language Quotient, Expressive Language Quotient and Combined Language Quotient, as well as the Receptive-Expressive Quotient (difference) scores for subgroups of children with four different types of clefts for each of the first three years of life. The data reveal some trends related to type of cleft, particularly for achieving a small R-E language difference. One subject with a cleft of the primary palate only had a substantial Receptive-Expressive Language level difference accounting for most of the negative difference score in years 1 and 2 for this small subgroup. Such differences indicate a functional delayed expressive language use related to environmental rather than physical causes. Since previous research found similar delayed

Table 11-6

Mean receptive language quotients (RLQ), expressive language (ELZ), combined language quotients (CLQ) and receptive-expressive language differences (Dif) found for four types of cleft subgroups in the first three years of life.

	Quotients	Primary palate only (N=3)	Secondary palate only (N=13)	Unilateral complete (N=19)	Bilateral complete (N=7)
Year 1	RLQ	150.0	107.2	115.5	108.2
	ELQ	125.0	97.6	105.4	94.0
	CLQ	137.5	102.4	110.1	101.2
	Dif	−25.0	−9.6	−10.0	−14.2
Year 2	RLQ	127.5	117.4	115.3	101.5
	ELQ	85.0	101.9	103.7	90.0
	CLQ	106.5	109.6	109.7	95.7
	Dif	−42.5	−15.5	−11.6	−11.5
Year 3	RLQ	100.0	98.3	101.5	107.5
	ELQ	110.0	94.0	90.0	100.3
	CLQ	109.0	96.7	95.7	103.8
	Dif	+10.0	−4.3	−11.5	−7.2

expressive language problems in children with cleft lip only, this possibility should be anticipated and language counseling and home stimulation programs initiated for this subgroup along with children with cleft palate. Interestingly, the one child in this subgroup with oblique facial cleft had above average language scores for the first two years of life but had large R-E language level differences. Children in this subgroup tested in the third year had slightly lower but normal language scores and a marked decrease in the R-E difference.

The children with a unilateral complete cleft of primary and secondary palates (n=19) had normal and above normal scores for all three years. Children with bilateral complete clefts of the primary and secondary palates (n=7) showed lower expressive scores than those with other cleft types in the first two years, although the scores were near normal. The R-E differences decreased but did not diminish in the third year. Expressive and receptive quotients remained in the normal range.

Two final factors thought to be related to delayed language development are (1) age at which complete primary reconstructive surgery is completed and (2) family socioeconomic level. No statistically significant differences were found for either factor. However, a trend based on the small sample subgroups for timing of surgery was thought to be worthy of describing for the purpose of this chapter. **The children in this sample who had clefts involving the secondary palate and who had complete reconstructive surgery between 7 and 12 months of age (n=26) all had excellent language level scores with small R-E language differences.** Subjects who had their surgery completed between 13 and 18 months of age had excellent (above 100) receptive language quotients but decreased (although within normal range) expressive language scores. They tended to have large R-E language differences in each of the first three years. Both a slight decrease in receptive language quotients and a more marked decrease in expressive language quotients were characteristic of the group (n = 7) who had primary palatal reconstructions after 19 months of age.

Findings from Audiology Test Data. A summary of the percentages of occurrence of hearing loss, abnormal impedance results and otologic abnormalities as a function of type of cleft indicates a marked difference in the frequency of pathologic findings for subjects with clefts limited to the primary palate. Aural pathology ranged from 25-33 percent. The overall incidence of aural pathology on the first examination was 60 percent; on the final examination it was 63 percent. Clefts of the secondary palate only, submucous clefts and combined clefts of primary and secondary palates maintained a high degree of hearing loss, abnormal tympanograms and aural pathology from the first to the last examination. Although there was only one individual with congenital velopharyngeal insufficiency from the first and last examinations, this individual went from abnormal hearing loss, tympanogram and aural pathology to no difficulty in any category.

The results of audiometric evaluation and aural pathology as a function of age at surgical repair from the last examination appear to indicate a trend for reduction of hearing loss or aural pathology that can be related directly to the earlier age at surgical repair.

Goal of Achieving "Normal" Early Speech and Language Development. The recent speech and hearing program in the craniofacial clinic at the University of Florida, as has been described, emphasizes many factors, all of which have contributed to the large number of subjects treated recently having normal and even above normal speech and language development early in life. These factors include the need for early and frequent evaluations, parental counseling regarding language development, routine audiological testing and encouragement of early palatal surgery and further reconstructive surgery when indicated, as early as possible in the life of each child.

Early and frequent speech, language and hearing evaluations are most helpful in order to inform parents about the effects cleft lip and palate can have on early language and speech development. Often, if this is postponed until surgery has been completed, as in the past, important months of development can be affected by poor stimulation due to lack of information given to the parents.

Frequent evaluations, at least every six months for children under 5 years of age, can monitor progress and are effective in solving individual problems that may arise. Waiting one year between evaluations does make intervention less effective.

Parents need and appreciate the guidance and reinforcement provided by professionals. Analysis of clinical data reported here indicates early intervention results in a significant decrease in delayed language development in preschool children with cleft palate. A team program emphasizing early complete surgical treatment and frequent professional speech, language and audiological consultation almost routinely can eliminate the occurrence of "cleft palate speech."

REFERENCES

1. Bzoch KR: Categorical aspects of cleft palate speech, in Grabbe WC, Rosenstein SW, Bzoch KR (eds): *Cleft Lip and Palate: Surgical, Dental, and Speech Aspects.* Boston, Little Brown & Co, 1971, pp 713-734.
2. Bzoch KR (ed): *Communicative Disorders Related to Cleft Lip and Palate,* ed 2. Boston, Little Brown & Co, 1979, pp 161-191.
3. O'Shea MB: *An Analysis of Two Indexes of Hypernasality,* thesis. University of Florida, Gainesville, Fla, 1982.
4. Lively MA, Emanuel FW: Spectral noise levels and roughness severity ratings for normal and simulated rough vowels produced by adult females. *J Speech Hear Res,* 13:502, 1970.
5. Reese M: Some variables affecting harshness. *J Speech Hear Res,* 1:155, 1958.
6. Sansone FE, Emanuel FW: Spectral noise levels and roughness severity ratings for normal and simulated rough vowels produced by adult males. *J Speech Hear Res,* 13:489, 1970.
7. Bzoch KR, League RL: *Assessing Language Skills in Infancy.* Baltimore, University Park Press, 1971.
8. Zimmerman V, Steiner G, Evatt R: *Preschool Language Scale.* Columbus, Ohio, Charles C Merrill Pub Co, 1971.
9. Bangs TE, Garrett SD: *Birth to Three Scale,* exp ed, Houston, Tex, Speech and Hearing Institute, 1973.
10. Coplan J, Gleason J, Ryan R, et al: Validation of an early language milestone scale in a high-risk population. *Pediatrics,* 70:677, 1982.
11. Bzoch KR, Kemker FJ, Wood VL, Dixon: The prevention of communicative disorders in cleft palate infants. *Adv Basic Res Prac,* 10:59, 1984.
12. Northern JL, Downs MP: *Hearing in Children.* Baltimore, Williams & Wilkins, 1979.
13. Hodgson WR: Testing infants and young children, in Katz J (ed): *Handbook of Clinic Audiology,* ed 2. Baltimore, Williams & Wilkins, 1978, pp 397-425.
14. Faircloth SR, Faircloth MA: Delayed language and linguistic variations, in Bzoch KR (ed): *Communicative Disorders Related to Cleft Palate.* Boston, Little Brown & Co, 1971, pp 734-740.
15. Fox D, Lynch J, Brookshire B: Selected developmental factors of cleft palate children between two and thirty-three months of age. *Cleft Palate J,* 15:239, 1978.
16. McWilliams BJ, Bluestone CD, Musgrave RH: Diagnostic implications of vocal cord nodules in children with cleft palate. *Laryngoscope,* 79:2072, 1969.
17. Trost JE: Articulatory additions to the classical description of the speech of persons with cleft palate. *Cleft Palate J,* 18;193, 1981.
18. Wilson D: *Voice Problems in Children.* Baltimore, Williams & Wilkins, 1972.
19. Westlake H, Rutherford D: *Cleft Palate.* Englewood Cliffs, NJ, Prentice-Hall, 1966.
20. Bluestone CD, Felder H: The role of the otolaryngologist in secondary surgical management of the cleft palate patient, in: *Trans Am Acad Opthalmol Otolaryngol,* 73:715, 1969.
21. Hess DA: Pitch, intensity, and cleft palate voice quality. *J Speech Hear Res,* 2:113, 1959.
22. McDonald ET, Baker HK: Cleft palate speech: An integration of research and clinical observation. *J Speech Hear Disord,* 16:9, 1951.
23. Morley ME: *Cleft Palate and Speech.* Edinburgh, Livingstone, 1962.
24. Moore GP: *Organic Voice Disorders.* Englewood Cliffs, NJ, Prentice-Hall, 1971.

25. Brackett IP: Parameters of voice quality, in Travis LE (ed): *Handbook of Speech Pathology and Audiology.* New York.
26. Darley F: *Diagnosis and Appraisal of Communicative Disorders.* Englewood Cliffs, NJ, Prentice-Hall, 1964.
27. Olson DA: *A Descriptive Study of the Speech Development of a Group of Infants with Cleft Palate,* thesis. Northwestern University School of Speech, Evanston, Ill, 1965.
28. Phillips BJ, Hanison RJ: Language skills of preschool cleft palate children. *Cleft Palate J,* 6:108, 1968.
29. Bzoch KR, Morley M, Fex S, et al: Development of speech and language in cleft palate children, in Fogh-Andersen (ed): *Proceedings of the Second International Congress on Cleft Palate.* Copenhagen, American Cleft Palate Association, 1973.
30. Swanson JF: *Language Development in Young Cleft Palate Children,* thesis. University of Florida, Gainesville, Fla, 1973.
31. Smit BL: *The Predictive Value of the Receptive-Expressive Emergent Language Scale,* thesis. University of Florida, Gainesville, Fla, 1975.
32. Dunn L: *Expanded Manual for the Peabody Picture Vocabulary Test.* Circle Pines, Minn, American Guidance Service Inc, 1965.
33. Boehm A: *Boehm Test of Basic Concepts.* New York, Psychological Corp, 1971.
34. Lee L: *Developmental Sentence Analysis.* Evanston, Ill, Northwestern University Press, 1974.
35. Kremenak, Wada, et al: *Factors Affecting Postsurgical Maxillary Growth: Age at Surgery.* Read before the 42nd Anniversary Meeting, American Cleft Palate Association, Miami, Fla, May 13, 1985.
36. McWilliams BJ, Lavorato AS, Bluestone CD: Vocal cord abnormalities in children with velopharyngeal valving problems. *Laryngoscope,* 83:1745, 1973.

AUTHOR INDEX

F

G

H

T

U

V

SUBJECT INDEX

D

E